Case Studies in Emergency Medicine

CASE STUDIES IN EMERGENCY MEDICINE

Third Edition

Howard A. Freed, M.D.
Associate Professor of Emergency Medicine and Surgery and Associate Director, Department of Emergency Medicine, Albany Medical College, Albany; Director, Emergency Services, Nathan Littauer Hospital, Gloversville, New York

Dan Mayer, M.D.
Theme Leader, Comprehensive Care Case Studies Course, Office of Medical Education, Albany Medical College; Attending Physician, Emergency Department, Albany Medical Center, Albany, New York

Frederic W. Platt, M.D.
Clinical Professor of Medicine, University of Colorado School of Medicine; Attending Physician, Presbyterian/St. Luke's Hospital, Denver, Colorado

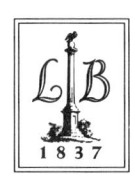

Little, Brown and Company
Boston   New York   Toronto   London

Copyright © 1997 by Little, Brown and Company (Inc.)

Third Edition

Previous editons copyright © 1974 by Little, Brown and Company (Inc); 1991 by Frederic W. Platt and Howard A. Freed

All rights reserved. No part of this book may be reproduced in any form or by any electronic or mechanical means, including information storage and retrieval systems, without permission in writing from the publisher, except by a reviewer who may quote brief passages in a review.

Library of Congress Cataloging-in-Publication Data

Freed, Howard A.
    Case studies in emergency medicine / Howard A. Freed, Dan Mayer, Frederic W. Platt. — 3rd ed.
       p.   cm.
    Includes bibliographical references and index.
    ISBN 0-316-29470-5
    1. Medical emergencies — Case studies.   I. Mayer, Dan.
II. Platt, Frederic W.   III. Title.
    [DNLM: 1. Emergencies — case studies.   2. Emergency Medicine — case studies.   WB 105 F853c 1996]
RC86.7.F74   1996
616.02'5 — dc20
DNLM/DLC
for Library of Congress   96-25824
                                                       CIP

Printed in the United States of America
COM

Editorial: Tammerly J. Booth, Joanne S. Toran
Production Editor: Katharine S. Mascaro
Copyeditor: Kevin Sullivan
Production and Design: Cate Rickard

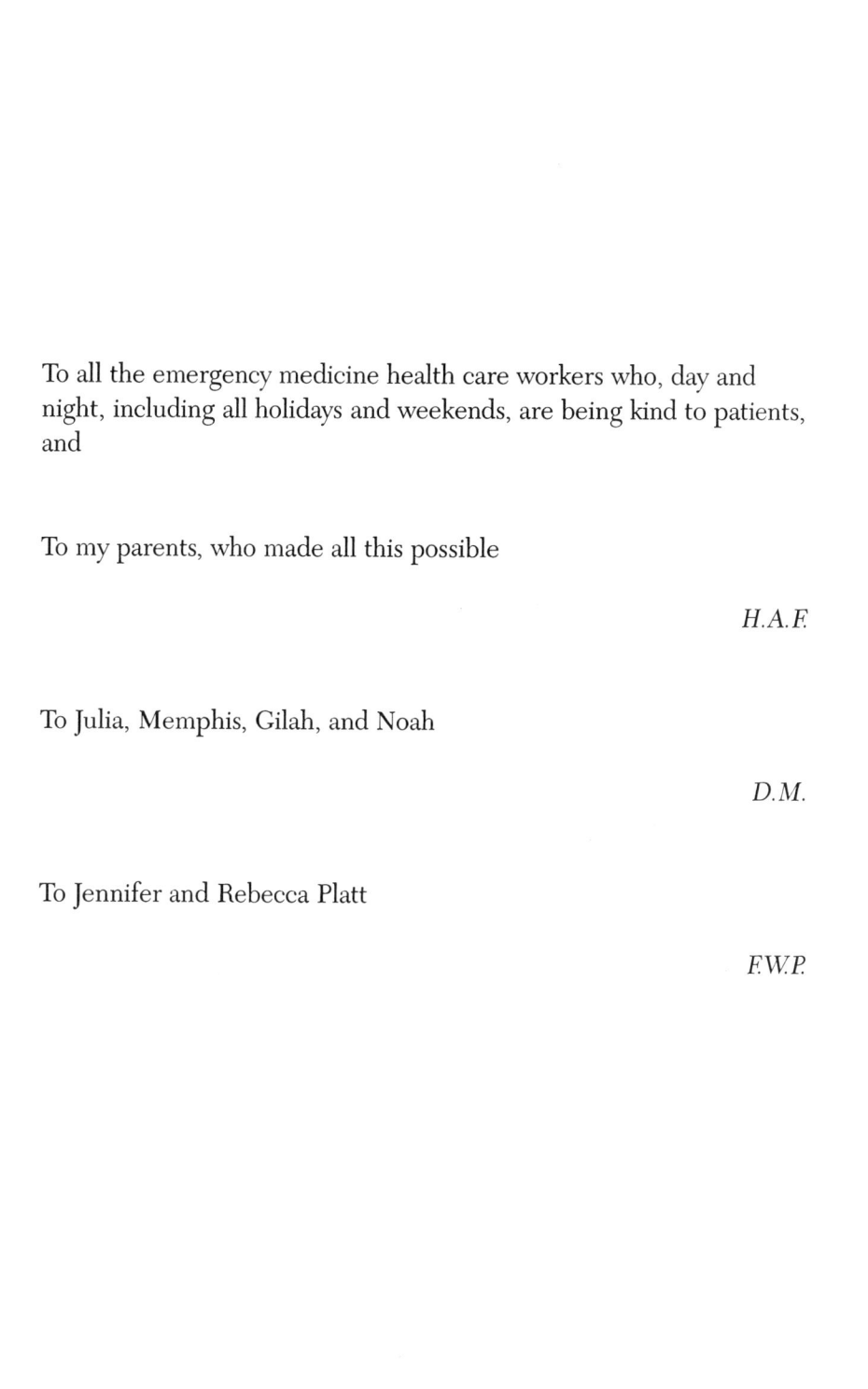

To all the emergency medicine health care workers who, day and night, including all holidays and weekends, are being kind to patients, and

To my parents, who made all this possible

H.A.F.

To Julia, Memphis, Gilah, and Noah

D.M.

To Jennifer and Rebecca Platt

F.W.P.

Contents

Preface   *xi*
Abbreviations   *xiii*

1.	Stabbing Victim with Hostile Entourage	1
2.	Multiple Somatic Complaints	4
3.	Sprain?	9
4.	Vital Signs Stable, Speaking Italian	12
5.	Terrible Sore Throat	15
6.	Seventy-Nine Years Old and Confused	18
7.	"Don't Make Me Stay in the Hospital"	20
8.	"Sick All Over"	22
9.	Sexual Assault	25
10.	Five Sick Siblings	29
11.	Suicidal	31
12.	Left Lower Quadrant Pain	35
13.	Drowned Child	38
14.	An Otherwise Well Infant	41
15.	Before the Accident	44
16.	Eighteen Years Old, Stopped Breathing	47
17.	Honking Horn on the Ambulance Ramp	51
18.	Monoarticular Arthritis	55
19.	They Had Never Seen Anything Like It Before	58
20.	Asthma	61
21.	A Request for Methadone	65
22.	Twenty-Eight Year Old with Chest Pain	67
23.	Nosebleed	71
24.	"Lockjaw"	74
25.	Hyperventilation: The Anxious Divorcée	77
26.	Rescued from a Fire	80
27.	The Morning After a Snowstorm	84
28.	A "Fainter" Under a Doctor's Care	87
29.	Motorcycle Accident	90
30.	Headaches	93

31.	"DTs"	98
32.	Blunt Trauma	101
33.	Rectal Explosion	105
34.	Lost Lab Tests	107
35.	Diabetic in Automobile Accident	110
36.	Unequal Pupils	114
37.	Shaky, Pale, and Drinking	117
38.	Leopard Bite	121
39.	Coma	124
40.	Coughing Up Blood	127
41.	Repeat Visits	130
42.	Seventy-Two Years Old, Feeling Faint	133
43.	Falling Down Stairs	137
44.	Probably Drunk	140
45.	Pain on Urination	143
46.	Mental Status: Confused	147
47.	Seeing Zebras	150
48.	OD	153
49.	Walking Away from a Car Accident	156
50.	Hand Laceration	160
51.	The Weekend Toothache	163
52.	"No Fracture"	166
53.	A Shooter with Vomiting	169
54.	Woman with Abdominal Pain	173
55.	The Blue Bruise	177
56.	Mistaken Identity, Shot in the Head	180
57.	EMS Radio Call	183
58.	Chronic Schizophrenic on Drugs	187
59.	Acute Myocardial Infarction	191
60.	Facial Trauma	195
61.	Laceration	198
62.	Constipation	201
63.	Difficulty Swallowing	203
64.	Allergic to Shrimp	206
65.	Pediatric Head Injury	209
66.	Pregnant and Bleeding	212
67.	Trouble Breathing	215
68.	Gunshot Wound	219

CONTENTS

69.	Pleuritic Pain	224
70.	Looked "Too Drunk" to the Police	227
71.	Hearing Aids	230
72.	No Pulse	233
73.	Three Days of Cough/Cyanotic	236
74.	Seizure	239
75.	Money Troubles	243
76.	Flank Pain	247
77.	Tricyclic Antidepressant Overdose	250
78.	Acting Weird	256
79.	Diarrhea	259
80.	Syncope	263
81.	Respiratory Infection	266
82.	Sudden Shoulder Pain	269
83.	Hit by a Car	271
84.	Kicked in the Groin	274
85.	Child with a Barking Cough	277
86.	HIV Positive	280
87.	Child with Small Toys	283
88.	Child After a Seizure	286
89.	Abscess	289
90.	Cardiac Arrest	292
91.	Bounce Back	298
92.	Recent Bypass Surgery	300
93.	Patient Who Became Loud and Abusive	303
94.	Multiple Shooting Victims	307
95.	Refusing Treatment	311
96.	The Exploding Car Battery	315
97.	Broke the Steering Wheel with His Chest	318
98.	VD	321
99.	Cerebrovascular Accident	325
100.	Medical Malpractice	329
101.	Rule Out MI	332
102.	The Liar	336
103.	Do Not Resuscitate	340
104.	"The Worst Headache of My Life"	344
105.	"I Think I Have Pneumonia"	347
106.	Keyhole Medicine	351

Appendixes
   A. Nursing Literature References   354
   B. Prehospital Care References   376

Index   395

Preface

In the years since 1971, when the first edition of *Case Studies in Emergency Medicine* by Frederic W. Platt, M.D., appeared in print, the field of Emergency Medicine has emerged as a medical specialty.

As emergency medicine has grown as a physician specialty, so have the roles of emergency nurses and the specialists in prehospital care—EMTs and paramedics. In fact, by one recent survey, for each emergency department in the United States there are approximately 5 full-time emergency physicians, 15 emergency nurses, and almost 100 full- and part-time emergency medical technicians at various levels of training. This edition of *Case Studies in Emergency Medicine* reflects the marked growth; the third edition includes more cases highlighting the contributions of these non-physician professionals and the subtle and important interactions they have with emergency physicians.

This book was written for all students and practitioners of emergency medicine. One reason we have written it is to try to convey to those considering any aspect of emergency medicine as a career what it is like to practice our specialty. The cases are arranged not by body system, but in a random sequence similar to what one might encounter working in a busy emergency department. Like bedside teaching, we have tried to link concepts with interesting cases and have not attempted to be encyclopedic. More detailed information can be found in the references cited.

References are provided throughout this book for each of the 106 cases. Nevertheless, physicians, nurses, and prehospital care providers each have their own medical literature. As a new facet of this third edition, we have included two new appendixes that offer references of particular interest to nurses (Appendix A) and to prehospital care providers (Appendix B).

In addition to the editors, several authors contributed work to earlier editions of this book. Revisions of their contributions are included in this edition as well. They are George Cooper, R.N., M.D.; William Fisher, M.D.; Charles Graffeo, M.D.; Bilal Kattan, M.D.; Peter Kelly, M.D.; Rachel Michaud, M.S.; Greer Pomeroy, M.D.; Philip Rabinowitz, M.D.; Kevin Reilly, M.D.; Richard Salluzzo, M.D.; David

Salo, M.D.; Howard Snyder, M.D.; Leonard Teitz, M.D.; and Shari Welch, M.D.

Additionally, Richard Salluzzo, M.D., Chairman of Emergency Medicine at Albany Medical College; Rachel Michaud, M.S., and the editors contributed new material to this edition. Thanks also to Wendy DeFazio, RoseMarie Lupoli, Marian Bush, and Carole Sweet for their patient help with the preparation of the manuscript.

Our biggest thanks and appreciation go to Frederic Platt, M.D.—a gifted physician, writer, and teacher.

H.A.F.
D.M.

ABBREVIATIONS

a-A	Alveolar-arterial
ABC	Airway, breathing, circulation
ABG	Arterial blood gas (oxygen, carbon dioxide) analysis
ACE	Angiotensin I converting enzyme
ACE inhibitors	A new class of medications for high blood pressure and congestive heart failure
ACLS	Advanced cardiac life support
AIDS	Acquired immunodeficiency syndrome
ALS	Advanced life support
AMA	Against medical advice
ANA	Antinuclear antibody, a blood test for *autoimmune* disorders such as Lupus
A-P	Anterior-posterior
AV	Arteriovenous; atrioventricular
aVF	Augmented vector, front. One of the 12 leads of an ECG; looks electrically at the front of the heart
aVL	Augmented vector, left. One of the 12 leads of an ECG; looks at the heart electrically from the viewpoint of the left shoulder
AZT	Azidothymidine, a commonly used medicine against HIV
BHCG	A pregnancy test that assays the *beta* subunit of the placenta-made human chorionic gonadotropin hormone
bid	Twice a day
BP	Blood pressure
BUN	Blood urea nitrogen, a test of kidney function
CBC	Complete blood count
CHF	Congestive heart failure
CNS	Central nervous system
COBRA	Comprehensive Omnibus Budget Reconciliation Act of 1988
COPD	Chronic obstructive pulmonary disease; often used in lieu of the term emphysema

C-PAP	Continuous positive airway pressure
CPK	Creatine phosphokinase, an enzyme found in muscle and released into the bloodstream when the muscle is damaged
CPK-MB	The myocardial (heart) form of the muscle enzyme CPK
CPR	Cardiopulmonary resuscitation
CSF	Cerebrospinal fluid
C-spine	Cervical spine
CT	Computed tomography, a computer analyzed x-ray test
CVA	Cerebrovascular accident (i.e., stroke); *also* costovertebral angle (in the back, where the lowest rib joins the spine)
CVP	Central venous pressure
DIP	Distal interphalangeal joint—the farthest out "knuckle" of each finger
DKA	Diabetic ketoacidosis
DNR	Do not resuscitate
DT	Delirium tremens
DVT	Deep vein thrombosis
ECG	Electrocardiogram; *also* EKG
ED	Emergency department
EEG	Electroencephalogram, a brain wave test
EGD	Esophagogastroduodenoscopy (i.e., visualizing the digestive tract down through the stomach to the duodenum using a flexible tube with a lens)
EMD	Electromechanical dissociation, electrical activity of the heart without the normally associated pumping activity
EMS	Emergency medical services
EMT	Emergency medical technician
ENT	Ears-nose-throat
EOA	Esophageal-obturator airway
ESR	Erythrocyte (red blood cell) sedimentation rate
ETA	Estimated time of arrival
FDA	Food and Drug Administration

# ABBREVIATIONS

GI	Gastrointestinal
HCG	Human chorionic gonadotropin; *see also* BHCG
HEENT	Head-eyes-ears-nose-throat
HIV	Human immunodeficiency virus
HMO	Health maintenance organization
IM	Intramuscular
INH	Isoniazid, the most common drug for tuberculosis
IV	Intravenous
IVP	Intravenous pyelogram
KUB	An x-ray which includes the kidneys, ureter, and bladder
LBBB	Left bundle branch block, a partial electrical blockage in the heart
LP	Lumbar puncture
LSD	Lysergic acid diethyamide, a hallucinogen
LWBS	Leaving the ED without being seen
MAST	Military anti-shock trousers
MAO	Monoamine oxidase, an enzyme involved in the chemistry of depression
MAO-inhibitors	A class of antidepressant drugs
MI	Myocardial infarction, i.e., heart attack
MRI	Magnetic resonance imaging
NG	Nasogastric
NSAID	Nonstreoidal anti-inflammatory drug, such as aspirin or ibuprofen (e.g., Motrin, Advil)
OD	Overdose
P	Pulse
P-A	Posterior-anterior
PAT	Paroxysmal atrial tachycardia, a rapid heart rhythm originating in the upper chambers of the heart
PCP	Phencyclidine, a hallucinogen; *Pneumocystis carinii* pneumonia
PID	Pelvic inflammatory disease
PR	The time interval between the contraction of the top and bottom halves of the heart
PT	Prothrombin time, a blood clotting study
PTT	Partial thromboplastin time, a blood clotting study
PVC	Premature ventricular contractions

qid	Four times a day
QRS	The main electrical impulse causing the heart to contract and pump
RA factor	A protein found in the blood of patients with rheumatoid arthritis
RBBB	Right bundle branch block, a partial electrical blockage in the heart
RBC	Red blood cell
REM	Rapid eye movement
Rh	A protein on the surface of some people's red blood cells
RMA	Refusal of medical attention
RSI	Rapid sequence intubation. Rapid sedation or paralysis of the patient followed by insertion of a tube down into the trachea to assist breathing
SAH	Subarachnoid hemorrhage
SIDS	Sudden infant death syndrome
ST	The part of the electrocardiogram that reveals ischemia (inadequate blood supply)
STD	Sexually transmitted disease
SVT	Supraventricular tachycardia; *see also* PAT
TCA	Tricyclic antidepressant
tid	Three times a day
TPA	Tissue plasminogen activator, a clot-disolving drug
T-wave	Part of the electrical pattern shown on an electrocardiogram
2-PAM	Pralidoxime
URI	Upper respiratory infection
UTI	Urinary tract infection
VD	Venereal disease
VDRL	A blood test for syphilis (developed by the Venereal Disease Research Laboratory)
V/Q	Ventilation-perfusion
VT	Ventricular tachycardia, a life-threatening abnormality in the heart's electrical activity
WBC	White blood cell
WPW	Wolff-Parkinson-White, a syndrome of congenitally acquired tendency to very rapid heart rates

This book is not fiction. All of the following were real cases.

Case Studies in Emergency Medicine

Notice. The indications for and dosages of all drugs in this book have been recommended in the medical literature and conform to the practices of the general medical community. The medications described do not necessarily have specific approval by the Food and Drug Administration for use in the diseases and dosages for which they are recommended. The package insert for each drug should be consulted for use and dosage as approved by the FDA. Because standards for usage change, it is advisable to keep abreast of revised recommendations, particularly those concerning new drugs.

Case 1 — STABBING VICTIM WITH HOSTILE ENTOURAGE

A 22-year-old man walked into the emergency department loudly saying that he had been stabbed in the abdomen. He was accompanied by several very large friends. He was brought to the trauma room, but the physician and nurse there were unable to approach his bedside because his friends, who were now quite agitated, were protesting loudly that everyone should "stay cool" and keep away from their friend, whom they were there to protect. In their words, "No one comes near him, OK?" When they were finally ushered out, the patient was noted to have a 1-inch long abdominal stab wound in the middle of his left upper quadrant.

What should be done first for the patient?

How do you distinguish a life-threatening stab wound from a worrisome but trivial cut?

Discussion

This group ritual is fascinating and its significance is still unclear. Is there really a need for protection? Is a rival gang about to burst into your emergency department (ED) and cut or shoot up the patient and your staff? It has been known to happen. More frequently, the group bluster is a face-saving gesture and is best dealt with by gestures of respect but firm policy statements. We seldom lose by adopting a posture of respect and honor toward our patients and their family or friends.

Should someone present a case to you in emergency medicine and ask "What should you do first?" a good answer is always "ABCs" (airway, breathing, and circulation) regardless of what the case is about. In this case, after the ABCs were checked, the physician scanned the patient for any other signs of serious trouble: tachypnea, tachycardia, diaphoresis, cyanosis, ashen appearance, or distended neck veins. (Elevated jugular venous pressure is important in trauma since there are two syndromes that can kill the patient rapidly and show markedly elevated venous pressure: pericardial tamponade and tension pneumothorax.) In this case, ignorant as we are of the length of the knife or the direction it took, we need to consider the very real possibility that the heart, lung, or aorta may have been injured in addition to the intra-abdominal organs. The best emergency physicians always consider the worst possibilities. If you diagnose the patient's condition as being relatively benign each time a relatively benign-looking patient presents to you, you will almost always be right, except when you are very wrong.

Since this patient showed no signs of systemic or serious injuries, the physicians were left considering the problems of a young man with a stab wound that might have violated the peritoneal cavity. Trauma centers vary in the care of this kind of case. We anesthetize the area and do a "miniexploration." If the wound is clearly superficial, and we can see the bottom of the wound and are convinced that the peritoneal cavity has not been entered, we suture and discharge the patient. If we get deeper into the wound and are not sure how deep it goes, we abort the procedure and do a diagnostic peritoneal lavage. There are a number of techniques for peritoneal lavage, but all include infusing 1000 ml of Ringer's lactate or normal saline into the peritoneal cavity and then measuring the concentration of red blood cells (RBCs) in the fluid after it is drawn off. In penetrating trauma our primary question is "Has the peritoneum been entered?" Our cutoff for a positive tap in this setting is 10,000 RBCs per mm^3 in the lavage fluid. In our institution all patients with trauma that has penetrated into the abdomen are admitted for serial examination or explored. If the patient has been hemodynamically unstable, we bypass the wound exploration and lavage and send the patient directly to the operating room for a laparotomy.

For blunt abdominal trauma, the diagnostic peritoneal lavage plays a different role. If the patient has sustained major blunt abdominal trauma and is hemodynamically unstable, again the proper path is to the operating room. On the other hand, if the patient is awake and alert and repeatedly has no signs or symptoms of any abdominal injury, then the lavage is again unnecessary. The role of peritoneal lavage is in the equivocal patient—where there has been a significant history of trauma but we are unsure if there is serious injury. Examples include patients who are intoxicated, difficult to evaluate, comatose from head injury, or have unexplained hypovolemia or falling hematocrit. We often find the peritoneal lavage clarifying in such patients.

REFERENCES

Review Article

Proctor, J. H., and Wright, S. W. Penetrating abdominal trauma: A state-of-the-art review. *Emerg. Med. Rep.* 1994;15:223–232.

Additional References

Thompson, J. S., et al. The evolution of abdominal stab wound management. *J. Trauma* 1980;20:478–484.

Marx, J. A. Penetrating abdominal trauma. *Emerg. Med. Clin. North Am.* 1993;11:125–135.

Feliciano, D. V. Diagnostic modalities in abdominal trauma: Peritoneal lavage, ultrasonography, computed tomography scanning, and arteriography. *Surg. Clin. North Am.* 1991;71:241–256.

Henneman, P. L. et al. Diagnostic peritoneal lavage: Accuracy in predicting necessary laparotomy following blunt and penetrating trauma. *J. Trauma* 1990;30:1345–1355.

Case 2: MULTIPLE SOMATIC COMPLAINTS

A 38-year-old woman presented to the triage nurse complaining of fatigue. She stated that this had gone on for several years on and off but had worsened over the past few days. The triage nurse correctly determined that the patient had no immediate threat to life or limb, and had her register with the clerk while assigning her an empty stretcher in a booth. Shortly after this, another nurse began to perform a nursing assessment of the patient. After this had been completed, the nurse told a junior medical resident that this patient had multiple problems and that the nurse could not quite figure out what her main problem was. She looked anxious but not sick otherwise.

The resident went in, introduced himself to the patient, and obtained the following history: The patient had muscle aches and fatigue for the past ten years. She noted no specific pattern to these but thought that they frequently were related to certain foods, and she wondered about an allergy to wheat or eggs. She had intermittent chest pain, dull in nature and related to neither rest nor exertion and sometimes associated with shortness of breath. Occasionally she was short of breath without chest pain. She also had frequent headaches that were frontal in nature and could be relieved, usually, by acetaminophen, but she occasionally required an injection of a painkiller in the emergency department. Her vision had been changing over the past two or three years, and she had a syncopal episode a few months before but did not tell anyone about it (at the time she had no physician or health insurance). She had frequent nausea and thought this also might be related to food ingestions, although not clearly to wheat or eggs. She also had occasional crampy abdominal pain associated with either diarrhea or constipation but occasionally with normal bowel movements. She had urinary frequency without dysuria and complained of missing periods and of heavy periods but ascribed this to a fibroid tumor she was told about eight years prior. She noted a weight gain and loss on and off during these years, but never more than 4 or 5 pounds at a time. She admitted to having swelling of her abdomen and occasionally her feet and hands. She took many vitamins and a thyroid pill every other day and

2. MULTIPLE SOMATIC COMPLAINTS

a water pill three times a week. She had been to various doctors over this period, but none of them had ever been able to help her for any period of time. She said she was sick of being sick.

The resident's examination showed no abnormalities.

The puzzled resident ordered a CBC, glucose, BUN, electrolytes, and also drew a computerized profile, thyroid function studies, and a rheumatoid profile (ANA, VDRL, RA factor, ESR). The first tests came back normal, and he was about to send the patient out with a follow-up appointment to the medical clinic (not his own) when the nurse asked him if he thought that the patient was depressed. A brief argument ensued during which the resident told the nurse that the patient was a "crock." The attending physician on duty was asked his opinion.

He questioned the patient briefly about sleep patterns and depressive symptoms. She admitted difficulty in getting to sleep, early morning waking, and periods of crying easily. She also admitted to job stress and marital problems with her husband. She had been depressed about her illness and occasionally felt like she wanted to die by taking a bottle of pills, and admitted that she felt that way earlier in the day.

The attending reassured her that all steps would be taken to look for an organic cause of her illness, but meanwhile a pressing need was for a psychological evaluation to be performed, and the effects of the multiple symptoms on her emotional state needed to be treated. She agreed to be seen immediately by the psychiatry resident.

What is a "positive review of systems"?

How do you evaluate and treat a patient with a masked depression?

What is the role of the laboratory in the emergency department evaluation of patients with multiple somatic complaints?

Discussion

Some patients will claim to have an astounding number of symptoms. Sometimes they only bring forth this array of symptoms when specifically asked. Terms we use to describe such patients are *multiple somatic complaints* and a *positive review of systems*. As physicians, we should avoid name calling. It does no good to label the patient a "crock"; it serves no useful therapeutic purpose for the patient and makes effective patient care almost impossible.

Patients with these types of complaints are obviously hard to diagnose. In a young person, these may be due to depression, overwork, failing relationships, major unresolved decisions, chronic anxiety, malingering, or the psychiatric syndrome known as somatization disorder. Some other illnesses will produce a multiplicity of symptoms. Infections such as mononucleosis or hepatitis, rheumatic or endocrine disorders, toxic exposures, and occasionally tumors may present with multiple vague symptoms, but these can usually be referred to one or a group of organ systems. In geriatric patients, vague multiple complaints can also be the presentation of cardiac, renal, or hepatic failure, drug effects, or anemia. Drug abuse, common among many young adults, may cause fatigue or other vague symptoms. The examiner must use the correct contemporary terminology to obtain an accurate history. Patients who deny drug use may admit to the use of analgesics, sedatives, tranquilizers, birth control pills, and laxatives. A patient who denies "using drugs" may later admit to "doing coke or smack" (cocaine or heroin) or "popping pills."

Although true medical emergencies can exist in this setting, a more common emergency is the depressed and suicidal patient who presents with organic symptoms and may at first deny psychopathology.

To help rule out organic illness in a patient like this, it would be reasonable to obtain laboratory studies such as a chest x-ray, ECG, urinalysis, complete blood count, biochemical survey (e.g., for hepatic enzymes, calcium, potassium, bilirubin, BUN), and a sedimentation rate. If these are all negative, the patient can be reassured that there is no sign of life-threatening systemic disease.

It should also be explained to the patient that correct therapy must await correct diagnosis. Too often patients are sent home without therapy, sometimes being told or given the impression that "nothing is wrong," or that "everything is all right." This is a disservice to the patient and the medical profession. The principle that correct treatment requires correct diagnosis, and that sometimes this takes more examinations and lab studies, must be explained to patients. At the same time, the physician must be alert for signs of depression and possible suicide risk in patients who present with these symptoms.

The resident physician in this case was misled by the patient's rambling history and thought that he should be able to discover the diagnosis. He became frustrated when this seemed impossible. The attending physician was able to recognize the apparently aimless nature of the patient's complaints, and focused on questioning for somatic symptoms of depressive illness. The common early symptoms of depression include anxiety, insomnia (especially early morning wakening, difficulty getting to sleep, or waking frequently during the night), fatigue, change in appetite (either increase or decrease), crying spells, and an overtly depressed feeling. The patient should have been asked if she felt depressed or if she felt like killing or hurting herself. A common misconception is that by asking these questions, it may "give the patient an idea" and render him or her more likely to commit suicide. In truth, most of these people want help and just need someone to ask the right questions.

Any patient who is depressed and for whom you have any doubts about suicide risk should be referred to a psychiatrist for an immediate evaluation. We tell our patients that this is a rule in our department and does not mean that they are crazy (a common misconception), but only that we feel there is a psychological component to their illness. It helps to emphasize to the patient that the psychiatric evaluation does not mean a diagnosis of mental illness is being made, but it serves as an entry into a counseling setting.

REFERENCES

Review Article
Purcell, T. B. The somatic patient. *Emerg. Clin. North Am.* 1991;9:137–160.

Additional References
Monson, R. A., and Smith, G. R., Jr. Somatization disorder in primary care. *N. Engl. J. Med.* 1983;308:1464–1465.

Pounds, R. A review of the medical and social consequences of generalized anxiety and panic disorder. *J. La. State Med. Soc.* 1992;144:479–483.

Margo, K. L. et al. The problem of somatization in family practice. *Am. Fam. Physician* 1994;48(8):1873–1879.

Wilson, A. et al. The treatment of chronic fatigue syndrome: Science and speculation. *Am. J. Med.* 1994;96(6):544–550.

Case 3 SPRAIN?

A 30-year-old male schoolteacher arrived in the emergency department complaining of having sprained his left wrist while playing tennis two days earlier. He was rather proud of his tennis game and stated that he had been reaching for a "winner" when he fell forcibly onto the outstretched palm of his hand. He had moderate swelling and there was pain with any movement of the wrist joint. The pain was most severe when he attempted to write anything on the blackboard.

The patient was a pleasant young man with physical findings limited to his wrist. On inspection, the left wrist showed diffuse swelling in comparison to the contours of the normal right side. The wrist felt spongy and full just distal to the end of the radius. The patient localized the area of maximum tenderness to a point distal to the radial styloid in the location of the "anatomic snuffbox." He had a great deal of pain when he tried to pronate or supinate his hand against resistance.

What is a sprain? A strain?

How should this patient be managed?

Discussion

A *sprain* is defined as an injury to one or more ligaments supporting a joint in which the joint retains its anatomic alignment. The sprain can be classified as first degree (mild ligamentous damage, moderate pain and swelling), second degree (moderate ligamentous damage, marked pain and swelling, but stable joint), or third degree (severe ligament damage and unstable joint). The degree of swelling and pain around an injured joint has a strong correlation with the amount of ligamentous damage.

The diagnosis of a joint sprain is really one of exclusion. It is diagnosed when all bony injuries in and around a specified joint have been excluded. When the location of maximum pain and swelling is over a known ligament, and a fracture has been ruled out, then a sprain can be diagnosed. Third-degree sprains can be differentiated from second-degree sprains with stress x-ray views of a joint. These views are usually too painful to perform in routine emergency department management and are usually delayed until the swelling has subsided three to four days later.

Most first-degree sprains have a benign course, but a missed third- or severe second-degree sprain can cause years of pain and disability. Operative management is sometimes necessary in these cases. All patients with sprains should be referred to a primary care physician or orthopedist for follow-up if discomfort persists.

The term *strain* describes overexercise or overstretch of a muscle or group of muscles resulting in pain and short-term disability. For example, the common presentation of back "strain" is usually a complex condition involving multiple muscles that support the spine. It can be precipitated by a single episode of heavy lifting lasting only seconds, by isometric contraction such as a "whiplash" injury, or by normal activity.

This case illustrates the necessity of performing a careful physical exam with a working knowledge of the underlying anatomy. The patient had maximum tenderness over the navicular (scaphoid) bone. A fracture in this bone is sometimes impossible to see on the standard x-ray views of the wrist, and a special "navicular view" should be requested. Nonetheless, even with the navicular view, fractures may only be detected seven to ten days later when persistent wrist pain leads to a follow-up x-ray, and bone resorption in the fracture site makes it visible on x-ray. Any patient with point tenderness over the navicular should be treated as a navicular fracture until follow-up evaluation rules it out.

In this case, the navicular view was requested in addition to the standard views, and a transverse fracture through the waist of the navicular bone was clearly seen. The patient was immobilized in a wrist and thumb cast for six weeks and had good union of the fracture site with no development of the painful aseptic necrosis that can follow fractures of this bone.

Other common injuries masquerade as sprains. A neck or back "sprain" may be a vertebral compression fracture, metastatic disease in the spine, meningitis, or even a subarachnoid hemorrhage. A shoulder "sprain" may be an acromioclavicular separation, a rotator cuff tear, a humeral or sternoclavicular dislocation, or even a myocardial infarction. A knee "sprain" may be a medial or lateral meniscus tear, a septic joint, a Baker's cyst, a tibial plateau fracture, gout, or may be referred pain from some disease in the hip.

So, the moral of this story is be suspicious, take a careful history, and think and examine anatomically any patient who complains of a "sprained" anything.

REFERENCES

Review Article
Meldon, S. W., and Hargarten, S. W. Ligamentous injuries of the wrist. *J. Emerg. Med.* 1995;13:217–225.

Additional References
Dobyns, J., and Linscheid, R. L. Fractures and Dislocations of the Wrist. In C. A. Rockwood and P. Green (eds.), *Fractures In Adults.* Vol. 1. Philadelphia: Lippincott, 1984. Pp. 411–420, 450–509.

Harris, T. H., and Harris, W. H. Hand and Wrist. In *The Radiology of Emergency Medicine*, 2nd ed. Baltimore: Williams & Wilkins, 1981. Pp. 250–292.

Dettori, J. R., et al. Early ankle mobilization, Part II: A one year follow-up on acute lateral ankle sprains. *Mil. Med.* 1994;159:20–24.

CASE 4 VITAL SIGNS STABLE, SPEAKING ITALIAN

We received a radio call from a local rescue squad telling us that they had picked up a male in his forties from a one-car automobile accident. His vital signs were "stable," and they had fully immobilized him to prevent head, neck, or body movement. They added that he had been unconscious and unresponsive to all stimuli, but after ten minutes he had awoken and spoken in Italian. The rescue squad brought him into the emergency department with two large-bore intravenous lines that they had started running at a "wide open" rate. The damage to his car was severe.

In the trauma room, the patient's vital signs were normal. His blood pressure was 110/60, pulse 104, and respirations 20. He was alert and answered questions in English. His eyes were open and his pupils were equal and reactive to light. A strong odor of alcohol was on his breath. He complained of chest and abdominal pains. He stated that he was 48 years old and in excellent health with no medical problems. Whenever asked for details about the accident, he began speaking in an unintelligible language. When the paramedics heard this, they identified it as the speech that they had called "Italian."

His chest was tender over the sternum, but his heart and lungs were normal. Abdominal exam showed diffuse tenderness. He was awake and alert, and other than some bruises, the rest of exam was entirely normal. X-rays were obtained and all were negative.

Blood samples were sent for arterial blood gas, complete blood count, glucose, electrolytes, BUN, amylase, clotting profile, type and crossmatch for 6 units, alcohol level, and drug screen. He was removed from restraints after his neck and back x-rays were read as normal. Although he was quite coherent during the evaluation, questions about his accident still led to incomprehensible answers, and when queried he admitted to be speaking in tongues. With further questioning about his religious beliefs, he became angry and agitated. After fifteen minutes of lying quietly on the stretcher, he suddenly jumped up and pulled out his intravenous lines. He tore one intravenous line in the middle of the tubing, and as he ran naked from the room he dripped a trail of blood.

4. VITAL SIGNS STABLE, SPEAKING ITALIAN 13

Five security guards subdued him and tied him to his bed. The staff psychiatrist was asked to see him, and he told of having driven into a tree because God had told him to kill himself.

Is forcible treatment of a trauma patient ever justifiable, and how should it be done?

How much training do emergency medical technicians (EMTs) have before they are allowed to infuse large amounts of intravenous fluid prior to the patient being evaluated by a physician?

DISCUSSION

Basic level EMTs (Emergency Medical Technicians) are trained to recognize most obvious life-threatening emergencies and to provide immediate stabilization. Advanced EMTs are trained to recognize more subtle presentations of emergencies and provide treatments such as intubation, defibrillation, initiation of intravenous therapy with fluids and drugs, and needle thoracostomy for tension pneumothorax. Basic EMT training requires about 100 hours, and advanced EMTs may spend up to 2000 hours in training.

Most victims of automobile accidents are initially treated at the scene by EMTs. Treatment usually includes splinting with a rigid cervical collar, and straps or sandbags keep patients from moving their necks. They are often strapped onto a long spine board. Many emergency medical services (EMS) systems also have standing orders that if the patient is hypotensive or if the mechanism of injury suggests a high likelihood of serious internal trauma, the Military Anti-Shock Trousers (MAST) should be placed on the patient. This may be done in the field for prophylactic reasons and then only inflated if the patient's blood pressure drops below 100 mm Hg. In addition to stabilization of the spine and a rapid infusion of fluids, this patient was given high-flow oxygen by the EMT who picked him up.

This case was complicated by the patient's violence toward the ED staff and his irrational behavior. Generally any patient whom the staff think *might* be suicidal can be held involuntarily and physically restrained if necessary. Patients who are unable to make a rational decision about their care due to acute organic brain syndrome risk death or disability if they leave the ED. Laws on involuntary treatment vary somewhat from state to state, but all accept the principle of well-intentioned therapeutic restraint.

To avoid staff injury, we recommend a team of at least six members when it is necessary to restrain patients who are overtly violent. Sedative medication should be used sparingly in the multiple-trauma patient. Violent trauma patients occasionally need to be paralyzed to undergo potentially life-saving procedures such as intubation or head computed tomography (CT) scanning, but paralysis should never be used as a form of behavior control.

As a last comment, the word *stable* means unchanging or enduring. It does not mean "normal." So we may find a patient's vital signs to be quite abnormal but stable (e.g., long-standing blood pressure of 240/120), or quite normal but unstable (e.g., blood pressure of 120/70 in a patient who is beginning to hemorrhage). If we mean normal, we should say normal. Saying "stable" sometimes acts to reassure us inappropriately.

REFERENCES

Review Articles

Koenig, K. L. *Quo vadis*: "Scoop and run," "stay and treat," or "treat and street?" *Acad. Emerg. Med.* 1995;2:477–480.

Schmidt, C. W., et al. Suicide by vehicular crash. *Am. J. Psychiatry* 1977;134:175–178.

Shuster, M., et al. Differential pre-hospital benefit from paramedic care. *Ann. Emerg. Med.* 1994;23(5):1014–1021.

Additional References

Feero, S., et al. Does out-of-hospital EMS time affect trauma survival? *Am. J. Emerg. Med.* 1995;3:133–135.

Stark, G., et al. Patients who initially refuse prehospital evaluation and/or therapy. *Am. J. Emerg. Med.* 1990;8:509–511.

Case 5 TERRIBLE SORE THROAT

A 26-year-old woman came to the emergency department at 7 P.M. with the following story: She had been ill for four days, suffering with a "terribly sore throat," fatigue, and fever. She felt "all in." There was no significant past history, and she had been well until four days before. The emergency physician examined her and noted large tonsils covered by purulent exudate. She had a fever of 101°F and the doctor thought that she might have slight splenomegaly. The upper cervical lymph nodes were large and tender, but she did not have significant lymphadenopathy elsewhere. The doctor said that he thought she had a streptococcal throat infection, but that mononucleosis was also a real possibility. He cultured her throat, obtained a Monospot test, and prescribed ampicillin four times a day for ten days.

Two days later she returned again to the ED and said that she felt even worse. Her fever had not subsided, the throat was only marginally better, and worst of all, she thought that her entire body was swelling up. The physician checked her throat culture from two days before and told her that she did indeed have strep, that she would surely feel better in a day or two, and encouraged her to continue with the ampicillin. He told her that nothing was wrong with her skin and that the sensation of "swelling up" was probably nothing to worry about.

Three days later she made an emergency appointment to see a physician in the community. She said that she thought she was dying and that she was worse and worse each day. The fever had risen to 104°F, she was very weak, and her skin was bright red. On examination the most remarkable finding was indeed her skin. It was markedly edematous, red, and hot all over her body. She was 20 pounds over her usual weight, and the doctor surmised that it was all fluid. She appeared very toxic and was, in addition, very angry about what she considered to be cavalier treatment by the ED doctor who had "refused to hear her complaint of swelling" on the previous visit. The physician called the hospital laboratory and found that indeed the throat culture had been positive for group A, beta-hemolytic streptococci, but that the Monospot test was also positive. He stopped her ampicillin and placed her on high-dose corticosteroids. She made an uneventful recovery over the next week.

What is the relationship between mononucleosis and ampicillin?

What should your strategy be when your patient is very concerned about a physical finding or a symptom that you cannot see on your exam? Or when you and the patient disagree about the diagnosis or the treatment?

Discussion

Patients with mononucleosis frequently develop rashes when treated with ampicillin or one of its derivatives. Some authors show that as many as 95% of such patients develop erythema, pruritus, or a maculopapular rash when exposed to ampicillin. The drug has even been suggested, perhaps facetiously, as a diagnostic test for the disease. Because ampicillin is no more useful for streptococcal tonsillitis than penicillin and has this unfortunate complication in patients with mononucleosis, and because other bacterial infections of the tonsils (e.g., *Haemophilus influenzae*) are rare in adults, it should probably not be one of your favorite drugs for bacterial pharyngitis or tonsillitis. A newer derivative, amoxicillin and clavulinic acid (Augmentin), interferes with the bacterial beta lactamases that inactivate penicillin. This combination drug may have a role that ampicillin itself lacks, but we would still not recommend it for routine treatment of exudative pharyngitis or tonsillitis.

This patient was convinced that her ED physician had refused to hear her complaint. She thought that he had treated her concern with disdain and that his arrogance had led him to continue her antibiotic several days further, causing more suffering. She was mad enough to sue. When patients report that their doctor did not listen to them, they are very often right: He or she has not listened. There is no excuse for such behavior, and neither patients nor our profession has to condone it.

Another possibility represents a situation that even careful, considerate physicians find themselves in frequently. The patient may tell you of a physical finding that you cannot find during examination. Then there is no satisfactory solution but to describe the trouble back to the patient. "We have a real dilemma here. You notice that your skin seems swollen, but I cannot identify it on my examination. You are probably sensing something that I can't pick up yet. I don't know what it means and may not be able to help until it gets even worse, so that even I can see it." It may help to tell the patient that such situations are common, that either they solve themselves by going away before the doctor can make a diagnosis, or they get worse and then we can figure them out. This is not really very different from the bind you find yourself in when your diagnosis or planned therapy differs from what the patient thought or expected. You have to say, "I know you thought that it would probably be wise to have a shot of penicillin for your cold. I think you are right about the diagnosis, but, unfortunately, this kind of infection doesn't respond to that sort of therapy." A discussion like this tends to leave patients not fully happy but with the feeling that their opinion has been considered, that they have been heard, and that even if they were right, it is reasonable to go with your opinion because you are the professional in the matter.

REFERENCES

Review Article
Heffelfinger, D. C. Gianotti-Croti syndrome in association with Epstein-Barr virus altered by ampicillin. *Ala. Med.* 1985;27:16–18.

Additional References
Pullen, H., et al. Hypersensitivity reactions to antibacterial drugs in infectious mononucleosis. *Lancet* 1967;II:1176–1178.

Pullen, H., et al. Hypersensitivity to the penicillins. *Lancet* 1968;II: 1090.

Case 6: SEVENTY-NINE YEARS OLD AND CONFUSED

A 79-year-old man with a previous diagnosis of organic brain syndrome was brought in by his relatives. They said that they had picked him up from his nursing home that morning to go to their annual summer picnic. He seemed fine except for his usual problem with memory. After lunch, he went to sit in the car to watch the softball game. Several hours later his relatives found him locked in the car, quite agitated and confused.

On physical examination, he was combative and irritable and had red, hot, dry skin. His rectal temperature was 42°C (107.6°F), pulse 160 and quite irregular, respiratory rate 24, and blood pressure 110/80. His neurologic exam showed no focal abnormality. His neck was supple. His venous pressure seemed slightly increased and he had bibasilar rales. A few petechiae were evident on his skin and, when a Foley catheter was inserted, it was noted that he had very little urine output.

What is wrong with this man?

What are the common risk factors for this disorder?

What are its major complications?

What are the most important therapeutic tasks?

DISCUSSION

Heat stroke is defined as hyperpyrexia (temperature above 105°F) with altered mental status. It is a true medical emergency and is often seen among the elderly, the very young, those who are mentally impaired, and those with defective sweating mechanisms. Sweating may be impaired in cystic fibrosis, brainstem or spinal cord injuries, and in the congenital absence of sweat glands. Certain types of drugs have been associated with heat stroke including anticholinergics, phenothiazines, antihistamines, tricyclic antidepressants, and amphetamines.

Complications can involve the cardiovascular system; heart failure and pulmonary edema may be secondary to the marked increase in cardiac output in this syndrome. The patient may suffer centrilobular necrosis of the liver or acute tubular necrosis of the kidneys. There may also be rhabdomyolysis and myoglobinuria leading to renal failure, especially if the heat stroke is exercise induced (as may be seen in young athletes). Pulmonary aspiration, seizures, and coma may occur.

Laboratory abnormalities in heat stroke may include thrombocytopenia and decreased clotting factors secondary to disseminated intravascular coagulation. One may find hypoglycemia, respiratory alkalosis, or metabolic acidosis. Hyperkalemia from cell breakdown and release of potassium stores is to be anticipated.

The treatment of heat stroke requires removing the patient from the hot environment, removing clothing, and allowing evaporative cooling by applying cool or cold water to the skin surface. Unlike *hypo*thermia, where rapid external warming can be detrimental, in *hyper*thermia, aggressive external cooling is exactly what is needed. Hypoglycemia is common in this syndrome, and dextrose should be given. Since many of these patients are alcoholic, thiamine is an appropriate accompaniment. Adequate hydration and alkalinization of the urine to protect against myoglobinuric renal failure are also important. Careful attention to the hydration state is essential. Most patients with heat stroke are volume depleted, but caution must be taken to avoid fluid overload. A central venous pressure monitor may be useful. Liver function and clotting studies should be monitored.

REFERENCES

Review Article
Tek, D., et al. Heat illness. *Emerg. Med. Clin. North Am.* 1992;10:299–310.

Additional References
Knochel, J. P. Environmental heat illness: An eclectic review. *Arch. Intern. Med.* 1974;137:841–864.

Shibolet, S., Lancester, M. C., and Danon, Y. Heat stroke: A review. *Aviat. Space Environ. Med.* 1976;47:280–301.

Drake, D. K., et al. Recognition and management of heat-related illness. *Nurse Pract.* 1994;19:43–47.

Case 7 "DON'T MAKE ME STAY IN THE HOSPITAL"

A 56-year-old woman was brought to the ED with a chief complaint of feeling faint. As the physician entered her booth for the first time and approached her to introduce himself, she took his hand in hers, pressed it to her forehead, and said emotionally, "Please doctor . . . don't make me stay in the hospital . . . please doctor . . . please . . ."

The history then given by the patient and her husband was as follows: They had been out shopping, as usual, one Saturday morning and had been in the check-out line of their supermarket when the patient began to feel faint. She did not actually pass out, but did fall to one knee and sustained a minor knee abrasion. An ambulance was called, and it arrived promptly. After lying down in the ambulance the patient began to feel better, and by the time the physician saw her she was back to feeling like her usual self. There had been no other associated symptoms.

Her physical examination was unremarkable. She had been placed on a cardiac monitor upon arrival at the ED, and no arrhythmias were noted at any time. After her normal examination and a period of observation, during which she continued to feel fine, she was discharged.

A few minutes later the husband telephoned the ED and said, "I think my wife is dead." An ambulance was dispatched, and the patient was found in full cardiac arrest. She could not be resuscitated. The husband stated that after discharge from the ED they had gone home, the patient had put her key in the door, stepped inside, said "I think it is happening again," and fallen down unconscious.

What went wrong here?

What else should have been done for the patient?

Discussion

The cause of this patient's death remains a mystery. Perhaps it would have been revealed if the patient had had a full workup in the ED. Every syncope patient deserves at least a review of current medications and an examination that includes vital signs (including orthostatics), an abdominal exam, a rectal exam including a test for occult blood, and an electrocardiogram.

One of the most important questions good emergency medicine specialists should ask themselves in *every* case is, "What is the worst thing that could be accounting for this patient's symptoms?" Sometimes one or two additional questions need to be asked of the patient, and the responses documented. Sometimes an additional test may need to be ordered. Sometimes discharge instructions need to be a little more complete or explicit, and sometimes nothing further will be done. Nevertheless, the most severe possibility needs to be given at least a moment's thought if disasters like the one in this case are going to be averted. If you ascribe the patient's symptoms to the most common, plausible diagnosis you will almost always be right—except when you are terribly wrong.

REFERENCES

Review Article
Daily, R. H. Approach to the Patient in the Emergency Department. In P. Rosen, et al. (eds.), *Emergency Medicine: Concepts and Clinical Practice* (3rd ed.). St. Louis: Mosby, 1992.

Additional Reference
Rosen, P., and Honigman, B. Life and Death. In P. Rosen, et al. (eds.), *Emergency Medicine: Concepts and Clinical Practice* (3rd ed.). St. Louis: Mosby, 1992.

Case 8 "SICK ALL OVER"

A 26-year-old woman came to the emergency department complaining of feeling "sick all over" and suddenly fainted in the triage area. She woke shortly after and was able to give the following history: She had been vomiting for several days and could not even keep water down. She also complained of a vague, diffuse abdominal pain.

On examination she was seen to be a very distressed woman who appeared to be breathing deeply but denied dyspnea. Her eyes were sunken, her skin turgor was decreased, and her mucous membranes were parched.

Her temperature was 99°F, pulse 120, blood pressure 100/50, respiratory rate 36, and her neck veins were flat, suggesting a very low central venous pressure. When asked to stand up, she became faint and pale. Her abdomen was soft and had normal bowel sounds. She had no abdominal or costovertebral angle tenderness, and the rest of her examination was normal.

What do you think about asking a patient who has just fainted to stand up?

What feature of this patient requires urgent therapy at this point without any further diagnostic testing?

What might be the underlying problem?

What diagnostic tests, some easy and available at the bedside, would you do?

Discussion

This patient has a low arterial blood pressure, and it will fall still lower when she sits or stands. Before standing her up, you should obtain a careful pulse and blood pressure in the supine position and then try it again in the seated position. If she has a significant fall in the mean arterial pressure or a rise in pulse rate when she sits up, there is no need to ask more of her. She might fall again and hurt herself.

8. "SICK ALL OVER"

Although it looks like a simple case of severe gastroenteritis, the patient actually has a rather classic picture of *new* diabetic ketoacidosis (DKA) with hypovolemia and dehydration. Abdominal pain, nausea, and vomiting are commonly seen in DKA. Her tachypnea is caused by her hypotension and her metabolic acidosis. Patients whose tachypnea is driven by metabolic acidosis may not sense shortness of breath. The feature of the disorder that demands urgent therapy is her hypovolemia. Eventually you will want to treat her with insulin, and perhaps with potassium, but right now she requires copious volumes of intravenous fluid.

Two bedside tests that could help confirm your diagnosis are Chemstrips (or Dextrostix) that give a rapid gross estimate of blood sugar, and a urine dipstick that will show sugar and ketones. Once you are giving the patient fluid, you should ask for more precise chemistry data, including electrolytes and an arterial blood gas determination. DKA patients usually present with hyperkalemia secondary to their acidosis. Once therapy has begun, they may quickly become hypokalemic as the acidosis corrects and insulin drives sugar and potassium into cells.

You need to search for the trigger event that put the patient into ketoacidosis. A focus of infection, inappropriate cessation of insulin therapy, trauma, a myocardial infarction, and maybe even emotional stress may trigger DKA. It is reasonable to obtain a complete blood count, urinalysis, blood cultures, chest x-rays, and an ECG. Unfortunately, in many cases we are unable to find the triggering event. It may be too subtle for us.

Normal saline is the fluid of choice and may be run in rapidly through a large-bore intravenous line. An initial hydration rate of 1000 ml over one-half hour is reasonable in a young adult. Once the potassium level begins to decline and is down into the normal range, potassium should be added to the intravenous fluid.

Insulin is usually given as a regular insulin drip at a rate of 6 to 10 units per hour after an initial bolus of 6 to 10 units. Patients with obvious infection require more insulin than those without such a disorder. When the blood sugar has decreased to about 250 mg per dl, glucose can be added to the infusion to prevent overshoot hypoglycemia. The insulin should be continued to clear circulating ketones.

REFERENCES

Review Article

Kitabchi, A. E., et al. Diabetic ketoacidosis. *Med. Clin. North Am.* 1995;79:9–37.

Additional References

Crane, E. J. Diabetic ketoacidosis: Biochemistry, physiology, treatment and prevention. *Pediatr. Clin. North Am.* 1987;34:935–960.

Forster, D. W., and Mcgary, J. D. The metabolic derangements and treatment of diabetic ketoacidosis. *N. Engl. J. Med.* 1983;309:159–169.

Tattersall, R., et al. Consequences of brittle diabetes: 12-year follow-up. *B.M.J.* 1991;302:1240–1243.

Case 9   SEXUAL ASSAULT

A 35-year-old woman was brought to the emergency department by two police officers at 2 A.M. for evaluation and treatment following a sexual assault. She stated that at about 11 P.M. she was abducted by two men who beat her with their fists and forced her to have oral and vaginal intercourse. She was not sure whether ejaculation occurred. Her complaints were of abdominal, perineal, and head pain. Her last voluntary sexual intercourse was three days previously.

On examination, the patient appeared preoccupied. Her hair was in disarray and her clothes spotted with mud. She had areas of abrasion and ecchymosis about the right eye. Oral examination was unremarkable, but samples were obtained for culture (gonorrhea and chlamydia), acid phosphatase determination (an enzyme present in semen), and a microscopic exam. She had scattered bruising over the forearms and abrasions over both knees. Her abdomen was soft with a mild, generalized tenderness. On pelvic exam, the external genitalia were normal, except for two small superficial posterior fourchette lacerations. The vaginal vault had scant amounts of white discharge that were also sampled for acid phosphatase and a microscopic examination. The bimanual exam showed mild discomfort with palpation of the uterus and adnexal structures, but no other abnormalities were found. On microscopic exam, the sample from the oral pharynx was negative, and the vaginal swab showed motile sperm.

What special steps need to be taken for legal documentation and evidence collection?

How should the problems of pregnancy and venereal disease prophylaxis be addressed?

What type of follow-up care should be arranged?

DISCUSSION

Care of the sexual assault victim in the ED should involve a team approach. The team should consist of the physician, a nurse, a rape counselor, a police officer (preferably specifically trained in rape intervention), and, when needed, a psychiatrist. Additionally, most cities have a rape crisis center with workers who can aid in the evaluation of rape victims and in early crisis management. The primary goal of the team should be care of the patient's medical and psychiatric needs. Secondary goals of evidence collection, documentation, and reporting the alleged assault to authorities should not take precedence over the patient's care.

The history should be as complete as possible without adding to the trauma of the incident by overemphasizing the details of the assault. Preferably, the history should be obtained by a single member of the team and not be repeated by other members. The date and time of both the assault and exam should appear on the chart. A brief description of the assault including the use of force, drugs, or foreign bodies, and the specifics of sexual contact (oral, vaginal, or anal penetration) need to be documented. Details of personal hygiene (urination, defecation, douching, and bathing) and any clothing change since the assault need documentation. Past gynecologic history (pregnancy, last menstrual period, and last vaginal intercourse) and medical history should be included.

The physical examination should be thorough and should document all injuries. The clothing worn during the assault should be placed in a paper bag by the patient. The mental status of the patient at the time should be noted, including whether she is mentally competent to consent to intercourse. Her pelvic exam should be documented in detail including external genitalia, vaginal vault, appearance of the hymen (or remnant), and presence of any discharge. Use of the Wood's lamp may facilitate location of dried semen, which will fluoresce.

Samples that should be gathered during the examination include:

1. Saliva from the patient on a small cotton cloth (to determine if the blood group antigens are secreted).
2. Blood sample for VDRL, pregnancy testing, and type/Rh.
3. Swabs from any orifice entered for acid phosphatase and a separate swab for a wet prep to be examined by the physician for sperm (motility should be documented).
4. Combings of the patient's hair and pubic hair for foreign material.
5. 10 pulled and 15 closely cropped hairs from the pubic region and a similar number from the head.

9. SEXUAL ASSAULT

6. Gonorrhea and chlamydia cultures.
7. Fingernail scrapings.

Each of these specimens must be labeled with the patient's name, the date they were obtained, the source of the sample, and the initials of the person obtaining the sample. All samples should be placed in a sealed envelope, and the chain of evidence should be documented on the envelope (date/time the evidence was obtained/transferred and your name/title).

Venereal disease prophylaxis should be offered to all patients who present with a history of sexual assault. Because 40 to 90% of patients do not return for follow-up, venereal disease prophylaxis should preferably be performed while the patient is still in the ED, instead of at a later date after culture results are obtained. Prophylaxis for gonorrhea, chlamydia, and syphilis should be initiated with standard therapy.

Counseling about human immunodeficiency virus (HIV) disease is always part of our rape treatment program. Depending on the nature of the assault, HIV blood testing *may* be recommended at 3 and 6 months after the encounter. Animal studies suggest that if the patient is seen within 24 hours of the assault, 6 weeks of treatment with AZT may be effective prophylaxis against the development of HIV infection.

Pregnancy prevention should be discussed with all patients. All forms of post-coital pregnancy prevention available at this time have a relatively high incidence of side effects. Treatment options include: (1) institute no therapy and wait for next menses, (2) repeat pregnancy test in 10 days and if positive consider therapeutic abortion, and (3) high-dose estrogen therapy such as two Ovral tablets bid every 12 hours for 2 doses plus an antiemetic such as Compazine for nausea. All "morning after" forms of therapy are effective within 72 hours of intercourse but are teratogenic to existing pregnancies; therefore, it is imperative that pregnancy be ruled out before initiation of therapy.

All patients should be offered follow-up through an established rape crisis center.

Follow-up examination should also be scheduled at 1 and 6 weeks, at which times repeat gonorrhea culture, syphilis serology, and pregnancy testing should be done. Psychiatric interventions and counseling at a rape crisis center should also be repeated as necessary at these times.

Sexual assault is a frightening experience that will change the victim's life forever. The expedient delivery of health care and the humanistic treatment of the patient at the time of presentation to the ED are important first steps in restoring order to a life in disarray.

REFERENCES

Review Articles

Kobernick, M. E., Seifert, S., and Saunders, A. B. Emergency department management of the sexual assault victim. *J. Emerg. Med.* 1985;2:205–214.

Dwyer, B. J. Rape: Psychological, medical, and forensic aspects of emergency management. *Emerg. Med. Reports* 1995;16:105–116.

Additional References

Elam, A. L., and Ray, V. G. Sexually related trauma: A review. *Ann. Emerg. Med.* 1986;15:576–584.

Tintinalli, J. E., and Holzer, M. Clinical findings and legal resolution in sexual assault. *Ann. Emerg. Med.* 1985;14:447–453.

Ranbow, B. Female sexual assault: Medical and legal implications. *Ann. Emerg. Med.* 1992;21:727–731.

Gostin, L. O., et al. HIV testing, counseling, and prophylaxis after sexual assault. *J.A.M.A.* 1994;271:1436–1444.

Cardello, D. Emergency department sexual assault assessment. *J. Emerg. Nurs.* 1993;19:450–451.

Sexual Assault. ACOG Technical Bulletin Number 172. *Int. J. Gynaecol. Obstet.* 1993;42(1):67–72.

Case 10 FIVE SICK SIBLINGS

On one hot summer afternoon, five of the seven children in one family visited a physician. They complained of abdominal pains of 2 days' duration. One child also had fever and diarrhea. The physician diagnosed viral gastroenteritis and suggested fluids and rest. There was no improvement during the next day, and by the following morning three of the children did not respond to voice, and the others were obviously ill. Later that day, all seven children were brought to a hospital emergency department. Two were in respiratory arrest, and the other five had various degrees of lethargy, increased respiratory secretions, increased salivation, and pupillary constriction. Two of the children died. The next day the laboratory reported that all the children had depressed serum and erythrocyte cholinesterase levels.

What sort of poisoning should have been suspected?

How is it best treated?

Discussion

The presentation of a cluster of cases of a similar illness should lead one to suspect an environmental toxic cause. Although it is common for all the children in a household to develop a viral gastroenteritis, it is unusual for them to all develop the symptoms simultaneously.

Food poisoning by staphylococcal toxin is the most common of the so-called common source illnesses that present this way. The common thread will be that all affected members ate the same food. Botulism will also present this way, with complaints related to muscular weakness, usually beginning with the ocular muscles. Carbon monoxide poisoning, another common source illness, may initially present with abdominal pain and headache before progressing to neurologic changes, coma, and death.

Serum and erythrocyte cholinesterase levels are depressed in acute organophosphate poisoning, but the results of that test may not be back soon enough to make the diagnosis. Additionally, the range of normal cholinesterase levels is so great that a level may actually be *significantly depressed from that patient's baseline* and yet be misinterpreted as "normal." Treatment with a test dose of atropine may make the diagnosis. Cholinergic poisoning is characterized by the SLUDGE (Salivation, Lacrimation, Urinary incontinence, Diarrhea, Gastrointestinal irritability, and Emesis) syndrome. There may be rhonchi and wheezes on the lung exam, the bowel sounds will be hyperactive, and bradycardia and profuse diaphoresis may be present. The most common cause of this syndrome is poisoning with any one of the common pesticides or insecticides of the organophosphate class. These agents, originally developed as instruments of war, bind to and inactivate acetylcholinesterase, causing a symptomatic build-up of acetylcholine and a rush of cholinergic discharge. The immediate treatment is with intravenous atropine titrated until signs of atropinization appear (the wheezing stops, the pupils dilate, and the heart rate increases). Huge doses of atropine, often 20 to 30 mg per hour, may be needed to control the symptoms. In severe anticholinergic poisoning, this is followed by pralidoxime (2-PAM), a drug that removes the organophosphate from the enzyme and allows acetylcholine to be degraded normally.

The source of the organophosphates in this case was never definitely identified. There was some dust on equipment used for spraying that the children were playing with. The adults, who had not touched the equipment, were unaffected. Organophosphates are rapidly absorbed through the skin, and they must be fully removed as quickly as possible to reduce the amount absorbed. The powder on the skin of a victim can also pose a hazard to the rescuer.

REFERENCES

Review Article

Mortensen, M. L. Management of acute childhood poisoning caused by selected insecticides and herbicides. *Pediatr. Clin. North Am.* 1986;33:421–445.

Additional Reference

Midtling, J. E., et al. Clinical management of field worker organophosphate poisoning. *West. J. Med.* 1985;142:514–518.

Case 11 SUICIDAL

A 32-year-old woman presented to the ED of a small rural hospital complaining of being very nervous and frightened. She was brought by a friend who thought the patient was suicidal. The patient had a history of suicide attempts and had been a psychiatric patient in the past. She also had a past history of alcoholism and had been treated in several rehabilitation programs. She had left the last rehabilitation program after being there for only a few days. She had abstained from drinking from that time until the night she was brought into the ED.

When asked what the problem was, the patient stated that she was having problems at home. She did not elaborate on this. However, when asked specifically if she was abused by her husband, the patient looked up without speaking, and her friend nodded in the affirmative. The patient denied having taken any overdoses or having a specific suicide plan. She did, however, state on several occasions that she "just wanted to get away" from her situation "forever."

A medical screening examination was normal and the only lab tests that were done were serum acetaminophen and aspirin levels. While waiting for these levels to be returned, the patient became somewhat anxious and agitated, and stated that she wanted to leave. She was told that she had to stay, and her friend agreed to keep an eye on her. The patient persisted in saying she did not want to go for psychiatric evaluation because she felt that she would be fine, and she just wanted to go home. Her friend told her that she would be better off in the psychiatric hospital, and was worried that the patient might try to kill herself if left at home.

A short while later the patient and her husband were seen leaving the hospital, walking very quickly to the parking lot. They drove off before they could be stopped. The local police department was contacted and an officer agreed to assist in finding the patient and returning her to the emergency department. Both the patient and her husband were well known to the police officer. He stated that they both had drinking problems and that the husband was very abusive of the wife. The officer had been called to their home on several occasions because of domestic violence.

The patient was finally located at her home and escorted back to the emergency department by the police officer and several fire department paramedics. She was then transferred to the local psychiatric facility for crisis evaluation.

What do we do when patients "elope" from the emergency department?

How do we recognize victims of domestic violence, and what should be the appropriate ED treatment for them?

DISCUSSION

All experienced members of the ED staff know that there are certain characteristic behavior patterns found in patients who come to the ED seeking help and then leave before they get it. Some patients simply walk in, see that the department is busy, and walk out without even registering for care. Others sign in, but leave before they can be seen (LWBS—leave without being seen). Some elope or disappear in the middle of their evaluation, and others object to some aspect of their testing or care and make an informed decision not to proceed (leaving AMA—against medical advice). The difference between eloping and going AMA is that the patient who goes AMA tells the ED staff that they are leaving and that they do not want the recommended testing or treatment. The patient who elopes just gets up and leaves without giving notice or signing the AMA form. They often don't discuss the pros and cons of treatment before leaving. They have simply "had it" for some reason, and then they are gone.

There are certain patients whom we want to keep in the emergency department for their own protection, and therefore we have an obligation to prevent them from eloping. These include patients who pose a risk to themselves because of suicide threats or attempts, who have severely altered mental status, who would be unable to care for themselves outside of a supervised setting, who are severely intoxicated, or who are severely incapacitated because of drugs.

Domestic violence is becoming more visible in society as well as in the emergency department. There has always been a large amount of domestic violence, but we are only now beginning to address it as a serious public health problem. Over 90% of the victims of domestic violence are women. Clues to domestic violence include injuries that are inconsistent with the history given by the patient, frequent visits to the ED for apparently very minor injuries, and psychiatric symptoms relating to a stressful home situation. We are also suspicious of domestic violence if the patient's spouse or significant other refuses to leave the room while the patient is being examined, or if he or she monopolizes the history and gives the information instead of letting the patient speak. In many cases the person being abused does not feel free to give a history of abuse to us unless we probe for it.

If we are dealing with a woman who has been abused, we offer her several things:

1. We treat her medical or psychiatric condition.
2. We give her a set of discharge instructions which do not refer to abuse. This is done because in many cases the husband will be searching through her purse to see what papers we have given her.
3. We offer to arrange to have her placed in a safe house. Almost all cities and rural areas have access to a shelter for battered women. In most cases this can be arranged through the local police department.
4. We also offer to call the police if she would like to press charges.

In this case, the patient's husband was an alcoholic (still actively drinking), well known in the community as someone who abused his wife, and in fact (although it sounds unprofessional), as they were leaving, both the police and firefighters who brought her to the hospital offered to "beat the living daylights out of him" if he didn't stop abusing her.

In any such case, it is crucial to let the woman know that she is not alone, that there are resources available in the community to assist her should she want help, and that help is readily available. We also should let her know that she would be much safer if she sought help, rather than stayed in the ongoing abusive relationship.

REFERENCES

Review Articles
Council on Scientific Affairs, American Medical Association, Chicago, Ill. Violence against women: Relevance for medical practitioners. *J.A.M.A.* 1992;267:3184–3189.

Dwyer, B. Strategies for recognizing and managing suicidal patients. *Emerg. Med. Reports* 1993;14(11):91–98.

Additional References

Stark, E., and Flitcraft, A. Killing the beast within: Woman battering and female suicidality. *Int. J. Health Serv.* 1995;25:43–64.

Johnson, L. A. Spurious assumptions about ED domestic violence victim caseloads. *Ann. Emerg. Med.* 1995;25:561–562.

Murphy, J. C. Legal protection for domestic violence victims: A guide for the treating physician. *Md. Med. J.* 1994;43:899–902.

Jackson, J. K. Understanding survival responses of battered women. *Md. Med. J.* 1994;43:871-875.

Loring, M. T., and Smith, R. W. Health care barriers and interventions for battered women. *Public Health Rep.* 1994;109(3):328–338.

Case 12 LEFT LOWER QUADRANT PAIN

A 35-year-old woman came to the emergency department complaining of low abdominal pain. The pain was bilateral but more marked on her left side. It had begun gradually the previous day and was not affected by anything she did. She denied having urinary problems, changes in her bowel habits, vaginal discharge, or vaginal bleeding except for a few spots of blood that had appeared on her pants the day before the pain began. She was ten days late for her period but had been slightly irregular in the past. She denied previous gynecologic problems.

On arrival she did not appear to be in any significant distress. She had normal respirations at a rate of 16, a pulse of 80, and a blood pressure of 120/80. Her abdomen had normal bowel sounds and was soft and nontender. There was no costovertebral angle tenderness. On pelvic examination she was found to have a normal parous cervix without any blood or discharge. Specimens of cervical mucus were obtained for chlamydia and gonorrhea cultures. She had a full, nontender bladder, mild cervical motion tenderness, and a moderately tender left adnexal region. The rectovaginal exam was normal and she had guiac negative stool.

The physician asked her to give a clean-catch urine sample and ordered a CBC and a serum beta–human chorionic gonadotropin (beta-HCG) pregnancy test. The patient walked to the bathroom and was found five minutes later crouched at the bathroom door, holding on to the doorjamb and about to collapse.

Her nurse and doctor lifted her onto a stretcher and noted that she was quite sweaty and had a pulse of 100 and a blood pressure of 80/50. They started two large-bore intravenous lines with lactated Ringer's solution and opened the stopcocks fully. They noted that her abdomen was more tender than it had been before, even to light palpation, and that bowel sounds were absent. A gynecologist was called and the operating room alerted. Her laparotomy began 20 minutes after her collapse. In the operating room, she was found to have 2000 ml of blood in the peritoneal cavity and a ruptured left tubal pregnancy.

What should be done when the diagnosis of ectopic pregnancy is first thought of?

What was there about her initial presentation that should have set off flashing lights in those caring for this healthy-looking patient?

DISCUSSION

Ectopic pregnancy is often difficult to diagnose, but it is increasingly common. The possibility of this diagnosis should spring to mind if any young woman presents with lateralized low abdominal pain. Patients with this condition often deteriorate abruptly.

This woman had lower abdominal pain, vaginal bleeding, a late period, and pain on adnexal palpation—all suggesting ectopic pregnancy. Her differential diagnoses, however, included salpingitis, ovarian cyst, appendicitis, and threatened abortion. After the history and physical exam, the first task in evaluating a woman with low abdominal pain of unknown origin is to determine whether or not she is pregnant.

This is not the first patient whose ectopic pregnancy ruptured after pelvic exam. Any patient whose history and physical suggest an ectopic pregnancy should be under observation with an intravenous line in place until the *serum* pregnancy test (more sensitive than urine) is known to be negative. If a urine specimen had been obtained prior to the examination, a urinary tract infection could have been ruled out and the bladder would have been empty, allowing a more accurate pelvic exam. Ectopic pregnancies generate lower levels of HCG than do intrauterine pregnancies, and occasionally the urine will be falsely negative.

If this patient had not worsened so dramatically and if the beta-HCG pregnancy test had been positive, then a pelvic ultrasound would have been ordered. If the ultrasound failed to show an intrauterine pregnancy, then she would have been admitted to the hospital for observation, serial HCG levels, and a repeat of the ultrasound. If this patient had arrived already in shock, rapid fluid resuscitation and immediate transfer to the operating room would have followed after a brief history and physical examination, intravenous line placement, and blood drawing for CBC, HCG, and crossmatching.

REFERENCES

Review Article
Jehle, D. Ectopic pregnancy. *Emerg. Med. Clin. North Am.* 1994;12:55–71.

Additional References
Gennis, P., et al. Cost effectiveness of an accurate and rapid assay for serum human chorionic gonadotropin in suspected ectopic pregnancy. *Am. J. Emerg. Med.* 1988;6:4–6.

Hockberger, R. S. Ectopic pregnancy. *Emerg. Med. Clin. North Am.* 1987;5:481–493.

Gaeta, T. J., et al. Atypical ectopic pregnancy. *Ann. Emerg. Med.* 1993;11:233–234.

Abbott, J., et al. Ectopic pregnancy: Ten common pitfalls in diagnosis. *Am. J. Emerg. Med.* 1990;8:515–522.

Brennan, D. F. Ectopic pregnancy. *Acad. Emerg. Med.* 1995;2:1081–1098.

CASE 13 DROWNED CHILD

The local rescue squad arrived at the emergency department ambulance ramp with a 16-year-old who had fallen into a nearby pond while ice-fishing with his father. The rescue worker said that it had taken them 35 minutes to retrieve him and that he was pulseless and apneic at the scene. Basic life support cardiopulmonary resuscitation efforts were begun immediately. He was ventilated using an esophageal-obturator airway (EOA).

At the ED, the boy was deeply cyanotic, cold, and without vital signs. His core body temperature was 28°C (83°F). His pupils were fixed and dilated.

Is there any point to going any further in this resuscitation?

What factors determine good outcome after prolonged submersion?

What is the esophageal-obturator airway (EOA)?

DISCUSSION

The longest documented submersion with full neurologic recovery occurred in a 2½-year-old girl who was submerged in ice water for 66 minutes. The factors that determine good or poor outcome after prolonged submersion in ice water are still unclear. The "mammalian dive reflex" has been credited as a mechanism, but no substantial evidence supports this hypothesis. The shunting of blood from other parts of the body to the heart and brain that occurs in seals and other diving animals has never been shown to be of any significance in humans. Protection of the brain by decreasing its metabolic needs for oxygen through the development of acute submersion hypothermia is a more plausible explanation.

Regardless of the protective mechanism, the implication is that prolonged and heroic resuscitation attempts after submersion in very cold water are of value. Anyone profoundly hypothermic should not be declared dead until they are rewarmed, hence the old dictum, "You are not dead until you are warm and dead."

The most important aspect of prehospital care is the immediate initiation of ventilation and oxygenation. Evidence of trauma should be noted, and cervical spine precautions taken if indicated. Contributing factors such as hypoglycemia, seizures, and child neglect or abuse need to be considered. There is no logic in attempting to drain water from the lungs in fresh water drowning since the hypotonic fluid is rapidly absorbed. The Heimlich maneuver should not be performed unless there is inability to ventilate the patient due to an obstructed airway. Pushing on the stomach only increases the potential for emesis and aspiration of gastric contents.

In the ED, critical patients should be intubated (going around the EOA, if necessary) and then hyperventilated. Continuous ECG and core temperature monitoring are needed. External rewarming modalities such as applying hot towels or heating lamps to the skin should be avoided because they produce peripheral vasodilation, allowing more cold, acidotic blood to enter the central circulation. The optimum rewarming method is extracorporeal blood rewarming, combining a heart bypass machine with a heat exchanger. When extracorporeal rewarming is unavailable, peritoneal, gastric, bladder, or thoracic cavity lavage can be performed. Normal saline warmed to 106°F can be used as the irrigating solution.

The EOA is not used frequently in the prehospital setting. It is one of a number of devices designed to be inserted down the throat and to occlude the esophagus, thus decreasing the likelihood of aspiration and allowing more effective bag-mask ventilation. Unfortunately, many complications are associated with its use, including accidental insertion down and occlusion of the airway, thus ensuring ventilation of the stomach!

Unfortunately, in spite of aggressive therapy, the teenager in this case died.

REFERENCES

Review Article

Olshaker, J. S. Near drowning. *Emerg. Med. Clin. North Am.* 1992; 10:339–350.

Additional References

Neal, J. M. Near-drowning. *J. Emerg. Med.* 1985;3:41–52.

Bolte, R. G., et al. The use of extracorporeal rewarming in a child submerged for 66 minutes. *J.A.M.A.* 1988;260:377–379.

Levin, D. L., et al. Drowning and near drowning. *Pediatr. Clin. North Am.* 1993;40:321–336.

Kyricon, D. N., et al. Effect of immediate resuscitation on children with submersion injury. *Pediatrics* 1994;94:137–142.

Feldman, K. W. When is childhood drowning neglect? *Child Abuse Negl.* 1993;17:329-336.

Case 14 AN OTHERWISE WELL INFANT

A young mother came running into the emergency department with her 4-month-old infant son, screaming, "He's not breathing, he's not breathing!"

The infant was cool, cyanotic, and without detectable pulse or blood pressure. He was intubated orally with a 3.5-mm endotracheal tube and was ventilated by bag as cardiac compression was begun. While efforts were made to start an intravenous line, 0.1 mg of epinephrine (1.0 ml of 1/10,000 solution) was given down the endotracheal tube, and an intraosseous line was placed in the anterior tibia for administration of medications and fluids. Despite 30 minutes of resuscitative efforts, there was no evidence of cardiac response, and he was pronounced dead.

His mother said that he had been well, had eaten a good supper of formula and cereal, and had gone to bed uneventfully. He had a little nasal congestion the prior week but otherwise was well. She remembered that once, about a month earlier, she had gone to look at him sleeping and thought that he was not breathing. She touched him and he woke, crying, much to her relief. She had told her husband, but he thought she was "just being a nervous mother."

The chaplain and a social worker were called to help console the family.

What is the most likely diagnosis?

What other diagnostic possibilities should be considered?

What is the primary event in pediatric cardiopulmonary arrest?

DISCUSSION

This is a classic presentation of sudden infant death syndrome (SIDS), commonly called "crib death." These infants are usually healthy and then suffer an unexpected cardiac and respiratory arrest. They are under 1 year of age, with the peak incidence at 2 to 4 months. The autopsy usually fails to define a cause of death. SIDS occurs more in the fall and winter months, and sometimes the death is preceded by a mild respiratory infection. There may be a familial association with sleep apnea or periodic breathing. SIDS seems to occur more in lower socioeconomic families, and boys are at greater risk than girls. Infants of low birth weight and those with cigarette-smoking mothers are also at increased risk. It is now known that the incidence of SIDS will be reduced if infants are always put down to sleep on their backs, not on their sides or their stomachs ("BACK to sleep"). The cause of SIDS is unknown. Over seventy theories have been proposed.

Pediatric arrests differ from adult arrests in that the primary event is usually respiratory rather than cardiac. After prolonged hypoxia, the heart rhythm deteriorates to a bradycardia, and then to asystole.

Therapy is usually unsuccessful. The attempts in this infant exemplify the usual difficulty establishing an intravenous line for medication administration. Once an airway has been established, generally using an endotracheal tube of the same diameter as the child's little finger, certain medications can be given down the tube: epinephrine, atropine, lidocaine, and naloxone (Narcan). Intraosseous cannulation of the anterior tibea can be used to administer medications intravascularly.

Although this case is typical of SIDS, the most common other diagnosis to look for is nonaccidental trauma or child abuse. We must be aware of the possibility of child abuse, but that awareness should not keep us from empathetic support of bereaved parents. SIDS support groups exist throughout the country, and parents of a child with SIDS should probably be referred to one for counselling and support.

REFERENCES

Review Article
Brooks, J. G. Unraveling the mysteries of SIDS. *Curr. Opin. Pediatr.* 1993;5:266–276.

Additional References
Oren, J., et al. Identification of the high risk group for sudden infant death syndrome among infants who are resuscitated from sleep apnea. *Pediatrics* 1986;77:495–499.

Kelly, D. H., and Shannon, D. C. Sudden infant death syndrome and near-sudden infant death syndrome: A review of the literature, 1964–1982. *Pediatr. Clin. North Am.* 1982;29:1241–1257.

Goldberg, J. The counseling of SIDS parents. *Clin. Perinatol.* 1992;19:927–938.

Lazoff, M. and Kauffman, F. Sudden infant death syndrome. Part III: Emergency department approach. *Acad. Emerg. Med.* 1995;2:1077–1081.

Case 15 BEFORE THE ACCIDENT

An 18-year-old man came to the emergency department following an auto accident. His car had hit a tree, and his forehead had hit the windshield, lacerating his right brow. Because of crowded conditions in the ED, he was seen only briefly by a nurse and then obliged to wait almost two hours before a physician could suture his wound. At the time of treatment, he claimed he felt fine, although he had been rather tired while waiting and appreciated the chance to rest. A cursory neurologic examination revealed no abnormalities. His laceration was debrided, cleaned, and sutured with 5-0 nylon. His eyebrow was not shaved. Because his last tetanus toxoid had been at age 8, he was given 0.5 ml of tetanus toxoid. The sutures were removed 4 days later, and his wound had healed well.

Four months later the man returned to the ED in the company of his mother. She claimed that he had been passing out since his injury. He had had about six episodes during which he stopped all activity, stared at the floor for several minutes, and once or twice fell to the floor. There were no associated involuntary movements and no incontinence. On close questioning, the patient recalled having a few spells during the year preceding his auto accident. He could not recall the exact events of his accident and never had been aware of striking the tree. After a faint, he usually would be a bit fatigued and sometimes momentarily confused. He denied dizziness, headache, or other symptoms. A thorough neurologic examination showed nothing abnormal, and there was no change of pulse or blood pressure when he changed from recumbent to standing position.

What is the matter with this young man?

Was his initial therapy correct?

Is there any significance to a "one–car accident"?

15. BEFORE THE ACCIDENT 45

Discussion

Occasionally, the situation surrounding an accident may be of more importance than the event itself. It is possible that a more prompt physician evaluation of the young man described here might have revealed significant confusion and lethargy, pointing to preexisting neurologic disease or concussion. The past history regarding lapses of consciousness is pertinent. In any case, the subsequent ED visit suggests that the patient is having recurrent losses of consciousness and that a seizure disorder may be present. An EEG and CT scan would be appropriate, and he deserves a follow-up evaluation by a neurologist. You should always consider six possible "S" causes of single car accidents: seizure, syncope, sugar (low), suicide, and the two most common "S" causes, sleep and sauce (booze).

This patient's initial evaluation should have included a thorough neurologic examination (not the cursory one noted in the case). If his neurologic examination (including a mental status exam) was in any way abnormal, a computed tomography scan of the head would have been ordered at that time to rule out an intracranial bleed (subdural or epidural hematoma) or a contusion of the brain. Patients with these injuries require admission and neurosurgical monitoring. On the initial visit, the patient should also have had an evaluation for cervical spine injury, since cervical spine injury should always be suspected in anyone having any head injury. It is often possible to "clinically" (without x-ray) rule out cervical spine fractures in a fully alert patient if there is no neck pain or tenderness and no pain on neck movement. Generally, x-rays are needed if the patient has any neck discomfort, any major distracting painful injury, or a mental status that is in any way abnormal.

The initial treatment of this patient's laceration was correct. Most authorities believe that eyebrows may not be shaved with impunity. If shaved, the eyebrow may not grow back normally. If no tetanus toxoid had ever been given to the patient, he would have been given 250 units of human tetanus immune globulin followed by a tetanus toxoid immunization program. When a patient has received tetanus immunization within the last 10 years, a booster dose of toxoid will call forth an adequate amnestic response.

The repair of facial lacerations such as this young man's should be done as quickly as possible after the injury, but, because of the excellent blood supply, the face may be primarily closed as long as 18 hours after the injury. Wound preparation should be preceded by adequate local anesthesia, generally with lidocaine (Xylocaine) buffered with sodium bicarbonate. If using an epinephrine-containing mixture, this injection provides hemostasis as well as anesthesia, and can be used on most areas of the face except the ears, tip of nose, and lips. The wound should be thoroughly cleaned and sutured with minimal if any debridement. Deep muscle and subcuticular tissues should be approximated with 5-0 Dexon sutures. The skin should be closed with fine nonabsorbable sutures such as 6-0 nylon. A plastic surgeon should generally be consulted if there is a large facial laceration with tissue loss or if there is a concern about the cosmetic result on the part of the patient or the physician.

REFERENCES

Review Article
Parsons, M. Fits and other causes of loss of consciousness while driving. *Q. J. Med.* 1986;58(227):295–303.

Additional References
Dushoff, I. M. About face (principles of wound repair). *Emerg. Med.* November 1974;6:24–77.

Alexander, E. A., et al. Multifactoral causes of adolescent driver accidents. *J. Adolesc. Health Care* 1990;11:413–417.

Mukart, D. J. Trauma: The malignant epidemic. *S. Afr. Med. J.* 1991;72:93–95.

Case 16 EIGHTEEN YEARS OLD, STOPPED BREATHING

An 18-year-old woman was brought into the emergency department in a wheelchair. She had been assisted from a car and into the chair, but by the end of her 100-foot ride into the ED, she had stopped breathing and her color was blue-gray. A pulse was present, although thready, at a rate of about 80. She was lifted onto a bed and began to vomit thin, green liquid. Her head was turned to the side, and her pharynx was suctioned with a rigid (Yankauer) sucker. An oral airway was placed, and her lungs were ventilated with a self-inflating bag for about 1 minute while one of the doctors readied an endotracheal tube and a laryngoscope. When he was ready, the bag was removed and he succeeded in placing an oral tube in her trachea within 1 minute. If it had taken longer, the resuscitation chief would have terminated the attempt and returned to the Ambu bag.

A nurse spoke with the patient's friend, who had brought the patient to the ED, and obtained information that the patient might have taken an overdose of propoxyphene (Darvon). A 2-mg dose of Narcan was given intravenously. The patient had a minor motor seizure involving the face and arms that lasted 1 to 2 minutes. An intravenous infusion of 5% dextrose in water was started. Four more brief seizures followed. Ventilation continued with a self-inflating bag attached to the endotracheal tube, and another 2-mg dose of Narcan was given intravenously 10 minutes after the first dose. The patient's breathing returned, and her color improved. A Foley catheter was placed in her bladder, and 300 ml of urine was sent to the lab for toxicology study. A blood sample was drawn (with H_2O_2, rather than isopropyl alcohol, used to scrub the skin) and sent to the laboratory for alcohol, barbiturate, glucose, BUN, and electrolyte analyses, and for CBC. A portable chest film was obtained, and a brief examination was made for neurologic and other major abnormalities. An esophageal tube (large-bore, Ewald-type) was placed in the stomach, and the patient was lavaged with 2000 ml of tap water in 400-ml amounts. The endotracheal tube cuff was inflated during all these events.

The patient was transferred to the medical intensive care unit within 1 hour of her arrival at the ED. While she was being transferred to a cart for the trip to the intensive care unit, a marijuana cigarette fell out of her jacket pocket. She awoke 6 hours later and admitted to having taken about 60 Darvon capsules.

Her ED visit required the attention of three physicians and two nurses.

What are the most urgent activities in an overdose case such as this?

What do the seizures suggest?

Was the Narcan the only therapeutic maneuver responsible for her improvement?

Discussion

Amazingly, a fair number of patients seem to make it to the door of the ED and expire there. This patient was clearly dying on arrival. Only rapid, vigorous, knowledgeable, and well-coordinated care could help her. A 10-minute delay would have been fatal.

This patient arrived in acute brain and respiratory failure. The only appropriate therapy was to secure control of her airway and ventilate her. The airway is best controlled via an endotracheal tube, and a self-inflating bag is best for ventilation.

Emesis with aspiration is an ever-present danger during resuscitation and can be adequately guarded against only by obstructing the trachea with a cuffed tube. Intubation will take seconds to minutes, and ventilation usually should be obtained first with a face mask. Before attempting intubation, the physician must ready all equipment: laryngoscope, endotracheal tube and stylet, syringe to inflate the cuff, suction, tape to secure the tube in place, and connectors for attachment of the tube to the source of ventilation (e.g., a self-inflating bag). The intubator should try holding his or her breath while attempting intubation. When the intubator needs to breathe, the patient will also need to breathe and, if the tube is not yet in place, should be hyperventilated using a bag with a mask.

Intravenous access should always be established. This may prove difficult in intravenous drug abusers, and if no simple percutaneous access is available, a cutdown should be performed or a central line established. Any young patient in coma from an unknown cause, including suspected drug overdoses, should be given an intravenous "cocktail" of 50 cc of 50% glucose solution and at least two 0.4 mg amps of Narcan. Both are almost entirely safe and can cause a rapid cure for coma from hypoglycemia and narcotics, respectively. Larger doses of either can be used if required. Most centers with a high proportion of chronic alcoholic patients routinely give 50 or 100 mg of thiamine also. This is a relatively benign therapy and can prevent the Wernicke's encephalopathy that may occur if dextrose is given to a thiamine-deficient patient.

Seizures in an overdose patient are often the result of hypoxia. Certain drugs are notorious for causing seizures, even in the absence of hypoxia. These include propoxyphene hydrochloride (Darvon), meperidine (Demerol), antidepressants, theophylline, INH, cocaine, and other sympathomimetics.

Narcan is very effective in reversing narcotics overdose effects. When treating patients with narcotics overdoses, one must be aware that the duration of action of heroin or other narcotics is far greater than the duration of action of any available narcotic antagonist. A patient may wake up, pull out the endotracheal tube, talk to the attendant, perhaps even be discharged, and then return to coma and hypoventilation as the antagonist wears off.

The evaluation of this patient's overdose should have also included an acetaminophen level, because she could have taken a combination drug such as propoxyphene acetaminophen (Darvocet) or, as frequently happens, she could have taken other pills the providers were unaware of. Treatment can be begun early in the course of the case if it is known that the patient took a toxic dose of acetaminophen. N-acetylcysteine (Mucomyst) given orally is the antidote. Acetaminophen overdose is initially asymptomatic, but can produce fulminant and fatal hepatic failure days later if not treated.

References

Review Article
Olsen, K. R., et al. Seizures associated with poisoning and drug overdose. *Am. J. Emerg. Med.* 1994;12:392–395.

Additional References

Allbutt, C. On the abuse of hypodermic injections of morphine. *Practitioner* 1870;5:327–331.

Handal, K. A., Schauben, J. L., and Salamone, F. R. Naloxone. *Ann. Emerg. Med.* 1983;12:438–445.

Case 17 HONKING HORN ON THE AMBULANCE RAMP

A 55-year-old man was brought to the ambulance ramp in a car by his wife. She remained in her car and honked its horn continuously. Several seconds later a clerk, an aide, and two nurses ran out with a stretcher. They found the patient drenched in sweat, unable to speak, and leaning forward in his seat. His wife started screaming, "He can't breathe, he can't breathe, do something!"

The patient was immediately brought to a treatment area where he was attached to a cardiac monitor and placed on a nonrebreathing mask to deliver 100% oxygen. He kept pulling the oxygen mask off. An intravenous line of 5% dextrose in water was established. His blood pressure was 170/90, pulse 80, and respirations 36 per minute.

Examination revealed coarse rales throughout both lung fields, and the respiratory noise obscured his heart tones. Sitting up, his neck veins were distended to the angle of the jaw, and there was slight pitting pretibial edema. He was very agitated, and his skin was cool and very diaphoretic. He nodded when asked about chest pain but was unable to speak. He preferred to sit bolt upright and to lean slightly forward. Morphine sulfate 2 mg and furosemide 40 mg were given intravenously, and 1 nitroglycerin tablet 1/150 grain (0.4 mg) was given sublingually.

His wife said that her husband had suffered a "mild" heart attack about two years earlier and had hypertension. He also was under a doctor's care for an irregular heart rhythm, but his only medications were hydrochlorothiazide and propranolol. He had told her that he had been feeling a little short of breath with exertion over the past few days, and he had complained of chest pain about an hour before the acute onset of shortness of breath.

What are the priorities in treating acute pulmonary edema?

What further evaluation is needed in assessment and treatment of these patients?

Discussion

The patient presented in acute respiratory failure due to acute pulmonary edema. This is most often due to cardiac decompensation and left ventricular failure, but can also be from noncardiac causes such as smoke inhalation, near drowning, high altitude, trauma, pneumonia, aspiration, and heroin overdose. Optimally, a patient like this gets highly sophisticated advanced life support provided by paramedics in an ambulance, and luckily for all of us, this type of care is increasingly common. In this case, he was brought in a car by his wife. She was hysterical because she recognized the severity of his condition and was concerned for his life. On arriving at the emergency department, she used the car horn to summon assistance. Well-seasoned ED staff members are always alert to unusual commotions outside the doors of the department. Patients will frequently present in this manner.

One can gauge the severity of this patient's respiratory distress by his inability to speak. He was expending all his energy to breathe. The typical presentation of these patients is in the sitting position. This maximizes their ability to breathe by using gravity to aid diaphragmatic excursions. Lung sounds will usually be very noisy, with rales present throughout the lung fields.

There may be wheezes due to airway spasm and edema ("cardiac asthma"), and there is the potential for a serious diagnostic error if the wheezing of CHF is mistaken for asthma or COPD.

The blood pressure is frequently elevated, and there is usually tachycardia. Patients on beta-blockers may have normal heart rates because the usual sympathetic response is blocked. The heart sounds are usually inaudible because of the noisy lungs, but, if audible, S_3 and S_4 gallops may be present. The skin is usually cool and moist, reflecting decreased cutaneous perfusion. If the cardiac output is severely depressed, cyanosis and hypotension may be present. These are ominous signs. Pedal edema and jugular venous pressure elevation are signs of accompanying right heart failure, but they are not always present.

The immediate concern of the ED staff is to begin treatment and prevent complications such as hypoxia-mediated myocardial infarction or arrest. The initial treatment is high-flow oxygen delivered by a face mask with a reservoir bag attached. The patient is placed on a cardiac monitor and an intravenous line is established. The solution of choice is

17. HONKING HORN ON THE AMBULANCE RAMP

5% dextrose in water because salt will make the heart failure worse. Sublingual nitroglycerin can be given even before an IV is established or the blood pressure is elevated. Furosemide and morphine sulfate are given intravenously as soon as possible. Furosemide is a mild venodilator and a potent diuretic. Morphine is a sedative and a venodilator. Because of their hypoxia, these patients will be very anxious and may refuse to keep an oxygen mask in place. Providing a small amount of sedation will reduce the work of the heart.

Nitroglycerin will dilate veins and arteries and should initially be given in the sublingual form. It is a rapidly acting treatment for pulmonary edema and is especially helpful in the patient who is experiencing some coronary ischemia and having chest pain with the episode. In the prehospital area, paramedics can begin much of this treatment including the use of oxygen, nitroglycerin, furosemide, and in some areas morphine sulfate. Rotating venous constricting bands (incorrectly called rotating tourniquets) were frequently used in the past. They are still sometimes used as an adjunct measure in severe cases.

After the initial therapy has been begun, the patient's response can be judged by following his vital signs, ability to speak, subjective dyspnea, and by the severity of his diaphoresis. If his pulse decreases and he is able to speak a few words, the process may be improving. In very severe cases, the therapy mentioned above is either not sufficient or too late. A prompt decision to nasotracheally intubate frequently saves lives in this setting.

Few laboratory tests will be very useful in the acute management of this type of patient. A portable chest x-ray is required to show the degree of edema, although the patient's clinical improvement will precede the improvement on the x-ray. A complete blood count should be obtained (to look for anemia), as should baseline electrolytes, BUN, glucose, creatinine, and cardiac enzymes. An ECG should be obtained initially and repeated when the patient is more comfortable and has a slower heart rate. This may show signs of ischemia. None of these tests, neither the obtaining nor the interpretation of them, ever takes precedence over ensuring adequate ventilation.

A number of other pharmacologic interventions may help these patients. Beta-blockers are contraindicated in patients with heart failure and should be cut back immediately if a patient on them develops heart failure. Aminophylline or a bronchodilator via nebulizer can be given if there is thought to be a component of bronchospasm. Arrhythmias should be treated as needed (ventricular arrhythmias with lidocaine or countershock, and supraventricular arrhythmias with IV diltiazem, adenosine (Adenocard), or countershock). Digitalis preparations were widely used in the past but are less used now in the treatment of acute pulmonary edema. They are used to treat supraventricular tachycardia due to atrial fibrillation. Patients with pulmonary edema will almost invariably require admission to the coronary care unit because an acute myocardial infarction cannot be ruled out.

Occasionally patients will present early in the course of worsening heart failure. The early symptoms are increasing shortness of breath, paroxysmal nocturnal dyspnea, leg edema, and orthopnea. These are not always present, or the patient may not be aware of the significance of the sensations. Your interviewing style may help the patient correctly identify these symptoms. The patient should be asked about his level of exercise and if there was any recent change. Other useful questions include the number of pillows used at night, change in sleep patterns (especially midnight or early morning wakening), new onset of coughing, light-headedness, nausea, or changes in appetite. Commonly, a patient may have consumed an unusually large amount of salt in his diet or forgotten to take his medication. The sudden worsening of heart failure might also be signaling myocardial ischemia or infarction, even in the absence of chest pain.

REFERENCES

Review Article
Gropper, M. A., et al. Acute cardiogenic pulmonary edema. *Clin. Chest Med.* 1994;15:501–515.

Additional References
Sand, I. C., et al. Maintenance fluids in prehospital care: Crystalloid versus dextrose solutions—is there a difference? *J. Emerg. Med.* 1994;12:803–809.

Aldrich, J. Pulmonary edema. *Nursing* 1994;24:33.

Case 18 MONOARTICULAR ARTHRITIS

A 30-year-old man came to the emergency department at 2 A.M. complaining of pain and swelling in his left knee for several hours. He had previously been well, although on careful questioning he admitted to having had some burning on urination for a few days about two weeks earlier. He recalled no trauma to the knee and was on no medications.

Physical examination revealed that the patient had a warm, slightly erythematous, swollen left knee. The knee was tender, and attempts at flexion led to severe pain. All his other joints seemed normal. His conjunctiva were normal, and he had no urethral discharge. He had no heart murmur, no skin rash, no adenopathy, and no hepatosplenomegaly. He had no nodules, tophi, or other lumps and was afebrile.

He was given codeine for his pain and referred to the arthritis clinic in two days.

Is acute monarticular arthritis ever an emergency?

Would you advise any laboratory studies?

Is there any danger in handling this case in this fashion?

DISCUSSION

There are few true rheumatologic emergencies. An acute non-traumatic monarticular arthritis is one of these. If the patient has not traumatized the joint by twisting, falling, or hitting it, and if he is not on anticoagulants or a known bleeder, then two common causes of an acute monarticular arthritis should be suspected: acute gout or a septic joint. Either one may be excruciatingly painful, but the grave danger lies in missing the diagnosis of a bacterial arthritis, because a septic joint may be destroyed within 48 hours. Rapid diagnosis and initiation of correct therapy are required.

The diagnostic procedure is a joint aspiration. It is quite easy to tap the knee medially under the patella if there is any effusion. Sterile technique should be used, with care to avoid introducing bacteria into a previously sterile joint. The aspirate should be cultured, a sample should be placed in a heparinized tube to examine for crystals, a white blood cell count should be done with saline solution as a diluent, and a gram stain of a smear should be made. If the white cell count is attempted with the usual acetic acid diluent, the cells will clump in the precipitated mucus and the count will be falsely low. Someone experienced at looking for crystals should use a polarized light microscope to search for uric acid or for the calcium pyrophosphate crystals seen in pseudogout. Cultures should be carefully done and should include a specific culture medium for gonococcus. When evidence of gout or pseudogout is lacking, treatment for sepsis should be initiated without waiting for culture results if the joint leukocyte count is high.

Gonococcal arthritis should be suspected in any sexually active person who presents with a single hot joint. Skin pustules on a purplish or erythematous base may be present, and it may be possible to aspirate gonococci (for culture or gram stain) from these lesions.

A patient with a septic joint urgently needs hospitalization. Even if the correct diagnosis is gout, the patient deserves more rapid diagnosis and therapy than were given in this case. Most patients who come to the ED at 2 A.M. are in significant distress, and they deserve rapid, effective care.

On arrival at the rheumatology clinic 2 days after his ED visit, this man's knee was tapped. The aspirated fluid had a white cell count of 15,500 per µl, and uric acid crystals were seen in some of the leukocytes. His acute attack was subsiding, and follow-up care was arranged.

Acute gout may be best treated acutely with colchicine (0.5 mg hourly by mouth until the joint improves or diarrhea appears), with indomethacin (50 mg tid for 1 day and then 25 mg tid for subsequent days), or with another nonsteroidal anti-inflammatory agent in adequate (large) doses. Before therapy is begun, the patient should have a CBC, blood uric acid, and rheumatoid preparation. The joint should be x-rayed, and follow-up should be arranged.

REFERENCES

Review Article
Talbot-Stern, J. K. Arthritis, Tendinitis, and Bursitis. In P. Rosen, et al.

(eds.), *Emergency Medicine: Concepts and Clinical Practice* (3rd ed.). St. Louis: Mosby, 1992.

Additional References

Sternbach, G. L., and Baker, F. J. Emergency joint arthrocentesis and synovial fluid analysis. *JACEP* 1976;5:787–792.

Brown, D. G., et al. Magnetic resonance imaging in patients with inflammatory arthritis of the knee. *Clin. Rheumatol.* 1990;9:73–83.

Case 19: THEY HAD NEVER SEEN ANYTHING LIKE IT BEFORE

A 64-year-old man was brought to the emergency department at 8 P.M. by his wife because of her concern that his scrotum was swollen and tender. He was not too eager to obtain medical care and volunteered little history but claimed to have been well previously and to have had scrotal swelling for about two days. He had felt some chills but had not taken his temperature. He was not on any medications and emphatically did not wish to remain in the hospital as an inpatient.

On examination, the patient appeared slightly confused and irritable but in no other distress. His temperature was 38.8°C orally, pulse 110, respiration 18, and blood pressure 150/90. His scrotum was swollen, slightly edematous, tender throughout, and erythematous. There was no remarkable inguinal lymphadenopathy. The scrotum was so tender as to prevent careful palpation.

The patient was seen by a medical resident, who admitted that the problem looked like some sort of an infection but that he had never seen anything quite like it before. The man was also seen by a urology resident, who admitted that he too had never seen such a problem before. They elected to treat him with rest and oral antibiotics.

Two days later the patient had deteriorated further and was brought back to the ED by his wife. He was more obtunded and even less communicative than before. His scrotum was further swollen and darker in color—almost black in areas—and swelling extended up the thighs and lower abdomen. Slight crepitus in the scrotum was noted.

This time the man was admitted to the hospital, and initial laboratory studies indicated he was in diabetic ketoacidosis. Major surgical debridement of the scrotum was done in the operating room. His subsequent hospital course was very stormy, with an episode of acute renal failure.

What diseases predispose to bizarre infection?

19. THEY HAD NEVER SEEN ANYTHING LIKE IT BEFORE   59

What simple laboratory tests can be done in the ED to look for these predisposing disorders?

What organisms are most commonly responsible for gas gangrene?

DISCUSSION

Remarkable diseases should be remarked on. This case puzzled both the medical and the urologic consultants, yet they were content to treat him as an example of a less bizarre illness and obtained no laboratory studies to search for other underlying diseases. The patient paid a price for this error in judgment.

A major red flag in this case was that the patient presented with abnormal vital signs. The presence of fever over 101°F (38.3°C) in a person over the age of 60 is more worrisome and more likely to herald serious underlying infection than in younger persons. This man also had another clinical sign experienced clinicians rarely ignore—tachycardia in a patient who is at rest. Any abnormal vital sign must be investigated thoroughly, and a resting tachycardia is often the premonitory sign of an impending disaster.

Additionally, an altered mental status should always prompt a detailed investigation for an underlying cause. This man presented with slight confusion and irritability. A mental status examination should be performed on a patient exhibiting altered behavior. Clues to an organic cause for the confusion include disorientation (person, place, time, or purpose) and inability to name common objects or perform simple subtraction of serial sevens. The acute onset of an organic brain syndrome should always prompt a search for a metabolic cause (hypoxia, acidosis, infection, electrolyte abnormality, or drug or other intoxication).

Immunodeficiency, diabetes mellitus, and hematologic disorders lead the list of diseases predisposing to unusual infections. A CBC, blood sugar, and BUN would have adequately screened for and would have picked up this patient's diabetes. Even a simple urinalysis would have led to detection of the ketoacidosis. Missing this ancillary diagnosis surely allowed the infection to remain out of control despite antibiotic therapy.

Gas-forming bacteria are plentiful. The three most commonly seen are clostridia, bacteroids, and nonhemolytic streptococcus. Penicillin used with an aminoglycoside to cover for gram-negative infection is fine for antibiotic coverage, but third-generation cephalosporins can also be used. Surgical drainage and debridement are essential, as is control of such associated problems as ketoacidosis. Ketoacidosis is itself a serious disorder with a significant mortality. It is usually viewed as a medical emergency requiring hospitalization and urgent therapy.

REFERENCES

Review Article
Lindsey, D. Soft tissue infections. *Emerg. Med. Clin. North Am.* 1992;10:737–751.

Additional References
Keating, H. J., et al. Effect age has on the clinical significance of fever in ambulatory adult patients. *J. Am. Geriatr. Soc.* 1984;32:282–287.

Canoso, J. J., et al. Soft tissue infections. *Rheum. Dis. Clin. North Am.* 1993;19:293–309.

Weiss, L. D., et al. The applications of hyperbaric oxygen therapy in emergency medicine. *Am. J. Emerg. Med.* 1992;10:558–568.

Case 20 ASTHMA

A 23-year-old man was brought to the emergency department from the city jail one evening because he had become short-winded. He had suffered bronchial asthma since childhood and had been on corticosteroids in the past but not lately. His usual therapy consisted of oral bronchodilator tablets and an isoproterenol (Isuprel) inhaler. On the evening of his ED admission, he had been arrested for verbally abusing a police officer who was trying to get him to move his car from an illegal parking area at an outdoor rock music festival. While in jail, the man had become short of breath and begun to wheeze. His jailers had him taken to the ED.

On arrival he appeared in only minimal respiratory distress. He was afebrile and had bilateral musical wheezes in his chest. An occasional nonproductive cough was apparent. His vital signs were temperature 37.0°C, pulse 90, respiration 20, blood pressure 150/80.

Therapy was begun with oxygen by nasal prongs at a flow rate of 5 liters per minute, and an intravenous infusion of 500 mg of aminophylline in 500 ml of 5% dextrose solution was given over a 2-hour period. At the end of this period, the patient felt better, his wheezes were "less tight," and he was returned to the city jail.

During the next six hours he became dyspneic again and used his pocket Isuprel inhaler frequently in his jail cell. He was then returned to the ED, where he was seen almost immediately by a physician. His vital signs were temperature 37°C, pulse 110 and regular, respiration 22, blood pressure 154/82. His chest had diffuse wheezes but he did seem to be ventilating adequately. He was not cyanotic. His heart sounded normal, and he had no edema. He was given 0.4 mg of epinephrine subcutaneously and within three minutes suffered a cardiac arrest. Despite vigorous immediate attempts at cardiopulmonary resuscitation, he could not be resuscitated.

Is epinephrine usually considered to be the drug of choice in treating asthma?

If this patient's death was not due purely to chance, what could have been the physiologic state due to asthma, prior to the epinephrine injection, that predisposed him to a fatal arrhythmia?

What other disorders can present in the ED as "asthma"?

DISCUSSION

Asthma is an increasingly common serious disease that is associated with sudden death, especially in users of inhaled bronchodilator aerosols. Asthmatics may become either alkalotic or acidotic. Either of these may be injurious but, in the setting of hypoxia and sympathomimetic loading, acidosis is more dangerous. Acidotic hypoxic hearts are very vulnerable to arrhythmias when sympathomimetics are given. If a sympathomimetic must be given when the patient might be hypoxic, it may be best not to give it by intravenous push or by intramuscular or subcutaneous injection. The physician caring for the patient in this case may not have fully appreciated the patient's self-administered "bronchodilator" and the possibility of serious hypoxia and pH abnormality. Infrequent premature ventricular contractions may have been present but missed. Unlike isoproterenol and epinephrine, most modern inhaled bronchodilators have a selective beta-1 effect on the lungs without as much beta-2 effect on the heart. Metaproterenol (Metaprel) and albuterol (Ventolin) can be used in these patients with a higher degree of safety.

Only a young asthmatic given no prior therapy, with several hours of dyspnea at most, who requests the drug because it worked best for him or her in the past, and with no notable fatigue now, receives epinephrine in our ED. Epinephrine is an effective drug in asthma, but, in a patient already loaded with sympathomimetics, the discomfort of the injection and the hazard of a fatal arrhythmia lead us to use other drugs that can be given safely in much higher doses via inhalation.

There are many ways to treat asthma, and some variation from medical center to medical center. Our approach is to give oxygen nasally and then immediately give a nebulized bronchodilator treatment with an inhaled bronchodilator such as albuterol. Using higher doses than in the past, we now sometimes request these treatments every 15 to 20 minutes until three or four treatments have been given or until there is some improvement. Patients on theophylline should have a theophylline level drawn. The patient should be well hydrated to loosen secretions: a

400- or 500-ml bolus of fluid in a young patient is perfectly reasonable. Intravenous steroids should be initiated early in any patient who has been on steroids before or who is not improving after an hour or two of ED treatment.

The peak expiratory flow rate is a useful measurement of the patient's response to therapy. An improvement should be seen after the first treatment and is a good sign. Patients not improving after three nebulized bronchodilator treatments should be considered for admission. The use of transcutaneous oxymetry (i.e., "pulse oxymetry") is increasingly common. There is some evidence that a transcutaneous oxygen saturation of less than 95% after treatment is a marker for subsequent admission. Any oxygen saturation below 90% after treatment should be viewed as a sign of extreme respiratory distress.

Fatigue is very dangerous and argues for admission. Extreme fatigue is an indication for elective nasotracheal intubation. A skillfully inserted nasotracheal tube is usually well-tolerated and a great relief to a tired asthmatic. In this extreme situation, very small doses of intravenous isuproterenol or intravenous terbutaline have been life saving in well-monitored settings.

Some asthmatics are regularly harder to treat than others. The physician should suspect that the case may be difficult when the patient relates a past use of steroids.

The diagnosis of asthma is not always correct. Most commonly, the middle-aged or older patient who comes in claiming that his or her "asthma is giving trouble" is *not* an asthmatic but rather has an exacerbation of chronic bronchitis, emphysema, or heart failure. As usual, the key to correct therapy is correct diagnosis, and one must not accept the patient's own diagnosis as correct. Obviously, a patient in heart failure with "cardiac asthma" should not be given large amounts of fluids intravenously. A careful initial appraisal should seek evidence of heart failure, such as elevated venous pressure or edema.

REFERENCES

Review Article
George, R. B. Bronchial asthma. *Dis. Mon.* 1991;37:137–196.

Additional References

Rudnitsky, G. S., et al. Comparison of intermittent and continuously nebulized albuterol for treatment of asthma in our urban emergency department. *Ann. Emerg. Med.* 1993;22:1842–1846.

Tiffany, B. R., et al. Magnesium bolus or infusion fails to improve expiratory flow in acute asthma exacerbations. *Chest.* 1993;104:831–834.

Duke, T., et al. Asthma in the emergency department: Impact of a protocol on optimizing therapy. *Am. J. Emerg. Med.* 1991;9:432–435.

Case 21 A REQUEST FOR METHADONE

A 21-year-old man came to the emergency department requesting a prescription for methadone. He stated that he was a heroin addict and used $200 to $300 worth of street heroin a day. He claimed to have used heroin heavily for two years and was involved in burglary frequently to support his habit. Now he wished to stop taking the heroin and was feeling ill after having no drug for 12 hours.

On physical examination, no abnormalities were observed. The patient's veins were not scarred visibly, he had no round subcutaneous dimples (results of "skin popping"), and his pupils were midposition and reactive to light. His blood pressure was 130/50, pulse 95, respiration 16, and temperature 37.0°C.

The patient was given 40 mg of methadone (in 10-mg tablets) and left the ED. Six hours later he was returned to the ED deeply comatose but with adequate respiration and blood pressure. A friend stated that the patient had taken the methadone "to get high," that he had *not* been on heroin, and that he had drunk some vodka. His blood alcohol was 346 mg per deciliter (also called "346 milligrams percent"). Narcan (2 mg given intravenously) produced no notable change, and the patient was kept in the ED under observation for 12 hours to "sleep it off."

What are the signs and symptoms of heroin withdrawal?

How is it treated?

Discussion

Obviously, this patient was mainly drunk. However, the combination of methadone and alcohol is very dangerous, and the prescribing of methadone should be part of a maintenance program and not done in the ED unless enrollment in such a program can be proven and the dose verified. This patient was probably neither a heroin addict nor withdrawing from heroin.

Diaphoresis, dilated pupils, rhinorrhea, diarrhea, and colicky abdominal pain are early signs of narcotics withdrawal. Evidence of injection sites—usually needle tracks on arm veins—should be sought. People with inadequate veins (including chronic users in whom all available veins have thrombosed) may resort to "skin popping" or subcutaneous injection. In addition to AIDS, they are prone to local abscesses, cellulitis, hepatitis B, tetanus, endocarditis, pneumonia, strokes, and lesser complications such as constipation, neuropathies, and secondary amenorrhea.

Often street heroin, "horse" or "smack," is not truly heroin or contains only a small dose of heroin diluted with other drugs. Quinine, because it is white, powdery, bitter, and produces flushing when given intravenously, is often mixed with barbiturate (for narcosis) unbeknown to the addict. Such a drug might lead to heroin withdrawal symptoms in an addict and later to barbiturate withdrawal symptoms such as seizures.

Methadone is widely used in the United States in maintenance therapy for chronic heroin addicts to prevent heroin euphoria and withdrawal symptoms. In such a program, a tolerant addict is usually given a daily dose of 60 to 120 mg of methadone; although, to a nontolerant person, even 40 mg could be a very large dose. Mixed with alcohol or other sedatives, this amount of methadone can be fatal, acting as a respiratory depressant like any other narcotic.

In lieu of methadone and its problems in the acute setting, clonidine can also be used for the treatment of addicts who are displaying symptoms of withdrawal.

REFERENCES

Review Article
Freitas, P. M. Narcotic withdrawal in the emergency department. *Am. J. Emerg. Med.* 1985;3:456–460.

Additional References
Farrell, M., et al. Methadone maintenance treatment in opiate dependence: A review. *BMJ* 1994;309:997–1001.

Gutierrez-Cebollada, J., et al. Psychotropic drug consumption and other factors associated with heroin overdose. *Drug Alcohol Depend.* 1994;35:169–174.

Case 22: TWENTY-EIGHT YEAR OLD WITH CHEST PAIN

A 28-year-old man came to the emergency department one evening complaining of chest pain. He stated that the pain had begun about an hour earlier, was substernal and crushing in nature, and radiated into his left arm. He had never had any pain like this before and had not been exerting himself heavily before the pain had begun. He was a non-smoker and did not drink alcohol to excess. There was no family history of diabetes, hypertension, or heart disease.

His blood pressure was 154/96, pulse 112, respirations 18, and he was afebrile. He appeared extremely anxious. His neck veins were flat while he was lying at 20 degrees. His lungs were clear and his heart tones were normal. His abdomen was benign without organomegaly and his legs were nontender without edema. His deep tendon reflexes were slightly hyperactive and he had a fine tremor. An ECG showed "early repolarization" but was otherwise within normal limits.

He was placed on a cardiac monitor and given oxygen by nasal prongs while an intravenous line was started with 5% dextrose in water at a keep-open rate. A chest x-ray was normal. He was given sublingual nitroglycerin tablets for the pain. After 3 tablets had only decreased the pain from 10 to 3 on a scale of 10, he was given some morphine intravenously. This relieved his pain and allayed his anxiety.

Further history was obtained at this time. He admitted that he had just been at a party where he had some cocaine for the second time in his life. He had first tried cocaine several weeks earlier without any problem. That evening he had snorted two lines of cocaine and soon felt his heart pounding in his chest. The chest pain began shortly thereafter.

He was admitted to the coronary care unit where further work-up showed that he had sustained a small anterior myocardial infarction. He was subsequently discharged without sequela.

What are the effects of cocaine use?

What are the priorities in the treatment of sympathomimetic overdose?

In cocaine abuse, how is the treatment of a "body packer" different from that of a "body stuffer"?

DISCUSSION

The typical presentation seen with a cocaine overdose is euphoria followed by hyperexcitability, delirium, and tremors, terminating in generalized seizures, often followed by respiratory arrest and death. Overdoses occur in three common situations: the user who increases the dosage higher and higher in hopes of reaching the ultimate experience and instead reaches the maximum tolerable dose; the "stuffer" who, in an attempt to avoid arrest, ingests large quantities of drug; and the "body packer" who attempts to smuggle drugs into the country by swallowing numerous drug-filled condoms or other containers.

Distinguishing cocaine intoxication from other intoxications or psychiatric disease may at first be difficult, but, because of the short half-life of cocaine, the symptoms tend to decrease quickly. The psychotic reaction with hallucinations and violent behavior can resemble PCP intoxication, delirium tremens (DTs), or the "toxidrome"* from other sympathomimetics such as amphetamines ("speed") and phenylpropanolamine (found in diet pills).

Treatment in the overdose situation is primarily supportive. Strict attention to the ABCs is the initial goal. In the situation of the "stuffer," gastrointestinal decontamination is warranted because the drug is hastily ingested and inadequately packaged in the panic of being arrested. Whole bowel irrigation with a non-absorbable osmotic agent (such as Golytely) can be used. The "body packer," on the other hand, may require surgical intervention to remove the remaining packets of drug or, if asymptomatic, may be observed in the intensive care setting until the drug-laden packets pass. Seizures should be treated with diazepam (Valium) or lorazepam (Ativan).

Because of improved supply and market strategies, the abuse of cocaine has become commonplace. Crack, the crystalline form of the cocaine freebase, has made cocaine abuse available to even wider markets, and a rapid onset and then abatement of euphoric effects perpetuates its use. With the tremendous increase in the use and purity

---

*A clinically recognizable syndrome associated with a class of toxic ingestions.

of cocaine available to the consumer, the number of toxic side effects and related deaths is increasing.

The onset of effects from cocaine use vary with the route of administration. Crack smoking shows the most rapid onset, within seconds of use. Intravenous use causes peak effects within 3 to 5 minutes. When insufflated into the nasal mucosa, peak effects are within 20 to 60 minutes.

Toxicity related to cocaine use may affect any organ system. Cardiac toxicity may present as myocardial infarction in an otherwise healthy young person, and arrhythmias due to myocardial irritability may cause sudden death. Stroke syndrome, seizure, subarachnoid hemorrhage, and hyperpyrexia also may occur. Psychiatric changes include decreased rapid-eye-movement (REM) sleep, agitation, inability to concentrate, visual hallucinations, tactile hallucinations (cocaine bugs), delusions, and acute onset of psychosis that may outlast the intoxication. Nasal septal perforation, sexual dysfunction, and a myriad of assorted adverse effects have also been related to cocaine use. Toxic effects including death have been seen with a variety of dosages (even as low as 20 mg or the equivalent of one "line") and with all routes (including intranasal).

Hypertension, a common problem with overdose, has been treated with nitroprusside, phentolamine, and propranolol. Supraventricular tachycardia and ventricular tachycardia have been successfully treated with intravenous propranolol, but, because of the rapid degradation of cocaine, a shorter half-life agent such as esmolol may be more beneficial. Hyperpyrexia, which is an uncommon side effect, should be managed aggressively with rapid cooling.

REFERENCES

Review Article
Olshaker, J. S. Cocaine chest pain. *Emerg. Med. Clin. North Am.* 1994;12:391–396.

Additional References
McCarron, M. N., and Wood, J. D. The cocaine body packer syndrome. *J.A.M.A.* 1983;220:1417–1420.

Gawin, F. H., and Ellinwood, E. H. Cocaine and other stimulants. *N. Engl. J. Med.* 1988;318:1173–1182.

Derlet, E. R., and Albertson, T. E. Emergency department presentation of cocaine intoxication. *Ann. Emerg. Med.* 1989;18:182–186.

Hoffman, R. S., et al. Whole bowel irrigation and the cocaine body-packer: A new approach to a common problem. *Am. J. Emerg. Med.* 1990;8:523–527.

Merigan, K. S., et al. Adrenergic crisis from crack cocaine ingestion. *J. Emerg. Med.* 1994;12:485–490.

Case 23 NOSEBLEED

A 64-year-old man was brought to the emergency department because of a nosebleed. His nose had been bleeding on and off for two days. He had placed some cotton in the left nostril for a few hours the day before his ED visit but then removed it. He was on no drugs, denied alcoholism, and had no known hypertension. There was no trauma to the nose, and family members who brought in the patient reported that he had been complaining of feeling tired that day.

The patient was placed on a bed with his head elevated. His blood pressure was 124/76 and pulse 70. He had a slow ooze of blood from his left nostril and sat clutching a blood-soaked terry-cloth towel. When he was stood up, he became dizzy and his blood pressure dropped to 70 systolic. No diastolic pressure was recorded. His pulse did not speed up noticeably on standing briefly. The inside of his left nostril was sprayed liberally with 4% cocaine, and then 4% cocaine was applied by cotton (twisted on a wire) into the nose. The left nostril was suctioned, but no precise bleeding point could be identified. A nasal pack with petroleum jelly-impregnated gauze was placed, and the bleeding stopped. An intravenous infusion of normal saline solution was given through a large intracatheter in the patient's left arm; 2000 ml was given over 1 hour. Blood was sent for type and crossmatch (4 units were set up). The patient was admitted to the hospital for observation overnight.

How much blood is usually lost by epistaxis?

If bleeding stops after spraying phenylephrine (a vasoconstrictor) in the nose, should you pack the nose?

How long should the pack be left in place?

DISCUSSION

Epistaxis is probably the most common ear-nose-throat (ENT) emergency. Although nonphysicians usually overestimate blood loss, exsanguination via epistaxis can occur, and the physician should seek evidence of hypovolemia. Initial vital signs may be normal, but the physician should look for a drop in blood pressure or an elevation of pulse rate when the patient sits or stands from a lying position. The patient should immediately resume the supine position if light-headedness occurs. Prior to further evaluation of the bleeding source, intravenous access should be obtained if hypovolemia is present, and fluid resuscitation with normal saline or lactated Ringer's should be begun.

Epistaxis may be influenced by local and systemic factors. Local factors include nasal trauma (fractures, nose picking), ulcers from nasal dryness, nasopharyngeal tumors, foreign bodies, and even hereditary hemorrhagic telangiectasia (Osler-Weber-Rendu disease). Systemic factors include hypertension, arteriosclerosis, blood dyscrasias, and coagulation disorders including nonsteroidal anti-inflammatory drug use and anticoagulant therapy. A thorough history and physical examination should provide clues to the diagnosis. In young persons with no other medical problems, no testing may be needed, or a spun hematocrit may be the only test required, but full laboratory evaluation including platelet count, clotting studies (PT, PTT), hematocrit, and blood typing and crossmatch should be considered.

Examination is best done with the patient in the sitting position and with the head tilted forward to reduce swallowing and potential aspiration of blood. The nasal septum, roof, and lateral walls should be inspected for a source of bleeding using a nasal speculum, headlamp, and suction. Anterior epistaxis most frequently originates from Kiesselbach's plexus on the anteroinferior septum because of its rich vascularity and propensity for local trauma. Posterior epistaxis tends to cause bleeding into the nasopharynx.

You will often be successful at stopping anterior epistaxis simply by pinching the nose continuously for 15 to 20 minutes. If bleeding continues, a topical vasoconstrictor such as phenylephrine and a topical anesthetic such as 20% benzocaine or Cetacaine should be sprayed or applied topically to the nasal mucosa with a cotton pledget. Topical cocaine solutions provide both vasoconstriction and anesthesia but can cause toxic effects such as seizures or hypertension if too much is given. Large intranasal clots should be removed, or they will prevent effective compression of the bleeding sites. The bleeding sites can then be cauterized with silver nitrate, or have hemostatic materials (Surgicel, Gelfoam) applied to them. If the bleeding is not controlled at that point, anterior packing is performed using a hemostatic nasal balloon or petrolatum gauze. Gauze packing is inserted using bayonet forceps. Half-inch gauze strips are layered into the nostril beginning at the nasal floor until it is fully packed. Ampicillin or cephalosporin should be started to prevent sinusitis from obstructing sinus drainage. The patient with a unilateral anterior pack is usually sent home and asked to return for pack removal in 48 to 72 hours. Patients with multiple bleeding sites who require bilateral anterior packs deserve admission and observation.

Posterior epistaxis persists after anterior nasal packing and usually requires otolaryngologic consultation. Patients with posterior nasal packing, especially if elderly, require admission because of the risk of airway compromise and ventilatory impairment. Emergency treatment of posterior bleeding sites can be accomplished using a Foley catheter or a specially designed nasal balloon.

REFERENCES

Review Article
Josephson, G. D., et al. Practical management of epistaxis. *Med. Clin. North Am.* 1991;75:1311–1320.

Additional References
DeWeese, D. D., and Saunders, W. H. (eds.), *Textbook of Otolaryngology* (6th ed.). St. Louis: Mosby, 1982. Pp. 189–220.

Dann, L. Severe epistaxis. *Aust. Fam. Physician* 1994;23:153–155.

Case 24 "LOCKJAW"

A 34-year-old woman walked into the emergency department accompanied by her aunt. The patient was obviously very frightened, and tears were running down her face, but she spoke with very little movement of her mouth and claimed that she had "lockjaw." The aunt furnished the following information: the patient had been well until one week earlier, when she had had a cramping, low abdominal pain and nausea. She had seen her physician, who had given her some yellow capsules. The pain and nausea had lessened, but for the past two days she had had trouble using her mouth, and today it had "locked on her." She recalled no trauma or puncture wounds and denied any experimental "pill popping" or "shooting up" of drugs. The yellow pills were unavailable.

On examination the vital signs were temperature 37.0°C, pulse 100, blood pressure 140/85, and respiration 18. The patient's chest and heart were normal, as were her deep tendon reflexes. Her gait was unremarkable, and muscle tone seemed normal. Her jaw was tightly clenched, but on coaxing she could open it for examination. No pharyngeal, ear, or neck pathology could be found.

One of the examining physicians at first thought the patient had a peritonsillar abscess or, failing that, a hysterical conversion reaction. To add to the confusion, the woman's aunt was loudly chanting prayers for her relief. Fortunately, an alert nurse correctly diagnosed the problem. The patient was given an intravenous injection and immediately remarked that she felt better. Within five minutes the jaw tightness was entirely gone. The patient left for home within thirty minutes of her arrival in the ED.

What was the matter with this woman?

What was in the yellow capsules?

What drug was given to her in the ED?

Discussion

The patient exemplifies an acute onset of the extrapyramidal movement disorder known as acute dystonic reaction. This is usually due to phenothiazines and is essentially unrelated to the dose, being an idiosyncratic reaction. The differential diagnosis must include (1) tetanus, (2) a seizure disorder, and (3) hysteria. Indeed, the unsophisticated physician usually picks hysteria as an explanation for phenothiazine reactions. At one time almost all extrapyramidal diseases were thought to be hysterical because the movements are exacerbated by anxiety, improved by tranquillity, and *partially* under the patient's control.

These movement disorders can present as dystonias such as torticollis, oculogyric crisis (patients may complain that they cannot get their eyes off the ceiling), or total body writhing. The patient may have spasmodic movements with leg-jerking, head-bobbing, or choreiform total body hyperactivity. Localized muscle tone increases may vary from jaw tightness or tongue protrusion to opisthotonos and extensor rigidity throughout the body.

Probably any phenothiazine can lead to movement disorders, although Haldol (haloperidol) does so more commonly than most. The yellow capsules were probably prochlorperazine (Compazine). Given for nausea, it is a very common cause of acute dystonic reactions. Several effective therapies are available. The offending drug must be stopped. If the movement disorder is of recent onset, diphenhydramine (Benadryl) given orally or intravenously will rapidly reduce symptoms. We usually give 50 mg intravenously to produce a dramatic improvement that is very reassuring to the patient. Then we continue the patient on 25 to 50 mg orally bid for 2 or 3 days. This was the therapy used on the patient described.

References

Review Article
Lee, A. Treatment of drug induced dystonic reaction. *JACEP* 1979;8:453–457.

Additional References
Denetropoullos, S., and Schauben, J. L. Acute dystonic reaction from "street Valium." *J. Emerg. Med.* 1987;5:293–297.

Bailie, G. R., et al. Unusual treatment response of a dystonia to diphenhydramine. *Ann. Emerg. Med.* 1987;16:705–708.

Farrell, P. E., et al. Acute dystonic reaction to crack cocaine. *Ann. Emerg. Med.* 1991;20:322.

Case 25 HYPERVENTILATION: THE ANXIOUS DIVORCÉE

A 29-year-old woman came to the emergency department complaining of "hyperventilating." She had suffered for years from chronic anxiety and had previously had many anxiety attacks accompanied by rapid breathing and weakness. Sometimes she would have paresthesias, and she had learned to treat the attacks by breathing in a paper bag. Aside from a regular alcohol consumption of several drinks daily, she had no other known medical problems.

On the day before her ED visit, as she was driving home from the divorce court where she had just obtained a final divorce decree, she noted the onset of rapid breathing with a sense of dyspnea and within minutes noted the onset of a pounding, rapid heartbeat in her chest. She felt weak but continued driving home. Bag breathing gave her no relief. None of her previous episodes of hyperventilation had been accompanied by palpitations. Eighteen hours later, at 4 A.M., she became worried enough about the palpitations, dyspnea, tachypnea, and weakness to call for an ambulance to bring her to the ED. The paramedic tried to calm and reassure her during the ride without much success.

On arrival the patient was anxious and in some evident distress. She was afebrile and showed acrocyanosis with cool extremities. She had a deep, rapid respiration (a rate of 35), tachycardia (cardiac rate 160 and regular), and blood pressure of 150/85. Her jugular venous pressure seemed normal. She had a clear chest, unremarkable heart sounds, and no edema. A brief neurologic exam showed no abnormality. She had no facial twitching on tapping the facial nerve just anterior to the ear (Chvostek's sign) and no carpal spasm on placing a blood pressure cuff around the upper arm and holding it at 170 mm Hg for 3 minutes (Trousseau's sign).

An ECG showed a regular supraventricular tachycardia that the physician present thought was paroxysmal atrial tachycardia (PAT). Carotid massage and gagging maneuvers produced no change. An intravenous route was established, and the patient was given digoxin, 0.5 mg intravenously. This treatment did not lead to any change, even after the massage and digoxin dose were repeated. An arterial blood gas sample was obtained and showed a pH of 7.08, pCO_2 18, pO_2 110. The acidosis was noted and thought to be a lactic acidosis resulting from tissue hypoperfusion due to the tachycardia. Physostigmine (2 mg) was given intravenously, followed by ampules of $NaHCO_3$ (44 mEq each), with no change in her condition. Edrophonium (Tensilon) (10 mg) was given intravenously, and the patient's cardiac rate slowed from 160 to 130. This was thought to be remarkable—PAT always converts abruptly or does not change at all—and redirected attention to her acidosis. She denied ingesting methanol, antifreeze, or aspirin. A urinalysis was done and showed glucose (4+) and a large amount of acetone. She was admitted to the ward with the diagnosis of diabetic ketoacidosis in a previously undiagnosed diabetic. Later she recalled that her mother had adult-onset diabetes.

What possibilities did the arterial blood gas levels reveal?

Is there any danger in bicarbonate therapy of the acidosis?

What is the danger of digitalis in an acidotic patient?

DISCUSSION

Hyperventilation is too often identified as a psychological problem. The differential diagnosis of hyperventilation includes primary lung disorders such as asthma, congestive heart failure, pulmonary embolism (a very frequently missed diagnosis), and metabolic disorders. The presence of hyperventilation *with other abnormal vital signs* should suggest one of these nonpsychogenic disorders as the primary cause. Psychological hyperventilation is a diagnosis of exclusion made after organic causes have been ruled out.

A normal pCO_2 at sea level is about 40 mm Hg. A slight hyperventilation produces a slight decrease of the pCO_2 to about 37 mm Hg. This patient showed a marked decrease of the pCO_2 to 18 mm Hg and thus might have been expected to show an alkalosis. Because the patient was not only not alkalotic but was severely acidotic, she had a metabolic acidosis.

Metabolic acidosis has four main causes. One is diabetic ketoacidosis, and the cardinal error in this case seemed to be neglecting to do a urinalysis when presented with a hyperventilating patient. If a urine specimen had been examined, the diagnosis would have been apparent before costly time was wasted and potentially dangerous maneuvers undertaken. Other causes of metabolic acidosis are exogenous poisons (especially methanol and salicylate), renal disease with uremia or renal tubular acidosis, and lactic acidosis (usually with gross tissue hypoxia and often due to shock).

Treatment of severe metabolic acidosis with $NaHCO_3$ is reasonable and can lessen the risk of fatal cardiac arrhythmias. However, the HCO_3 is denied easy access to the cerebrospinal fluid (CSF), and the brief increase of pCO_2 by the reaction

$$H^+ + HCO_3^- \rightleftarrows H_2CO_3 \rightleftarrows H_2O + CO_2$$

will allow for an increased CSF pCO_2 and a paradoxical increase in H^+ concentration in the CSF—thus a decrease in CSF pH. This may produce coma or seizures, so bicarbonate therapy should be given sparingly and only if the pH is less than 7.1.

Digitalis is a dangerous drug. It can produce serious arrhythmias, especially if given in a setting of hypoxia or acidosis. Although useful in treating a patient with PAT, use of digitalis in a setting of sinus tachycardia and acidosis can be hazardous and not helpful. Adenocard (adenosine) or diltiazem IV are the drugs of choice in a hemodynamically stable patient. (Electrical countershock is the initial therapy of choice in the unstable patient.) Physostigmine and Tensilon have no place in the modern treatment of PAT.

REFERENCES

Review Article
Hanashiro, P. K. Hyperventilation: Benign symptom or harbinger of catastrophe? *Postgrad. Med.* 1990;88:191–196.

Additional References
Kitabchi, A. E. Diabetic ketoacidosis. *Med. Clin. North Am.* 1995;79:9–37.
Tommasini, N. R., and Federici, C. M. Recognition of panic disorder in the emergency department. *J. Emerg. Nurs.* 1992;18:319–327.

Case 26 RESCUED FROM A FIRE

A 53-year-old woman was brought in to the ED after having been pulled out of a burning apartment by fire fighters. She had been conscious after the rescue but had no memory of what had caused the fire. She had smoked cigarettes for almost forty years and admitted to having a chronic smoker's cough. She complained of pain in her arms and upper chest where her clothing was burned, but she denied any shortness of breath and said that, except for the pain, she felt completely well.

Her initial vital signs were blood pressure 156/84, pulse 96, and respirations 24. She had second-degree burns over her shoulders, upper chest, and anterior upper arms with surrounding first-degree burns down to the elbows. Her trauma exam was otherwise unremarkable, and the remainder of the physical exam showed only somewhat coarsened breath sounds with an increased expiratory phase.

The blisters were debrided and treated with silver sulfadiazine cream and sterile dressings. She was given 2000 ml of lactated Ringer's solution over a 3-hour period. The emergency department became quite busy, and she was mostly ignored for the next 5 hours, during which time another 1000 ml of intravenous fluid slipped in.

At this time the resident responsible for her care decided that she was well enough to go home. The attending physician, having just arrived on duty, spoke to the patient who volunteered that she was a bit short of breath. Her respiratory rate was 28 per minute and wheezes were audible. Despite the protestations of the resident, the patient was admitted to the surgical intensive care unit for observation. Forty minutes after arrival in the intensive care unit, the patient began to cough up frothy fluid and was diagnosed as having pulmonary edema. She was treated with diuretics and oxygen and was allowed to rest in a semiseated position. She was discharged eight days later to be followed in the burn clinic for outpatient treatment of her burns.

What are the priorities in burn management?

What burns can be treated in an outpatient setting?

26. RESCUED FROM A FIRE

What are the respiratory complications of burns, and how should they be treated?

DISCUSSION

The state of the airway is our first concern in a burn case, just as it is in other major emergencies. If there is any clinical evidence of an airway burn, the patient should either be intubated prophylactically or examined with direct laryngoscopy to assess damage to the airway. The signs of significant airway burns include severe burns in or around the mouth, singed nasal hairs, hoarseness or stridor, dyspnea, and expectoration of carbonaceous sputum. Burns from fires in a confined area and high-pressure steam burns to the face are likely to be associated with airway compromise.

The next priority is establishing intravenous access, usually with two large-bore intravenous lines. In most serious burns, large amounts of fluid are lost, and it is easy to get behind in the patient's fluid replacement. An estimate of the fluid requirements can be obtained by formula, but ongoing fluid management must be gauged by the urine output and the level of the central venous pressure assessed clinically or measured directly.

Burns in enclosed areas also produce smoke inhalation injury. A variety of direct pulmonary irritants can produce noncardiac pulmonary edema. For example, many synthetic materials release hydrogen chloride when burning, and this forms hydrochloric acid when it comes in contact with the moist mucus membranes of the respiratory tract.

Carbon monoxide may be formed, so carboxyhemoglobin levels should be obtained in anyone with altered mental status, especially if the burn occurred in a closed area. Elevated levels or signs of neurologic dysfunction should prompt consideration for emergency use of a hyperbaric chamber. Cyanide is formed whenever plastic or wool burns and should be suspected in any patient with an altered level of consciousness and a severe metabolic acidosis. Treatment is with a commercially available cyanide treatment kit.

The burn should be covered with a sterile, dry "burn sheet." The direct application of ice is not necessary and will actually risk increasing the depth of the burn. The extent of a burn is usually estimated by a chart using the rule of nines. In small children or persons with irregular burns, the body surface area involved can be estimated by using the patient's hand as a guide. One side of a person's hand is approximately 1% of their body surface area. If an extremity burn is circumferential, neurovascular compromise can result. Circumferential chest burns can result in respiratory embarrassment due to restriction of ventilation. In either of these cases, escharotomy may be needed on an urgent basis to allow expansion of the tissues.

Patients with high voltage electrical burns and inhalation injuries should be admitted to the hospital. Patients with burns over 20% of the body surface area, patients with serious burns of the hands, feet, or genitalia, and patients with accompanying injuries or serious medical conditions should also be admitted.

First-degree burns such as sunburn are superficial and cause only erythema. Second-degree burns are into the dermis and cause blistering. Third-degree burns go through the dermis and are characterized by insensate (numb) areas, which are blackened or covered with a hard, leatherlike eschar.

Small burns can be treated on an outpatient basis. First-degree and superficial second-degree burns can be treated with analgesics and cool water. We fill a basin with sterile water and a few ice cubes, and then let the patient self-treat by dunking the burned part into the cold on and off, as needed for comfort. This provides surprisingly effective analgesia. We give oral pain medication and anti-inflammatory medication (e.g., codeine and ibuprofen) and then cover the burn site with an application of antibacterial ointment or cream. Blisters can be left intact but should be peeled away if they have burst. A prescription for a short course of narcotic analgesics should be considered for pain relief. Third-degree burns and electrical burns, which are typically deeper and more extensive than they appear on the surface, usually require subspecialty consultation for definitive care.

REFERENCES

Review Article
Drueck, C. Emergency Department treatment of hand burns. *Emerg. Med. Clin. North Am.* 1993;11:797–809.

Additional References
Harvey, J. S., et al. Emergent burn care. *South. Med. J.* 1984;77:204–214.

Jones, J., McCullen, M. J., and Dougherty, J. Toxic smoke inhalation. *Am. J. Emerg. Med.* 1987;5:317–321.

Mosley, S. Inhalation injuries: A review of the literature. *Heart Lung* 1988;17:3–9.

Carrougher, G. J. Inhalation injury. *AACN Clin. Issues Crit. Care Nurs.* 1993;4:367–377.

Latarjet, J. Immediate cooling with water: Emergency treatment of burns. *Pediatrie* 1990;45:237–239.

Case 27: THE MORNING AFTER A SNOWSTORM

The morning after a snowstorm, a family of four presented to the emergency department. The father, a 30-year-old medical researcher, had headaches and passed out once for a few minutes. He also complained of abdominal pain and nausea and had vomited several times. His wife was very drowsy and had a severe headache. The children seemed fine. They lived in a rural area, and after their electricity had gone out in the storm they had switched on a small gasoline-powered generator.

The father's blood pressure was 150/90, his pulse 100, and respirations 24. Otherwise, he appeared entirely normal. His wife also had a completely normal examination. Their carboxyhemoglobin levels were 30% and 22%, respectively. These figures were extrapolated backward to the time of their exposure, estimating maximum exposure levels of 40% and 30%. They were both treated with 100% oxygen by face masks for 4 hours. Repeat carboxyhemoglobin levels were then 4% and 1%. They refused permission for blood gases to be drawn on the children since the examination of the children was completely normal.

Twenty-four hours later the wife called up and said that her husband was behaving violently and seemed to have lost his memory. The husband corroborated these symptoms and was very upset about them. The wife and children were acting normally. He was immediately referred to the nearest hyperbaric chamber (100 miles away) where he was given two "dives" to 3 atmospheres at 100% oxygen. This completely reversed his symptoms although he stated that it still took him a second or two more than usual to recognize persons he knew and to remember their names.

How would you recognize carbon monoxide poisoning?

What is the significance of elevated carboxyhemoglobin levels?

When is hyperbaric oxygen treatment required for carbon monoxide poisoning?

Discussion

Carbon monoxide is colorless, odorless, and tasteless, and poisoning by it has few pathognomonic symptoms or signs. Patients with mild intoxication complain of nonspecific symptoms such as headache, nausea, vomiting, and dizziness. It may be misconstrued as a flu-like illness by physicians, even when several members of the same family present to the ED simultaneously. A clue to carbon monoxide poisoning as the correct diagnosis in this case was that family members became sick at the same time. This is very unusual for a viral illness, where symptoms would most likely develop at different rates in each person.

A thorough environmental history may facilitate the diagnosis. Victims found in automobiles, residing in rooms heated by oil-powered furnaces, or using charcoal-powered hibachis or portable room heaters should be suspect.

Carbon monoxide binds to hemoglobin with an affinity 250 times greater than that of oxygen. The remaining oxygen molecules bind to hemoglobin more tightly, shifting the oxyhemoglobin dissociation curve to the left. The net result is tissue hypoxia and lactic acidemia from the body's attempt to compensate through anaerobic metabolism.

The carboxyhemoglobin level, a measure of the percentage of hemoglobin bound by carbon monoxide, can rapidly be obtained by most EDs. The level can be misleadingly low if significant time elapses between the exposure and the blood test, or if oxygen was administered. The symptoms of carbon monoxide poisoning can be roughly correlated with carboxyhemoglobin levels. Headache is the primary manifestation at levels of 15 to 30%; dizziness, nausea, and confusion occur at 30 to 40%; and coma develops at 50 to 60%. Death is likely at levels greater than 70%. Levels up to 10% may be seen in smokers.

Other tests can lead one to suspect carbon monoxide poisoning. A venous blood sample may appear more red than normal due to the binding of carbon monoxide to hemoglobin. The arterial blood gas may reveal a low pH due to lactic acidosis. The arterial pO_2 should remain deceptively high because it measures the amount of oxygen dissolved in the blood and not the amount bound to hemoglobin. Oxygen saturation as reported by most labs is calculated from both the measured PaO_2 and hemoglobin values and will also remain elevated because both these values are unaffected by carbon monoxide poisoning. In suspect cases, request that the lab *measure* the oxygen saturation. If the *measured* value is less than the *calculated* value, a "saturation gap" exists, giving a differential diagnosis of carbon monoxide poisoning, cyanide poisoning, or methemoglobinemia.

The immediate management of carbon monoxide poisoning is administration of 100% oxygen by nonrebreather face mask. This reduces the half-life of carboxyhemoglobin from 5 hours to approximately 80 minutes.

The husband in this case developed a delayed neuropsychiatric syndrome manifested by personality alteration and memory loss. This syndrome is estimated to occur in 3 to 10% of patients, and its mechanism is unknown. No clinical parameters reliably predict which patients will develop it, although those who lose consciousness and then later recover are at higher risk. The syndrome does not seem to occur in patients treated with hyperbaric oxygen.

Although indications for and the benefit of hyperbaric oxygenation remain controversial, some authorities recommend it if there has been a history or presence of coma, neurologic findings other than a mild headache, a carboxyhemoglobin level greater than 20% at any time, symptoms persisting longer than 4 hours, or signs of the delayed neuropsychiatric syndrome. Why hyperbaric oxygen therapy helps patients with the delayed syndrome is unclear, since carbon monoxide itself is long gone from these patients by then.

REFERENCES

Review Articles

Hardy, K. R., and Thom, S.R. Pathophysiology and treatment of carbon monoxide poisoning. *J. Toxicol. Clin. Toxicol.* 1994;32:613–629.

Reisdorff, E. J. Carbon monoxide poisonings: From crib death to pickup trucks. *Emerg. Med. Reports* 1993;14:181–190.

Additional References

Myers, R. A. M., Snyder, S. K., and Emhoff, T. A. Sub-acute sequelae of carbon monoxide poisoning. *Ann. Emerg. Med.* 1985;14:1163–1167.

Grace, T. W., and Platt, F. W. Subacute carbon monoxide poisoning: Another great imitator. *J.A.M.A.* 1981;246:1698–1700.

Olson, K. R., and Seger, D. Hyperbaric oxygen for carbon monoxide poisoning: Does it really work? *Ann. Emerg. Med.* 1995;25:235–237.

Case 28 A "FAINTER" UNDER A DOCTOR'S CARE

A 65-year-old man was brought to the emergency department by ambulance. He had passed out on a downtown sidewalk, and the ambulance was called by bystanders. On arrival, the patient insisted that he felt well. He claimed to be a "fainter." He had fainted over fifteen times in the last year. During these faints, which lasted no more than a few minutes, he was never incontinent and had no remarkable movements. There was no aura or warning, and he had never hurt himself in a fall. The man was visiting from another city, where he was under the care of a Veterans Administration hospital cardiologist for these faints. He was planning to return home the very next day and in fact had an appointment with his physician within a week. He denied any other symptoms and was on no medications.

The physical examination revealed nothing remarkable. Blood pressure was 140/80, pulse 80 and regular, respiratory rate 15, temperature 37.0°C, and jugular venous pressure seemed within normal limits. The patient was alert, well-oriented, and had no gross neurologic defects. An ECG showed right bundle branch block (RBBB) and first-degree atrioventricular (AV) block with a PR interval of 0.26 seconds.

The patient wanted no therapy and minimized the event. He was discharged to return to the care of his physician in his home city. Twelve hours later he was brought back to the ED, having expired suddenly. He was dead on arrival, and no resuscitation was attempted.

What is the significance of coexistent RBBB and first-degree AV block?

What other ECG abnormalities might have the same ominous portent?

What might best have been done for the patient when he came to the ED?

DISCUSSION

Syncope, a transient loss of consciousness, in most cases lasts less than five minutes and is caused by a decrease in delivery of oxygen or glucose to the brain or by seizure activity. Cardiac causes account for less than 10% of syncope but have a high degree of lethality (30% in one year).

This patient's history is classic for Stokes-Adams attacks: loss of consciousness that follows the development of complete heart block ventricular fibrillation, ventricular tachycardia, a profound bradyarrhythmia, or asystole. The arrhythmia may be intermittent, or the patient may die during an attack, as probably happened in this case.

Not all cardiac causes of syncope are signaled by the ECG. However, some ECG signs are important as probable progenitors of complete heart block or sudden death. These are RBBB with left anterior hemiblock (marked left axis deviation of the unblocked early QRS forces), Mobitz type-II block (complete sudden failure of a beat to conduct), alternating RBBB and left bundle branch block (LBBB), LBBB masquerading as RBBB, and some instances of either RBBB or LBBB with first-degree AV block. These ECG patterns reflect bilateral bundle branch disease. It may be a small step from such bilateral disease to complete heart block, and the history of syncope bridges this gap.

In rare instances the ECG will make the diagnosis of a myocardial infarction that was silent except for the syncope. Occasionally, myocardial defects or valvular lesions associated with loss of consciousness, such as aortic stenosis, may be found through patient history, physical examination, or ECG.

With a resting ECG abnormality suggestive of periods of severe AV block and with a history of many faints, this patient should have been admitted to the hospital and evaluated by clinical examination, serial ECGs, Holter or prolonged ECG monitoring, and, perhaps, sophisticated electrophysiologic studies of his conducting system.

Permanent pacing is indicated in intermittent or fixed asymptomatic AV (His bundle) *and* trifascicular block, symptomatic block at any site, and symptomatic bradyarrhythmic sinus node dysfunction.

One probably should assume that any fainter might die with the next faint. A pacemaker could be counted on to take over if the patient's own conduction system failed. The fact that he had not died with previous faints does not make further episodes of AV block less dangerous. The fact that he had experienced multiple episodes lulled the ED staff into suspecting a benign cause of the syncope and, thus, ignoring the significance of the ECG. The actual mechanism of death in this patient was not determined, but it seems most likely to have been a blockage of AV conduction.

Syncope is a common presenting problem in most EDs. Most patients have no suggestions of a seizure in their histories, and few have helpful ECGs. Perhaps more patients should be admitted to hospitals for monitoring purposes even with normal ECGs. (See also Case 7.)

REFERENCES

Review Articles
Hori, S. Diagnosis of patients with syncope in emergency medicine. *Keio J. Med.* 1994;43:185–191.

Edwards, F. J. Overcoming the diagnostic challenges of dizziness, vertigo, and syncope. *Emerg. Med. Reports* 1994;15:1–9.

Additional References
Falk, R. H., Zoll, P. M., and Zoll, R. H. Safety and efficacy of noninvasive cardiac pacing: A preliminary report [classic article]. *N. Engl. J. Med.* 1983;309:1166–1180.

Sobel, B. E., and Roberts, R. Hypotension and Syncope. In E. Braunwald (ed.), *Heart Disease: A Textbook of Cardiovascular Medicine*. Philadelphia: Saunders, 1988. Pp. 7–8, 884–894.

CASE 29 MOTORCYCLE ACCIDENT

A 20-year-old was riding his motorcycle too fast on a country road when he lost control and the bike fell over. He and the bike slid down the road 75 feet and smashed into a guard rail. The noise was heard by nearby neighbors, who soon called an ambulance. The volunteers arrived about fifteen minutes later, and since they had little training they provided the patient with a "scoop and run" transport that involved little medical care but did get him to the hospital promptly. On arrival, he was awake and screaming, "I am all right . . . Get me out of here . . . I can't breathe . . . Let me out of here . . . I can't breathe!" He had no apparent injury other than a bleeding cut over his eyebrow. Several minutes were spent trying to coax him to stay on the hospital stretcher and trying to obtain a blood pressure reading despite his lack of cooperation. He had no obvious chest injury, but auscultation of his lungs was difficult since he was still talking loudly and thrashing about. Shortly thereafter, the staff noticed that he was more cooperative with their attempts to start intravenous lines—in fact, he was soon not moving at all. Vital signs were noted to be absent, and cardiopulmonary resuscitation was begun. During the resuscitation, a chest x-ray was taken. After about twenty minutes of unsuccessful attempts at resuscitation, "the code was called," and the man was pronounced dead. Just then the x-ray technician returned with the chest film. It showed a tension pneumothorax.

What are the priorities in the initial evaluation of a multiple-trauma patient?

Discussion

This young man died in the hands of three physicians who were diligently working to save his life. These three, a surgeon, an emergency physician, and an anesthesiologist, all missed the diagnosis of an easily treatable and reversible condition. No one diagnosed a tension pneumothorax because no one looked for it. The patient probably would have

29. MOTORCYCLE ACCIDENT

been saved if an 18-gauge needle had been poked through his chest wall in the second interspace at the midclavicular line.

Preventable trauma deaths are surprisingly common: We estimate thousands of cases per year in the United States alone. There is a natural tendency on the part of the physician to make a treatment and stabilization plan for the patient based on the type of accident. With an infinite number of accident scenarios, plans for patient care can be quite varied, and this variation can lead to oversight. A better method stresses a standardized approach to the trauma patient, regardless of the mechanism of injury. The American College of Surgeons' Advanced Trauma Life Support course recommends four steps: a primary survey, including the ABCs; a primary resuscitation phase, including initial interventions such as oxygen, intravenous fluids, and treatment of immediately life-threatening injuries; a secondary survey, including a head-to-toe physical examination; and then definitive care.

A mnemonic for the necessary actions in the first few minutes of care is A, B, C, Strip, Hemorrhage, Shock, Splint Major Fractures, Survey.

A — Airway	If the patient is talking clearly, the airway is adequate, at least at that moment.
B — Breathing	We must not only look for adequate ventilation, but consider the three major injuries that can rapidly lead to patient deterioration: tension pneumothorax, sucking chest wound, and flail chest.
C — Circulation	Does the patient have an adequate pulse and blood pressure?
Strip	You cannot adequately evaluate a multiple-trauma patient who has his clothes on.
Hemorrhage	You do not have to stop every little cut from bleeding, but you do need to stem life-threatening hemorrhage rapidly. You should be able to stop bleeding from any blood vessel in the body with one or two well-placed fingers, although with some vessels, such as the aorta, getting your fingers in the right place is difficult.
Shock	At least two large-bore intravenous lines are needed. Eighteen-gauge is considered small bore in this setting.

Splint Major Fractures	Not every broken finger needs to be fixed at this time, but major unstable long bone fractures need to be immobilized early. Do not waste time here; quick stabilization will prevent further soft tissue injury and may decrease the incidence of acute respiratory distress syndrome from "fat embolism."
Survey	Two-minute head-to-toe initial survey.

During the first five minutes of care of a multiple-trauma patient there is always time to consider what should be done next.

And remember: It is very hard to check vital signs too often.

REFERENCES

Review Text
American College of Surgeons' Committee on Trauma. *Advanced Trauma Life Support Program.* Chicago: American College of Surgeons, 1993.

Additional References
Jackimcyzck, K. Blunt chest trauma. *Emerg. Med. Clin. North Am.* 1993;11:81–96.

Kulshrestha, P., et al. Chest injuries: A clinical and autopsy profile. *J. Trauma* 1988;28:844–847.

Wakabayashi, Y., and Bush, W. H., Jr. Pneumoscrotum after blunt chest trauma. *J. Emerg. Med.* 1994;12:603–605.

Paape, K., and Fry, W. A. Spontaneous pneumothorax. *Chest Surg. Clin. North Am.* 1994;4:517–538.

Cales, R. H., and Trunkey, D. D. Preventable trauma deaths. *J.A.M.A.* 1985;254:1059–1063.

CASE 30 HEADACHES

A 30-year-old man, a psychologist, came to the emergency department complaining of severe, left-sided, throbbing headaches over the preceding two weeks. His headaches involved the left face from brow to maxilla and centered about the left eye. During headaches that lasted for several hours, he often vomited, and this seemed to relieve the pain somewhat. He had no family history of headache, no juvenile carsickness or frequent nausea, and recalled no head trauma. He noted that one of his more severe episodes had followed an alcoholic drink, but usually he did not drink or smoke. Although one headache had awakened him, the rest had been during the daytime hours. About three years earlier he had suffered several similar headaches over a two-month period. He was on no drugs except aspirin, which gave him little relief.

On physical examination he appeared to be a normal man in no apparent distress. Vital signs were normal: temperature 37.0°C and blood pressure 130/80. His pain was now gone, and his conjunctivae were normal, although he thought the left eye was sometimes bloodshot with the pain. There was no tenderness over the sinuses, and his fundi and tympanic membranes were normal. His neck was supple, and the patient appeared entirely normal on a careful neurologic exam and a brief general physical exam.

What should be examined when a patient complains of headache?

What sort of headache syndromes are most common in the ED?

When does a patient deserve a spinal tap?

What is the diagnosis in this case?

DISCUSSION

The patient information needed to evaluate a case of headache includes the following: Where is the headache? Is it unilateral or bilateral? Does it pound with the pulse, or is it a steady headache? (It is important to avoid using the word "only" in discussing this matter with the patient, as in "Is your headache pounding or *only* steady?") Does the patient have a fever or chills? Has he or she been suffering from upper respiratory symptoms such as runny nose, stuffy head, earache, ringing in ears, sore throat, prurulent nasal discharge, or hoarseness? Was there any previous head trauma? Has the patient been having blurred or double vision, nausea, or vomiting? Has he or she had high blood pressure in the past? What drugs is the patient taking and what is he or she allergic to? Does coughing or sneezing exacerbate the headache? Is there photophobia? How does he or she try to relieve the pain? Are there any warnings before the headache? Have previous headaches ever been this severe? Is this the worst headache of the patient's life?

The important physical findings to elicit in any case of headache include the vital signs, a thorough head and neck exam, and a neurological exam. Be sure to check for tenderness of the skull and the maxillary and frontal sinuses. The frontal sinuses must be felt from under the supraorbital ridge, as opposed to the maxillary sinuses, which can be palpated directly. Check the equality of the pupils and their response to light. Evaluate the presence of nystagmus. Check flexibility of the neck by asking the patients to touch ears to shoulders and then to flex their chin on their chest. Observe the patient's gait and look for any lateralizing neurological signs. Examine the optic fundi for papilledema or hemorrhages.

Headache syndromes that present in the ED include the following:

1. Febrile headaches—usually bilateral, and present with a fever of at least 101°F. This headache may be steady but is often pounding. Of course, the source of the fever must be found, and this may turn out to be as simple as a respiratory tract infection or viral syndrome.
2. Muscular headache—usually bilateral and mainly in the back of the head. It is steady and worse in the evening. It may last for days. It is the most common headache syndrome seen and usually responds to salicylates or other mild pain medications and to adjunctive measures such as rest, relaxation, or heat to the back of the neck.
3. Vascular headaches—usually classified as (a) atypical or common migraine or (b) typical or uncommon migraine. The point of this is that the vascular headache usually seen does not have all the features

of classic migraine. The classic migraine headache is a unilateral, pounding headache with visual changes, nausea, and vomiting; it lasts for hours, and there is a strong family history of headaches. The more common varieties often lack some of these features and may have no prodrome. In addition, a vascular headache often eventually develops into a muscular headache. A number of drugs are being used with some success to treat these headaches prophylactically. Aspirin, propranolol, tricyclic antidepressants, metoclopramide (Reglan), and other drugs all have a role. Once the headache has progressed, the best treatment used to be strong analgesics, especially narcotics. A new, alternative treatment is a dose of prochlorperazine (Compazine) or chlorpromazine (Thorazine) given slowly intravenously. It is often surprisingly effective, and avoids the use of narcotics. Sumatriptan is very effective in treating true migraines, but it is expensive and may cause dangerous coronary artery spasm in susceptible patients.

4. Sinus headaches—rare. Many patients who come in complaining of sinus headaches are actually experiencing another type of headache. If the patient indeed has a fever and is tender over the sinuses, a set of sinus films should be obtained. In adults, sinusitis is usually caused by streptococcal infections or viral infections. *Haemophilus influenzae* is a common pathogen in children and adolescents and is becoming more common in adults. Treatment should, of course, include antibiotics if the physician suspects bacterial sinusitis. Usually the microbial etiology will be unclear and a broad-spectrum antibiotic, such as amoxicillin or Bactrim, is the antibiotic of choice. Important adjuncts in treatment are analgesics and decongestants.

5. Hypertension headache—generally in the back of the head and often worse in the morning. The diastolic blood pressure should be at least 110 mm Hg to make this diagnosis. The problem is increased by the fact that many people get a temporary elevation of the diastolic blood pressure with pain anywhere, including headache. Headache alone is not a sign of hypertensive emergency, although signs of central nervous system, renal, or cardiac decompensation should be looked for.

6. Post head-trauma headache—often involves the entire head. Patients who have been hit on the head (especially if they have suffered concussion) may have a syndrome consisting of headache, light-headedness, and malaise that can last for weeks. The patient's affect

may be depressed, and he or she may be "neurotic" and unable to do his or her usual work. As long as the patient is continuing to improve, the most important part of the therapy is reassurance. The patient should be told that this syndrome often occurs following head trauma and that it always goes away.

7. Although eye problems are often suggested, they are very rare as a cause of headache. Nevertheless, glaucoma should be kept in mind. The glaucoma patient may present with a headache and then parenthetically add that their vision has blurred and that they have seen rings around lights. Diagnosis can usually be made in seconds by noting a red eye with a poorly reactive pupil and a hazy or cloudy cornea. Immediate ophthalmology consultation can be sight saving.

8. Dental problems also can cause headaches in rare instances, but one first should consider trigeminal neuralgia or temporal mandibular joint arthritis.

Any headache patient who has remarkable physical findings and who does not seem to fit clearly into any of the above categories may have more serious organic brain disease. The physical examination recommended here for headache workup is actually quite brief and can be done in about four minutes. Headache patients may need further workup for disorders such as brain tumor and other intracranial pathology. Patients making *repeated* visits for severe headache without a clear diagnosis usually deserve to have at least one CT scan and a spinal tap. The adage "When you think of it, do it" holds most of the time for a spinal tap. A patient who says that his or her present headache is *the worst ever* probably deserves a tap to rule out meningitis or a subarachnoid hemorrhage. Another possibility, particularly in the era of AIDS (acquired immunodeficiency syndrome), is that the headache may be due to chronic meningitis or a mass lesion such as a brain abscess. A lumbar puncture (LP) in these patients can cause herniation and death. Consequently a very close look for papilledema, and preferably a CT scan, is essential before the LP in these cases.

In this case the patient probably had a vascular headache known as cluster migraine or Horton's histamine cephalalgia. Therapy with Cafergot (ergotamine plus caffeine) aborted many of his subsequent headaches, but he still eventually needed therapy with methysergide (Sansert).

REFERENCES

Review Articles

Thomas, S. H., and Stone, C. K. Emergency department treatment of migraine, tension, and mixed-type headache. *J. Emerg. Med.* 1994; 12:657–664.

Caesar, R., et al. Acute headache management. *Emerg. Med. Reports* 1995;16:117–128.

Additional References

Packard, R. C. What does the headache patient want? *Headache* November 1979;370–374.

Gower, D. J., et al. Contraindications to lumbar puncture as defined by computed cranial tomography. *J. Neurol. Neurosurg. Psychiatry* 1987;50:1071–1074.

Iserson, K. V. Parenteral chlorpromazine treatment of migraine. *Ann. Emerg. Med.* 1983;12:756–758.

Seymour, J. J., et al. Response of headaches to non-narcotic analgesics resulting in missed intracranial hemorrhage. *Am. J. Emerg. Med.* 1995;13:43–45.

Case 31 "DTs"

A 36-year-old man was brought to the emergency department by a concerned friend who promptly vanished. The patient claimed that he was "going into the DTs." He had been drinking heavily for about sixteen years and had been dry for no more than four months at a time during that period. His present binge had lasted three weeks. He had been drinking mainly vodka at a rate of over a fifth a day, but for the past few days he had been drinking wine, and today his money had run out. His last drink had been six hours before he came to the ED. Between binges he had worked as a laborer, dishwasher, and cook. He smoked two packs of cigarettes a day and admitted to having "a smoker's cough." During the preceding few days he had been nauseated and had vomited several times, most commonly in the mornings. The vomiting did not follow a coughing spell, and after taking a drink ("the hair of the dog that bit him"), he felt better. Now he felt shaky, nauseated, and generally very sick. He claimed to be hallucinating when left alone: "seeing animals on the wall." He said he "needed a drink" and asked for an injection of Librium.

On physical examination the patient was tremulous and anxious and looked ill. He was wasted and unshaven. His right hand had multiple cigarette tar stains. His clothes smelled of urine and other unidentifiable odors. Vital signs included blood pressure 160/110 in the right arm when recumbent, 140/100 standing, pulse 130, respiratory rate 25, and temperature 38.1°C. His venous pressure seemed normal. His eyes were bloodshot. His chest had audible bilateral coarse wheezes. His abdomen was diffusely moderately tender, and his legs and feet seemed inordinately sensitive to stroking or pressure. He would jerk his leg away when the sole of the foot was touched.

Why do alcoholics stop drinking?

Does this patient have delirium tremens?

Can alcohol withdrawal symptoms appear while the patient is still drinking?

Discussion

The *binge drinker* can be dry for months but is drunk for days or weeks when drinking. The binge is generally ended in one of three ways. He or she may be arrested by the police for "being drunk in a public place" or driving while under the influence of alcohol and, once in jail, begin to suffer withdrawal symptoms. He or she may suffer an attack of acute gastritis, pancreatitis, or pneumonia that will render him or her too ill to continue to drink. Most commonly, the binge drinker will run out of money. In this setting the binge may taper off over several days with wine or beer.

The earliest withdrawal symptoms are usually nausea and vomiting, notably the morning after a binge. These are treatable with alcohol or benzodiazepines and so represent withdrawal symptoms rather than gastritis or other intra-abdominal pathology. Then tremor, anxiety, and malaise become prominent. Many withdrawing alcoholics seem unable to define their symptoms beyond being "sick."

Fever is common, as is tachycardia, in alcohol withdrawal. However, almost all drinkers are heavy smokers and may be cross-addicted to other drugs, such as cocaine and sedatives. The alcohol suppresses the white blood cell count (folate deficiency and direct bone marrow suppression) and the pulmonary mucociliary apparatus. The cigarette smoke is a chronic irritant, making the patient prone to bronchitis, pneumonia, and tuberculosis. Gastrointestinal bleeding is common in alcoholics because of the increased incidence of peptic ulcers, Mallory-Weiss tears of the esophagus, gastritis, and esophageal varices. Such a patient should have pulse and blood pressure taken supine and upright to look for evidence of hypovolemia. The patient also must have a rectal examination and a stool test for occult blood.

Head trauma is common in alcoholics, and chronic or acute subdural hematomas are prevalent. Confusion and ataxia should not be ascribed to alcohol intoxication too quickly. With head trauma and alcohol intoxication (a very common combination), we always do a serum ethanol level to confirm that the patient's confusion or obtundation is consistent with, and therefore explained by, a measured serum level.

Hallucinations—deranged and distorted sensory perceptions—are common in alcohol withdrawal. They may begin as nightmares, then go on to appear when the patient is alone in a dark room. Next there may be visual (seldom auditory) hallucinations even in well-lighted rooms. All these are generally ego-alien to the patient: He or she recognizes them as frightening but unreal. Only after many days are the hallucinations ego-syntonic, and the patient is truly lost within them. Early alcohol withdrawal syndrome may also include tonic-clonic seizures and an increase in sympathetic tone (increased blood pressure, pulse, diaphoresis, and tremors), which is promptly and dramatically treatable with intravenous benzodiazepines.

Delirium tremens is a rare syndrome in a withdrawing alcoholic who does not also have an associated illness, such as pancreatitis, or some major trauma (accidentally or surgically incurred). DT patients are totally disoriented, agitated, and unable to remove themselves from their hallucinations. Visual and tactile hallucinations are common, and these patients may be seen "picking bugs" off themselves. They also have a tachycardia and often a very high fever. They do *not* arrive able to tell us that they are "going into DTs." DT requires intensive care.

This patient seems to have an alcohol withdrawal syndrome with tremor, nausea and vomiting, tachycardia, and focal hallucinations. He also has chronic bronchitis. The alcohol withdrawal syndrome may develop even while the person is still drinking as long as intake and blood alcohol level are dropping. One should not assume this patient's blood alcohol to be zero—he may have had several drinks more recently than he tells us.

Intoxicated patients with an abnormal mental status should never be allowed to leave the ED unless supervised by a responsible observer. Two of our patients once left the ED accompanied only by each other and were hit by a truck as they crossed the street adjacent to the hospital.

REFERENCES

Review Article
McMicken, D. B. Alcohol withdrawal syndromes. *Emerg. Med. North Am.* 1990;8:805–819.

Additional Reference
Simon, R. P. Alcohol and seizures. *N. Engl. J. Med.* 1988;319:715–716.

Case 32 BLUNT TRAUMA

A 74-year-old woman was brought to the emergency department after having been involved in a motor vehicle accident. The EMTs reported that she had turned into traffic and drove head on into another car that had been traveling at approximately 50 mph. The patient was awake, alert, and breathing shallowly at a rate of 40. She complained of anterior chest and abdominal pain and a sore right knee. Her blood pressure was 130/65 with a pulse of 138. She was given oxygen and a large-bore intravenous line was started. An initial evaluation revealed no other signs of injuries. After the initial evaluation, she was sent for x-rays of her chest, cervical spine, and right knee. While in x-ray she suffered a cardiopulmonary arrest and could not be resuscitated.

How do you recognize that a real emergency is present?

Discussion

Victims of multiple trauma may initially show little evidence of major malfunction, but the story of the accident or injury may suggest great violence, and that violence should lead us to expect to find serious damage. Events associated with serious injury include gunshot and stab wounds, falls from heights greater than 15 feet, and surviving an accident in which someone else died. Motor vehicle accidents with impact at greater than 20 mph or where the vehicle deformity is greater than 20 inches are also associated with a substantial risk of serious injury. Anatomic injuries that suggest severe internal injuries include two or more proximal long-bone fractures, pelvic fractures, and multiple rib fractures.

Once the patient is in our hands, we can often identify the true emergencies by attention to the patient's chief complaint, mental status, and vital signs. Immediately life-threatening emergencies present as problems in the central nervous system, the respiratory system, or the cardiovascular system. Dysfunction in one of these systems often quickly progresses to dysfunction in all three.

To appraise brain function, the physician must make a careful neurologic and mental status examination, but a few simple questions will elicit indications of the more urgent problems: Does the patient respond to me? Is the patient awake? Does the patient know where he or she is, how far it is from home, what day it is, and about what time of the day it is? Is the patient responding appropriately to my presence or struggling with and hostile to someone who is here to help? If the patient is confused, hostile, or asleep and not easily roused to full alertness, then this may be a true emergency.

Adequate evaluation of the respiratory system requires only a few simple observations. What is the patient's respiratory rate? To be accurate at least a full half-minute should be counted. A rate under 12 or over 20 per minute should be considered a bright-red danger signal. All too often tachypnea is written off as "hyperventilation," and the correct diagnosis of pneumonia, metabolic acidosis, serious cardiovascular or pulmonary pathology, or subarachnoid hemorrhage is delayed. While the respiratory rate is counted, the regularity of respiration should be noted. A chaotic or cyclic respiratory pattern is cause for alarm. Volume of ventilation may be difficult to ascertain by watching the patient's chest or listening to it. It is easier to estimate the volume of air moved by placing a hand loosely over the patient's nose and mouth during respiration. Again, either a low or a high volume of ventilation is a serious sign. The patient's color should be gauged, and if it is dusky gray or blue, especially around the lips, there is danger. Finally, the patient may complain of being short of breath, unable to get her breath, or of choking.

Problems involving the cardiovascular system may be signaled by the most awesome physical signs, such as no palpable pulse, or may present with a normal, healthy-appearing patient who says that any chest discomfort has now vanished. Chest pain or discomfort is ominous because of its association with sudden death and myocardial infarction.

The pulse and blood pressure, especially if taken supine, seated, and upright, provide a wealth of information. An irregular pulse, or one with a rate under 50 or over 120, is a danger sign par excellence. A low blood pressure (systolic blood pressure of 100 plus patient's age will give a first approximation of the patient's blood pressure) or one that falls significantly when the patient stands is, of course, very dangerous. The mean blood pressure can be approximated by the diastolic blood pressure plus one-third of the pulse pressure. This mean should not fall 10 mm Hg on standing. A fall of 15 mm is surely significant and one of 20 probably

32. BLUNT TRAUMA

dangerous. This maneuver will pick up hypovolemia, one of the most common pathologic processes seen in an ED as a true emergency.

There is no such thing as "just a little bit of shock." Shock is a serious problem. A drop in blood pressure after bleeding indicates a loss of at least one-third of the total blood volume. By the time blood pressure drops, the patient is in severe shock. The initial sign of occult shock in the supine patient may be the presence of a metabolic acidosis (e.g., an initial arterial blood gas of pH 7.24, pO_2 90, pCO_2 36). Tachypnea and tachycardia, altered mental status (usually agitation), light-headedness, and thirst are later signs. Narcotics, of course, can add to the hypotension by vasodilation and should be used with *great* care if at all in a case such as this.

Fluid repletion must be done quickly with crystalloid, colloid, or blood. If the patient is in extremis, type O-negative or type-specific uncrossmatched blood should be infused until type-specific fully crossmatched blood is available. Large intravenous lines are needed. A central venous pressure catheter is helpful, but it should be a short line inserted through the internal jugular or subclavian vein if fluid is to be infused rapidly through this route. The resistance of a tube is proportionate to the fourth power of its radius, so a large catheter with a diameter about twice that of a medium one can infuse fluids sixteen times as fast.

The evaluation of abdominal injuries in blunt trauma is a major challenge. Abdominal examination may be difficult for many reasons. Blood, by itself, is not immediately irritating to the peritoneum, and significant internal bleeding may be initially present with only mild local tenderness. The unconscious patient may show no sign of peritoneal irritation. Additionally, patients who are intoxicated may show either increased or decreased perception of painful injury. Patients who exhibit significant abdominal tenderness, who are intoxicated and have a significantly serious mechanism of injury, or who have major alterations of their mental status should be considered for either a diagnostic peritoneal lavage or CT of the abdomen.

Peritoneal lavage is performed with local anesthesia, usually inferior to the umbilicus. A small incision is carried down to the peritoneum, and a trochar is then gently poked through. A catheter is slipped over the trochar and aspirated. The presence of 5 ml or more of gross blood in the aspirate reveals major bleeding and is an indication for laparotomy.

If there is no blood grossly, a liter of saline is infused into the abdomen and then drained out. The fluid is then sent for cell count and is considered positive if it contains more than 100,000 red blood cells per mm^3, 500 white blood cells per mm^3, or any bile, food particles, or fecal material. Great debate still continues in the literature regarding the role of CT and lavage in evaluating blunt abdominal trauma. Certainly CT is better at assessing an organ injury that is bleeding and much better at assessing the retroperitoneum (aorta, pancreas, kidneys, and duodenum). Lavage is better at picking up hollow viscus injury such as intestinal perforations and can be performed without moving the patient.

REFERENCES

Review Text

Committee on Trauma of the American College of Surgeons. *Advanced Trauma Life Support*. Chicago: American College of Surgeons, 1989.

Additional References

Cales, R. H., and Trunkey, D. D. Preventable trauma deaths. *J.A.M.A.* 1985;254:1059–1063.

McCabe, C. J., and Warren, R. L. Trauma: An annotated bibliography of the recent literature. *Am. J. Emerg. Med.* 1995;11:652-655.

Trunkey, D. D. Trauma. *Sci. Am.* 1983;249:28–35.

CASE 33 RECTAL EXPLOSION

A 24-year-old man was brought to the emergency department by ambulance. He had placed a firecracker in his anus and lit it. The explosion brought him to the attention of bystanders, and he was brought in with a small amount of blood leaking from his anus. He had a past history of many psychiatric hospitalizations for schizophrenia and for "sexual deviancy." He had come to the ED previously with self-inflicted razor cuts of the scrotum. He had been in the state psychiatric hospital for two years for child molestation.

On physical examination the patient appeared well. There was a small mucosal tear of the anal canal and no further pathology on proctoscopic examination. Vital signs were normal.

How does one treat rectal injuries?

What parts of the treatment are most often overlooked?

DISCUSSION

We have removed from rectal ampullae a variety of foreign bodies, including pop bottles, razor blades, and electric vibrators. The trauma done to the rectum is often underestimated. A tear may lead to retroperitoneal abscess, which has a high mortality Tears can be difficult to diagnose. A stool hematest is mandatory in these cases; fiberoptic sigmoidoscopy or even gastrografin enema should be done if there is sufficient injury potential (e.g., an explosion or deep penetration). In this case the damage was limited to the anal canal and was trivial. Sitz baths alone were adequate therapy.

There is considerable rectal fascination in nonschizophrenics, and one ought not to jump to the diagnosis of schizophrenia in all patients who introduce foreign objects into the rectum. Evaluation of such patients must include attention to both ends. Careful proctoscopy must be done. If the foreign body cannot be removed with the examining finger(s), passage of a Foley catheter beyond the object and inflation of the balloon will frequently help. Care must be taken not to do more damage. Removal of large foreign bodies may require insertion of a gloved hand with near-general anesthesia.

Preoccupation with the rectal lesion can cause the physician to forget to consult a psychiatrist, and this may be the most serious omission possible. Some attempt should be made by the emergency physician to determine if the aberration in behavior is of psychotic or organic origin. No single test is absolutely reliable in this setting, but a mental status exam will help. Three hallmarks of an organic process are *disorientation, loss of a basic fund of knowledge* (name of the president, governor, or other important person), and *loss of the ability to do simple mathematical calculations*.

This incident was triggered by the patient's failure to take his antipsychosis medications, which resulted in the reactivation of his psychosis. Returning him to his usual therapy was enough to achieve control of his psychotic behavior.

REFERENCES

Review Article
Burnstein, M. Managing anorectal emergencies. *Can. Fam. Phys.* 1993;39:1782–1785.

Additional References
Darby, C. R. et al. Management variability in surgery for colorectal emergencies. *Br. J. Surg.* 1992;79:206–210.

Bernner, B. E., and Simon, R. R. Anorectal emergencies. *Ann. Emerg. Med.* 1983;12:367–376.

Case 34 LOST LAB TESTS

A 39-year-old woman came to the emergency department complaining of abdominal pain and vomiting for two days following a day of rather heavy drinking. She denied any significant past ills but admitted that she would get an "acid stomach" if she drank two or more beers. On physical exam she appeared entirely normal except for slight diffuse abdominal tenderness. Blood pressure was 116/84 supine and 106/80 seated. Her pulse was 120 supine or seated. One ounce of Mylanta antacid gave her relief from pain, and a finger-stick hematocrit was 53%. A complete blood count and a set of electrolytes were sent to the lab but were lost there. After two hours the patient said she felt well and was sent home on a regimen of antacid, propoxyphene (Darvon) for pain, and fluids, with instructions to return if she remained ill.

Four days later she returned in severe distress. Her blood pressure was 75 systolic. Her abdomen was tense and tympanitic. Her temperature was 38.6°C. An x-ray showed free air under the diaphragm. She was hyponatremic, hypokalemic, and dehydrated. Central venous pressure was zero, and the patient was treated with high-flow intravenous fluids. After four hours she had exploratory surgery. The findings included a perforated duodenal ulcer, peritonitis, and several areas of near-necrotic bowel. Despite heroic emergency measures, *Escherichia coli* and clostridial sepsis developed, and the patient died one week after exploration.

Had the ulcer perforated at the time of the patient's first ED visit?

How does one make the diagnosis of an acute abdomen requiring surgical attention?

Discussion

We cannot tell retrospectively whether the patient's ulcer had perforated on her first visit. However, pain from a distended viscus may briefly decrease when the organ perforates. The tachycardia suggests that she was sicker than she seemed. No patient should be lightly discharged with an unexplained abnormal vital sign. That is often your only clue to an impending catastrophe. Often, nurses are the caregivers most conscious of abnormal vital signs. A good general rule is that every abnormal vital sign should be repeated before discharge. If there is still an abnormality, this should be brought to the attention of the ED physician, and further evaluation and/or observation planned. They are vital *signs*, and it is dangerous to downplay them.

The classic features of an acute abdomen are distention, rigidity, and pain, although all three need not be present. Distention is often written off as unimportant "gas" by patient and physician alike. Indeed, gaseous distention is a sign of underlying disease. Rigidity occurs secondary to peritoneal inflammation in patients with serious acute abdominal states such as pancreatitis, appendicitis, cholecystitis, or a perforated viscus. It decreases with diminished alertness and may lessen when the patient's attention is diverted. Severe abdominal pain out of proportion to physical findings in an ill-appearing individual flags an abdominal catastrophe. Remember that acute mesenteric ischemia or ruptured abdominal aortic aneurysm may present in this manner.

Sometimes an acute abdomen can present in obscure ways, but an alert physician with a high index of suspicion can make the diagnosis. Especially careful assessment should be given to older, alcoholic, debilitated, diabetic, leukemic, and steroid-treated patients. In these patients, the classic signs and symptoms of acute abdomen might be absent. The combination of accurate history, physical examination, nasogastric tube placement, upright film of the abdomen or chest showing both diaphragms (to look for free air), CBC, and amylase will help in the majority of these patients. The onset of pain before other symptoms may be an important early hint of the presence of an acute abdomen. Whenever there is doubt, a surgeon should be consulted.

A positive hemeoccult test on rectal examination, or fresh blood or "coffee grounds" on nasogastric tube placement, would have been helpful and indicative of acute upper gastrointestinal bleed necessitating further workup. Antacid therapy is good for symptomatic relief, but narcotic analgesics should be given sparingly. The analgesic given to this woman masked her abdominal pain, and the patient returned in septic shock.

REFERENCES

Review Article
Jordan, P. H., and Morrow, C. Perforated peptic ulcer. *Surg. Clin. North Am.* 1988;68:315–329.

Additional References

Rokkas, T., et al. Eradication of Helicobacter pylori reduces the possibility of rebleeding in peptic ulcer disease. *Gastrointest. Endosc.* 1995;41:1–4.

Bretagne, J. F. Management of nonsteroidal anti-inflammatory drug induced upper GI bleeding and perforation. *Dig. Dis.* 1995;13 Suppl. 1:89–105.

Case 35 DIABETIC IN AUTOMOBILE ACCIDENT

A 50-year-old man was involved in an auto accident. Seemingly unprovoked, he drove his car down a hillside into a creek. The car rolled over, and the man bounced around but stayed in the car. A police car arrived, and the officers extricated the patient. After the ambulance arrived, the EMT was able to learn from the patient that he was a diabetic. The patient was then brought to the emergency department, and the EMT told a passing nurse that he had a diabetic who had rolled his car. The nurse glanced at the patient and, deeming him "in not too bad shape," went on about her work in another room. The EMT returned to his ready room.

The patient became more confused and by the time he was seen by a physician fifteen minutes later was stuporous and could give no history. The physician arrived with a blank encounter form and an ambulance trip report that stated only "auto accident—possible injuries." The patient had no obvious signs of head injury and no focal neurologic signs but was clearly confused and stuporous. Fortunately, a youth who was in the room waiting for his girlfriend on the next bed to be sutured remarked that the man was a diabetic: "I heard the ambulance driver say so." A blood sugar was drawn, and 50 ml of 50% glucose solution was given intravenously. The patient became much more alert, and the blood sugar was later reported at 30 mg per dl.

What sort of information does the physician need to learn from the ambulance crew, firemen, policemen, or other on-the-scene observers?

If focal neurologic signs developed in the patient, would they rule out hypoglycemia?

Discussion

Patient history information is of great value to the emergency physician. All too often the patient is confused or comatose or becomes so shortly

35. DIABETIC IN AUTOMOBILE ACCIDENT

after arrival. Often no one is present who can give information about the patient. Relatives may never arrive at the ED even though they tell the ambulance attendant they are coming in, or they may leave before the physician can talk with them.

We like our EMTs to try to determine the following information and include it in the trip report for each case:

A. Trauma Patient
   1. What happened before the event? Was the patient acting strange? Did he or she pass out, become confused, fall, become dizzy? Did the patient complain of any symptoms? Was he or she on any drugs or other treatment? Alcohol?
   2. Description of event: If a weapon was involved, what size and sort? If a fall, how far and in what position? If an auto accident, was the victim seat-belted? Where was the victim seated? Was he or she thrown out? Did he or she hit any secondary objects? How did the accident occur? How much damage was noted on the automobile?
   3. What did the victim then do? Was he or she unconscious? Was there retrograde amnesia? Could the patient move his or her extremities? Did he or she complain of pain or shortness of breath? What has been the course of consciousness since the event?
   4. Other information: Are there any family members coming in? Whom can we contact for further information regarding the accident (an observer of the event)? Whom for background on the patient? Is he or she on any drugs? Allergic to any drugs? Is the patient being cared for by a physician for any chronic illness? What is the name of the physician? When did the patient last eat? (This must be asked should any emergent surgery be required.)
   5. How does the patient now feel? What hurts (the major injury may not be the most apparent)? Trouble breathing? Confusion? Amnesia? Weakness? Dizziness?
B. Nontrauma Patient
   1. Describe major symptoms: A history taken by a neophyte tends to accept as important information the patient's own diagnosis or suggested therapy. This must be bypassed and the patient's symptoms elicited.

2. *Why now?* What led the patient to pick this moment to seek help? Sometimes this is obvious, but, if not, the question must be answered.
3. Is the patient being treated for chronic illness? Again, what is the name of the physician? What drugs is the patient taking, including over-the-counter medicines? (It is helpful to have the EMTs bring in any medications found in the house.) Any allergies to drugs? Who can give us more information?
4. What events occurred (and when) during ride into the ED?

The treatment of many medical emergencies can be safely begun in the field. Most EMS systems have medical control mechanisms in place that help guide the prehospital care providers. The initial care is begun under standing orders. The EMT or paramedic then contacts a base station emergency physician by radio for further orders. Remember that paramedics are trained to start intravenous lines and administer drugs, under protocol, by intravenous, endotracheal, intramuscular, subcutaneous, and oral routes. EMT training is more basic and emphasizes airway management, spinal and extremity immobilization, and rapid transport. This patient's treatment should have been started in the prehospital phase. Most EMS systems require paramedics to give intravenous glucose, Narcan, and thiamine to any young patient found with a depressed level of consciousness. Many EMS systems also equip their ALS (advanced life support) ambulances with glucose meters to get rapid values of blood sugar. Basic EMTs cannot start an intravenous line but may be able to administer glucose orally if the patient is adequately responsive.

Hypoglycemia may present in many ways. Confusion, anger, fighting, ataxia, anxiety, stupor, diaphoresis, tachycardia, or focal neurologic findings all may be present in diabetics. Hypoglycemia is indeed a medical emergency and should be treated promptly. The nurse involved in this case did not realize the significance of an auto accident for a person with diabetes.

Hypoglycemia may mimic alcohol intoxication and, in a busy city hospital ED, is often confused with alcohol intoxication. To further confuse the issue, alcoholics with depleted hepatic glycogen stores may develop hypoglycemia even without insulin or other drug therapy. One may always draw a blood sugar and a blood alcohol, but if the diagnosis of hypoglycemia is being entertained, there is almost never any harm in giving a bolus of sugar (orally in a conscious patient or intravenously in a comatose one). We usually give 25 gm of glucose intravenously (50 cc of 50% glucose) and may repeat it once or twice. We start an intravenous infusion of 5% dextrose in water and feed the patient in the ED. The hypoglycemic action (especially with certain oral hypoglycemic drugs) may long outlast the effect of the glucose given, and the patient may lapse back into coma. Careful observation, oral sugar once awake, and instructions regarding future therapy are necessary.

Differentiating between a metabolic encephalopathy (e.g., hypoglycemia, anoxia or postanoxia, uremia, hyponatremia), a traumatic encephalopathy (e.g., postconcussion, subdural hematoma), and a toxic encephalopathy (e.g., alcohol, sedative, other drugs) can test the most adept neurologist. The patient history, as in this case, can save the day.

REFERENCES

Review Article
Service, F. J. Hypoglycemia. *Med. Clin. North Am.* 1995;79:1–8.

Additional References
Adler, P. M. Serum glucose changes after administration of 50% dextrose solution: Pre- and in-hospital calculation. *Am. J. Emerg. Med.* 1986;4:504–506.

Callure, A., et al. Comparison of intravenous glucagon and dextrose in treatment of severe hypoglycemia in an accident and emergency department. *Diabetes Care* 1987;10:712–715.

Yamashiro, E. Informative usefullness of age, sex, and vital signs in the differential diagnosis of disturbed consciousness among 175 emergency outpatients. *Fukuoka Igaku Zasshi* 1994;85:353–360.

Case 36 UNEQUAL PUPILS

A 51-year-old man was brought to the emergency department by ambulance. He was found lying on the street, and one observer said that he may have had a seizure. On arrival in the ED, he had a pulse of 120, blood pressure 150/80, respiration rate 18, and was somnolent. He responded to deep pain by withdrawing but did not respond to voice commands. His right pupil was slightly larger than the left. He had no asymmetry of reflexes or tone, and plantar responses were flexor (a normal Babinski reflex). "Doll's eyes" (oculocephalic responses) were not evaluated because of the possibility of a cervical spine injury. He was given 50 gm of glucose (100 ml of 50% glucose solution) by vein, and blood sugar, BUN, and electrolyte samples were drawn. There was no improvement, and shortly thereafter the patient had a generalized seizure, during which he seemed to be looking to the right. A skull film showed a probable fracture, and a CT scan was done but was normal. The following laboratory data were then returned: a BUN of 3 mg per 100 ml, blood sugar of 480 mg per 100 ml (unfortunately drawn after the bolus of sugar was given), and electrolytes showing a sodium concentration of 98 mEq/L; chloride, 62 mEq/L; potassium, 3.4 mEq/L; and bicarbonate, 16 mEq/L. Treatment with 3% saline solution and potassium chloride led to arousal and then pulmonary congestion. The patient was admitted to the hospital.

What is the significance of unequal pupils after a seizure?

How low must the serum sodium drop before seizures or confusion can be ascribed to it?

What causes hyponatremia?

Discussion

Seizures may lead to unequal neurologic signs in the postictal period. Todd's paralysis or anisocoria is not unusual. The postictal findings may help define the focus of the seizures in the brain. In this case the physicians were concerned about the possibility of impending cerebral herniation due to a subdural or epidural hematoma, and an emergency CT scan was needed to rule out the presence of an evacuatable mass lesion.

The evaluation of a seizure patient should include blood sugar and serum sodium analyses. Hypoglycemia or hyponatremia (sodium concentration under 120 mEq/L) may cause seizures. The cause of hyponatremia is not always clear but usually includes excessive sodium loss or excessive water intake and may include an excessive, inappropriate antidiuretic hormone secretion. This has been associated with acute and chronic diseases of the lung and the brain. Young people may develop hyponatremia after vigorous exercise that involves heavy sweating and repletion of volume with water but not salt. They usually present first with muscle and abdominal cramps but may progress to seizures.

Hypertonic saline treatment is indicated when the serum sodium is below 120 mEq per dl and the patient has shown significant neurologic symptoms. Replacement should be done slowly in order to avoid pulmonary congestion from fluid overload. Other electrolyte abnormalities such as hypocalcemia and hypomagnesemia can cause seizures. Hypomagnesemia is frequently found in alcoholics, and the decision to order serum calcium and magnesium levels is always reasonable in the workup of a new seizure patient.

Needless to say, a blood sugar obtained after giving glucose has little value. In this case, a few seconds spent obtaining a sample before therapy would have been worthwhile. Nevertheless, treatment with 50% glucose solution prior to knowing the serum glucose is generally accepted for a young, acutely obtunded or seizing patient because it virtually never does harm (except perhaps in the patient who is having a stroke). If the patient has more than a slight probability of being alcoholic, thiamine should be given with or before the first carbohydrate (i.e., glucose) load to prevent Wernicke's encephalopathy.

REFERENCES

Review Articles
Tardy, B., et al. Adult first generalized seizure: Etiology, biological tests, EEK, CT scan, in an ED. *Am. J. Emerg. Med.* 1995;13:1–5.
Pellegrino, T. R. An emergency department approach to first-time seizures. *Emerg. Med. Clin. North Am.* 1994;12:925–940.

Additional References

Einser, R. F., et al. Efficacy of a "standard" seizure workup in the emergency department. *Ann. Emerg. Med.* 1986;15:33–39.

Messing, R. O., and Simon, R. P. Seizures as a manifestation of systemic disease. *Neurol. Clin. North Am.* 1986;4:563–584.

Culpepper, R. M., et al. Hypertonic saline: Patterns of and guidelines for use. *South. Med. J.* 1994;87:1203–1207.

Turnbull, T. L., et al. Utility of laboratory studies in the emergency department patient with a new onset seizure. *Ann. Emerg. Med.* 1990;19:373–377.

Case 37 SHAKY, PALE, AND DRINKING

A 35-year-old man had been drinking heavily until two days before he came to the emergency department. When he arrived he complained that he had become shaky and felt sick. He appeared pale, had tremors, and was perspiring but afebrile. The man was alert and gave no evidence of hallucinations. He appeared somewhat dry. He was treated with intravenous fluids and sedation. During the next three hours he began to feel much better and largely lost his tremors. He was discharged, but, as he got out of the bed to leave, he collapsed on the floor. He was then found to be hypotensive, and his hematocrit was 13%. Subsequent evaluation showed massive upper gastrointestinal bleeding—probably from a duodenal ulcer or an acute gastritis. The patient was hospitalized for further therapy.

In evaluating a withdrawing alcoholic, what history and physical examination data should be collected to rule out the most common serious associated illnesses?

If you think you are dealing with an upper GI bleeder, what should you do in the ED?

What was the significance of this patient's diaphoresis (sweatiness)?

Discussion

The following workup is very helpful in identifying patients who are withdrawing from alcohol but are too ill for a simple detoxification (drying-out) facility to handle. The serious diseases picked up include acute head trauma, acute or chronic subdural hematomas, epidural hematomas, pneumonia, tuberculosis, GI bleeding, and severe hypovolemia.

Case 37 was adapted from Platt, F. W. More than DTs. *Emerg. Med.* 1972;4:167.

Evaluation of Alcohol Withdrawal Patients
A. History
   1. Chief complaint—main symptom. Duration of symptoms. Alleviating and worsening factors. COMMENT: These patients often cannot clarify this more than "sick."
   2. Drinking how much? _____ of what? _____
      Last drink when? _____ How long this binge? _____
      When last on detox ward? _____
   3. Smokes _____ packs/day.
      Cough _____ oz. _____ (color) sputum/day.
      Tuberculosis history? _____ Chest pain? _____
      Short of breath? _____
   4. Head trauma recently? _____
      Seizures? _____ Hallucinations? _____
   5. Vomiting blood? (how much) _____
      Black, tarry stools? _____
   6. Taking medications? _____ Allergic to medicines? _____
      Any other serious illnesses? _____
   7. Other: _____
B. Physical Exam
   BP _____ P _____ right arm, recumbent
   BP _____ P _____ right arm, standing or sitting
   Temp _____ Respiration _____ Weight _____
   HEENT—(jaundice, evidence of head trauma).
   Neck, Nodes—
   Chest—
   Cardiovascular—(cardiomegaly, edema, gallops, . . .)
   Abdomen—(tenderness, liver size, . . .)
   Rectal—Stool to hematest
   Neurologic—(gait, nystagmus, mental status, tremor, focal sign)
C. Lab
   Chest x-ray _____ CBC _____
   Urinalysis _____ Blood alcohol _____

Upper GI bleeding is a life-threatening problem. We try to determine whether the patient is significantly hypovolemic and, if so, expand his blood volume with saline or lactated Ringer's solution. We pass a nasogastric tube and, if any evidence of bleeding is obtained, initiate gastric lavage with saline. We obtain blood for typing, crossmatch at least 4 units of RBCs, and do a hematocrit. Initial treatment is with intravenous fluids, intravenous H_2 blockers (e.g., cimetidine or ranitidine), blood replacement as needed, and nasogastric suction. NG lavage with iced saline is not effective therapy. Occasionally angiography is needed to embolize bleeding vessels. Esophagogastroduodenoscopy (EGD)/GI endoscopy may help to localize bleeding and cauterize the bleeding site.

Patients with evidence of voluminous blood loss (by history) or of hypovolemia (by examination) are admitted, usually to the medical service. Tarry stools or a low hematocrit usually lead to admission. An occasional patient will complain of vomiting blood but will have normal vital signs with no postural change, a normal hematocrit, and negative stool and gastric aspirate. Such a patient may be sent home.

Lower GI bleeding usually presents with red blood passed by rectum. Proctoscopy should be done to locate the bleeding site and evaluate the rectal mucosa although it does not need to be done on an emergency basis in the ED. Hemorrhoidal bleeding is, of course, most common and is usually less significant than bleeding from the rectum or higher.

When this patient presented to the ED, he was afebrile but perspiring (diaphoretic). Diaphoresis usually means hypoglycemia, shock, extreme expenditure of energy such as in a laboring asthmatic, or a very hot environment. It is also frequently seen in patients with acute myocardial infarctions, acute pulmonary edema, or severe abdominal or back pain such as renal or biliary colic. True diaphoresis is a significant clinical finding and should always be considered a sign of significant organic disease.

REFERENCES

Review Article
MacMath, T. L. Alcohol and gastrointestinal bleeding. *Emerg. Med. Clin. North Am.* 1990;8:859–872.

Additional References
Steer, M. L., and Sile, N. W. Diagnostic procedures in gastrointestinal hemorrhage. *N. Engl. J. Med.* 1983;309:646–650.

Klerman, G. L. Treatment of alcoholism (editorial). *N. Engl. J. Med.* 1989;320:394–395.

McMicken, D. B. Alcohol withdrawal syndromes. *Emerg. Med. Clin. North Am.* 1990;8:805-819.

Case 38 LEOPARD BITE

A 54-year-old zoo keeper was bitten by a leopard. Some sort of illness had killed one leopard in the zoo, and the others were being treated with parenteral tetracycline prophylactically. The zoo keeper was trying to hold the leopard down for its shot when it bit him on the hand. He was seen in the employees' health clinic where he was given a shot of tetanus toxoid. The following day he came to the emergency department complaining of a painful, swollen hand. He was afebrile. There were no red streaks on his arm, and he had only one small, nontender lymph node in the right axilla. Two small, closed puncture wounds were evident. The patient was taken to the operating room where incision and drainage were done under regional anesthesia. Copious pus was drained and cultured.

What organism is most likely to be cultured?

Should the patient be started on rabies vaccine?

Are any other animal bites handled differently?

Is it true that the bite of the leopard is the most dangerous known to humans?

Discussion

Leopards are unusual in that they have frequent bouts of *E. coli* septicemia. Therefore, we might expect an *E. coli* septic abscess in this case. Nonetheless, the organism cultured was *Pasteurella multocida*. This organism is present in large amounts in the saliva of domestic cats and often in that of dogs. Because of this organism, cat bites are notorious for rapid accumulation of pus and rapid swelling. Fortunately, *P. multocida* is very sensitive to almost any antibiotic and responds well to a 10-day course of penicillin, erythromycin, or tetracycline. With cellulitis, one may occasionally do without incision and drainage if drug therapy is begun before an abscess forms. In this case, initiation of antibiotic therapy one day earlier might have eliminated the need for surgery. It remains controversial whether prophylactic antibiotics given shortly after the time of the bite are effective. Studies have shown that they are effective in cat bites but not effective in dog bites; yet prophylactic antibiotics are usually used in both dog and cat bites when the wound is significant. If antibiotics are to be given, then, based on the usual flora, we think reasonable first-line drugs are dicloxacillin in dog bites and penicillin V in cat bites.

Rabies vaccination is not appropriate in this case. The question of rabies prophylaxis usually comes up in connection with a dog bite. Even then, unless there is particular reason for suspicion, no therapy need be done if the animal can be observed. A rabid dog is a sick dog and will either die shortly or be so ill as to warrant sacrificing and autopsy. The local animal control officer can be notified through the police and will usually handle the matter. We treat dog bites with copious irrigation, debridement if needed, tetanus toxoid, and antibiotics. We generally suture such wounds, although some physicians do not. When cosmesis is not a consideration, these wounds are probably best left unsutured to freely drain and granulate in. When cosmesis matters, we suggest suturing loosely (to allow for drainage) and giving antibiotics orally. When suturing bites, ensure close follow-up in case an infection develops.

Skunks and bats should be assumed to carry rabies. Other wild mammals may also carry rabies, although for unknown reasons rodents (mice, rats, squirrels, etc.) almost never do. The local health department is the best resource for determining the potential presence of rabies among the various types of animals in your area. Suspicious bites are treated with rabies immune globulin (half is given into the wound and half intramuscularly) and human diploid cell vaccine (given in five intramuscular injections spread over 28 days). This course of therapy is more effective and less painful than the older, dreaded series of 23 injections of duck embryo vaccine into the skin of the abdomen.

Snake bites are benign—unless of course the snake is poisonous! Pit vipers (e.g., rattlesnakes) are found throughout most of the United States. These cases will announce themselves by a painful, rapidly developing, local reaction. Treatment is with horse serum antivenin intravenously. Luckily, the only poisonous snake bites in the United States that do not develop such an obvious local reaction are the rarer neurotoxic (elapid) envenomations seen only in zoos (e.g., cobra) or a few isolated parts of the country such as the California desert and the southeast coastal waterways (coral snake). Serious poisonous arthropod bites are rare in most parts of the country. Black widow spider bites cause painful muscle contractions that can be treated with intravenous calcium. Brown recluse spiders can cause severe local ischemic damage, and their bites are sometimes excised to prevent extensive necrosis. Scorpion stings can cause severe hypertension and anxiety, but most cases are mild except for the increase in the stress level of the person bitten.

Human bites are probably the most serious that we see. They should be cleaned, debrided, and copiously irrigated. They must be observed closely and hospitalization urged at any serious sign of infection. Prophylactic antibiotics are appropriate with human bites that "break the skin" (i.e., cause bleeding) and probably should be begun with penicillin.

Hand infections must be aggressively diagnosed and treated to avoid functional disability. Remember that a human "bite" to the metacarpophalangeal joint is often produced by a punch to the mouth. The intra-articular nature of the wound may only be seen if the wound is examined in the fully flexed position, and the patient may not eagerly tell how the joint injury was sustained.

REFERENCES

Review Articles

Goldstein, E. J. Bite wounds and infection. *Clin. Infect. Dis.* 1992;14:633–638.

Dire, D. J. Cat bite wounds. *Ann. Emerg. Med.* 1991;20:973–979.

Additional References

Galloway, R. E. Mammalian bites. *J. Emerg. Med.* 1988;6:325–331.

Callaham, M. Controversies in antibiotic choices for bite wounds. *Ann. Emerg. Med.* 1988;12:1321–1330.

Kauffman, F. H., and Goldmann, B. J. Rabies. *Am. J. Emerg. Med.* 1986;4:525–531.

Cohle, S. D., et al. Fatal big cat attacks. *Am. J. Forensic Med. Pathol.* 1990;11:208–212.

Case 39 COMA

A 50-year-old man was brought to the emergency department by ambulance. He had been found lying in the street unconscious. There was no obvious evidence of trauma.

On arrival the man was comatose. He appeared unkempt, unshaven, and dirty. There was a distinct alcohol odor mingled with several less well-defined odors. He moved away from painful stimuli but would not respond to verbal communications. Vital signs included a pulse rate of 100, respiratory rate of 15, blood pressure of 160/90, and temperature of 37.5°C rectally. He had normal oculocephalic reflexes ("doll's eyes"). His muscle tone was normal throughout. Deep tendon reflexes were symmetric, although ankle jerks could not be elicited. The plantar responses ("Babinski reflexes") were normal and the pupils were equal. An intravenous route was established, and 50 ml of 50% glucose solution was given. No response was noted. The patient was thought to be in alcoholic stupor. Blood sugar, electrolyte, and blood alcohol analyses were ordered. The patient was laid flat on his back, tied with gauze restraints, and left to sober up. Two hours later he vomited and aspirated some of the vomitus. He did not suffer a respiratory arrest but was thought to have an aspiration pneumonitis and was admitted to the medical ward.

What is the preferred position in which to place comatose patients?

Discussion

Coma position should ensure patency of the airway. If the patient vomits (not uncommon in an unconscious patient), the emesis should be able to pour out by gravity and not remain in the pharynx to cause obstruction or be aspirated into the lungs. The standard position is semiprone, lateral decubitus with the mouth pointed down near the edge of the bed. Vomitus will then tend to pour off the bed. The patient can be tied in such a position and be relatively safe.

Of course, nothing is better than close observation, but all too often a patient is well observed in an ED until a patient in worse shape arrives, and then attention is diverted from the first patient. Some emergency units have attached observation wards with monitoring facilities and a separate nursing staff. Even when such an intensive care observation unit is maintained, observation may be inadequate when the system becomes overloaded.

Observation should include looking for signs of increasing intracranial pressure—checking for arousability, pulse, blood pressure, and pupillary size and reactivity. A comatose patient who clearly is not more alert in 4 hours should be admitted to the hospital.

Coma is an emergency with metabolic, toxicologic, and neurologic causes. A history of trauma or the presence of an asymmetric neurologic deficit suggests a mass lesion such as a subdural or epidural hematoma. Venous blood sampling may reveal hypoglycemia, hyperglycemia, hepatic or renal failure, or ethanol or other toxic ingestion. Arterial blood sampling may reveal an unsuspected hypoxia or metabolic acidosis (from shock or poison).

When presented with a comatose patient, it is necessary to act before all the data (e.g., blood tests) are back. Except when a stroke is thought to be the likely diagnosis, all coma patients should promptly be given oxygen, 25 gm of glucose, 0.8 mg or more of Narcan, and 50 to 100 mg of thiamine. This empiric therapy should be given unless the cause of unconsciousness is clear. A complete neurologic examination must be performed on all comatose patients. This includes pupillary size and reactivity, best motor response, deep tendon reflexes, and checking for the presence of an abnormal Babinski response. Any lateralizing neurologic signs mandate an emergency head CT, as does an unexpectedly prolonged unconscious state (e.g., a seizure patient who does not wake up) or a coma that is unexplained.

Once a patient has aspirated, severe chemical pneumonitis may develop. Steroids are no longer used for treatment of aspiration pneumonitis. Antibiotics should be used if signs of infection, such as fever and purulent sputum, develop.

REFERENCES

Review Article
Ropper, A. H., and Martin, J. B. Coma and Other Disorders of Consciousness. In E. Braunwald et al. (eds.), *Harrison's Principles of*

Internal Medicine (11th ed.). New York: McGraw-Hill, 1987. Pp. 114–120.

Additional References

Pennza, T. T. Aspiration pneumonia, necrotizing pneumonia, and lung abscess. *Emerg. Med. Clin. North Am.* 1989;7:279–307.

Yamashiro, S., et al. Informative usefullness of age, sex, and vital signs in the differential diagnosis of disturbed consciousness in 175 emergency outpatients. *Fukuoka Igaku Zasshi* 1994;85:353–360.

Plum, F., and Posner, J. B. *The Diagnosis of Stupor and Coma* (3rd ed.). Philadelphia: F. A. Davis Company, 1980.

CASE 40 COUGHING UP BLOOD

A 23-year-old man came to the emergency department complaining of shortness of breath, fatigue, and coughing up blood. He claimed that he had been suffering these symptoms for about ten months and denied any remarkable recent worsening. He admitted smoking one pack of cigarettes daily. His cough produced about 1 ounce of almost pure blood daily. He could do very little without suffering dyspnea and had quit his job about one year earlier because of dyspnea and fatigue. He slept flat, but several times a week he awoke with choking and walked about the house, drank water, and even went outdoors before settling back in bed. He denied any chest pain and had no history of rheumatic fever or heart murmur.

This night, he called for help when he awoke from an afternoon nap in a state of panic. He was confused and terrified. The confusion quickly disappeared, but the panic remained. He had recently been having marital difficulties and was separated from his wife. In the past, there had been several episodes of panic, but none had been as severe as this day's.

On physical examination, the patient appeared anxious and tremulous. His pulse was 100, respiration 24, blood pressure 150/80, and temperature 37.5° C. His chest was clear, jugular venous pressure was normal, and he had no edema. Pulses were normal. His cardiac impulse was forceful but not sustained and was localized at the fourth intercostal space in the midclavicular line. He had no abnormal gallops, a loud S_1 and S_2, and a faint short systolic murmur at the aortic area. On being asked to cough, he produced bloody saliva by sucking at a bleeding gum around a carious tooth. He had no adenopathy and no thyromegaly. The patient appeared otherwise normal. A chest x-ray was normal.

What should be done next for this patient?

In what order should organic and psychiatric symptoms be pursued in the ED?

DISCUSSION

This young man presented clear, organic-sounding symptoms and clear emotional symptoms. Of the two, the reason for this arrival at the ED was an emotional symptom, acute panic, and this should be addressed. Physicians are often loath to approach psychiatric problems because of their own insecurities. Nonetheless, the ED must attend primarily to the problems bringing the patient to the hospital. Often, as in this case, a combined approach works best.

This man was told that he had several problems, that his lungs and heart seemed to have nothing seriously wrong with them, but that he should be seen in the medical clinic. He was told that an interview with one of the psychiatric staff was essential and then given some mild sedation (5 mg of Valium, 2 to 4 times a day). After the initial psychiatric interview, the patient was calmer and returned home.

This case was grossly unfinished as the patient left the ED; however, several things were begun. An appraisal had been made of possible life-threatening cardiac or pulmonary diseases, and none were found. The importance of the emotional features of the illness had been stressed to the patient, and arrangements had been made for follow-up. The obvious features of malingering (sucking on a bleeding mouth lesion and claiming the bloody saliva as hemoptysis) did not go unnoticed, but the patient properly was not punished for this. In fact, this unusual behavior—producing more symptoms in order to be heard—should be viewed as a cry for help.

In general, one should work up what appears to be most prominent. A barber once told me that his technique was "to cut off whatever sticks out." This is the most fruitful ED approach—that is, examine whatever sticks out. If psychopathology stares you in the face, evaluate it. Fear of labeling the patient a neurotic should not lead the doctor to avoid dealing with emotional symptoms that the patient desperately wants to discuss.

Hemoptysis can be an acute medical emergency when massive but more frequently presents as small amounts of blood-tinged sputum, such as with tracheobronchitis. A complete examination should rule out malignancy, pneumonia, hypertension, and mitral stenosis as the cause.

Benzodiazepines are useful agents for the treatment of acute anxiety, but must only be used for short periods of time until proper medical and psychiatric follow-up can be arranged. The importance of psychiatric evaluation must be stressed to the patient before the underlying emotional problems can be addressed and corrected. The evaluation in the ED must include an assessment of suicide potential, as will be shown in Case 41: Repeat Visits.

REFERENCES
Review Article
Goldmann, J. M. Hemoptysis: Emergency assessment and management. *Emerg. Med. Clin. North Am.* 1989;7:325–337.

Additional References
O'Shea, B., et al. Factitious hemoptysis. *Arch. Intern. Med.* 1984; 144(2):415–419.

Rudzinski, J. P., and delCasciall, J. Massive hemoptysis. *Ann. Emerg. Med.* 1987;16:1561–1564.

Purcell, T. B. The somatic patient. *Emerg. Med. Clin. North Am.* 1991;9:137–160.

Margo, K. L., et al. The problem of somatization in family practice. *Am. Fam. Physician* 1994;48:1873–1879.

CASE 41   REPEAT VISITS

A 20-year-old woman was brought to the emergency department on a Saturday night with a laceration. She had cut herself with a razor blade and was brought in by ambulance. The EMT had placed a pressure dressing on her superficial wrist laceration, which was bleeding slowly. The patient was relatively uncommunicative but admitted she felt depressed.

During the preceding eighteen-month period, the woman had spent a total of over thirteen months hospitalized on several psychiatric wards with the diagnosis of depression. During the preceding week, she had appeared at the ED five times. She had been discharged from the psychiatry inpatient unit on Tuesday and that same evening returned to the ED with slashed wrists. The wounds were irrigated and sutured, and she was referred to the psychiatry team, who interviewed her and judged her to be not suicidal. Two days later, on Thursday, she arrived at the ED to discuss her worsening depression with the psychiatry team. After her interview she went out—only to return four hours later with a new laceration of the left wrist. On Friday she was brought in with a presumed overdose of aspirin, Librium, and Thorazine. She refused to wait for a physician to see her and left within an hour of her arrival. The ED had been very busy with major trauma cases, and both nurses and physicians viewed her as a nuisance rather than as a challenging new problem. On Saturday night she returned with her latest laceration. She was again sutured and referred to the psychiatry team. She announced that she was now under the care of an outside private psychiatrist. When he was called, he responded by stating that she was no suicide risk and that he was getting disgusted with her. Her parents had both killed themselves when she was 3 years old.

Is this patient suicidal?

One of the physicians claims that the patient is in the running for the "Turkey of the Year Award." How do you believe she should be handled?

DISCUSSION

All patients who have taken an overdose, are intoxicated, have made a suicidal gesture, have made threats against themselves or others, or wish to sign out of the ED against medical advice must have a careful mental status examination performed. This should include orientation (to person, place, time), content of thought, and the presence of hallucinations or of suicidal or homicidal ideations. (Patients who have hallucinations that consist of commands of any sort are at the highest risk for suicidal or homicidal actions and usually should be hospitalized in a psychiatric facility.) Abnormalities should be carefully documented on the medical record for serial examinations. Any potentially suicidal or acutely psychotic patient should be seen by a psychiatrist prior to leaving the ED. In some rural areas, a mental health worker may perform a screening examination and discuss the findings with a supervising psychiatrist. Intoxicated patients should be held in the department until they have "sobered up" unless they are taken home by another responsible person. Patients in these categories who are allowed to leave without proper supervision represent a threat to themselves and a risk of malpractice suit against the ED staff for negligence in allowing them to leave.

A successful suicide is by definition a disastrous event. In general, when a patient admits to depression, he or she should be queried about suicidal thoughts or plans. These should be taken seriously. Viewing the gamut of patients who have made a suicide attempt and failed, one finds some with serious depression and desire to kill themselves and others with far less emotional distress who intended a mere gesture or an appeal for help, love, attention, or even punishment. Unfortunately, it can be difficult to tell the difference, because serious intent does not always ensure success and a mere gesture may accidentally be fatal. In general, psychiatrists tend to put the most effort into aiding suicidally depressed patients and not into working with persons they judge to be immature gesturers. This patient may die by her own hand eventually, even though any one attempt is not likely to be a serious one.

This patient exemplifies an extremely difficult ED problem. It is not clear what she is getting from the ED, but it is hard to believe that she is in any way getting assistance. She has been labeled a "chronic underdoser." Her diagnosis is probably "borderline personality disorder," and she will continue to be very difficult for therapists of any sort. Harassing the staff seems to be part of a destructive game she plays—destructive to her and to those superficially appearing to help her. At the very least, she is "crying wolf" too often and might not be heard when she cries for real. She is becoming the victim of considerable ED staff hostility—perhaps the very thing she is trying to provoke. She interrupts and dilutes the care of other patients and makes the staff aware of its failure in dealing with her.

No one has been able to find a satisfactory approach to this sort of patient. She is chronically depressed and shows few signs of hope. She believes she can do nothing well, not even suicide attempts. Her more-or-less pathologic involvement with the ED may be all the human contact she can tolerate or obtain. An apocryphal tale relates that for a similar patient a collection was taken up one night by the ED staff. The collection bought a one-way bus ticket to a city 600 miles away and temporarily stopped the patient's visits. A more constructive approach for these patients is to involve staff from the ED, psychiatry, and social services in a meeting to work out an individualized patient treatment plan. In selected cases, we have had some success with this type of interagency team approach, at least in the short term.

REFERENCES

Review Article
Hofmann, D. B., and Dubovsky, S. L. Depression and suicide assessment. *Emerg. Med. Clin. North Am.* 1991;9:107–121.

Additional References
Ruben, H. L. Managing suicidal behavior. *J.A.M.A.* 1979;241:282–284.
Clayton, P. J. Suicide. *Psychiatr. Clin. North Am.* 1985;8:203–214.
Henneman, P. L., et al. Prospective evaluation of emergency department medical clearance. *Ann. Emerg. Med.* 1994;24:672–677.

Case 42 SEVENTY-TWO YEARS OLD, FEELING FAINT

A 72-year-old man was brought to the emergency department because he had become faint at a bowling alley. On arrival at the ED he felt well. He was placed in the cardiac resuscitation room because that night it possessed the only working ECG. On examination, he denied faintness, shortness of breath, or chest pain. He was being cared for by an outside physician and was on no medications. He believed that he had suffered a "heart attack" five years earlier that consisted of "auricular fibrillation."

His blood pressure was 110/70. His pulse was counted at 104 and was noted to be irregular; an apical pulse of 120 was noted. He had no edema, rales, or elevation of jugular venous pressure. He had carotid bruits but no heart murmurs. The diagnostic ECG was normal except for the presence of atrial fibrillation.

While the patient was resting, still attached to the ECG monitor, he noted an unusual formation on the monitor oscilloscope and called it to the attention of the physician and nurse in the room. The formation appeared to be five ventricular beats in a row. These ended spontaneously and did not reappear. A defibrillator paddle was coated with electrode paste and placed under the patient's upper back. The other paddle was coated, and the capacitor charged with 200 watt seconds. An intravenous injection of lidocaine (100 mg) was given. The patient's physician was contacted. He agreed to take over the patient's care if he could be transferred to a nearby private hospital but questioned the wisdom of moving him at that time.

Did this patient have a run of ventricular tachycardia?

How do you treat ventricular tachycardia?

What might have led to this patient's arrhythmias?

Discussion

Ventricular tachycardia (VT) is usually a life-threatening arrhythmia because of the likelihood of its proceeding to ventricular fibrillation. In the ED, it should always be assumed to be a disastrous arrhythmia and not the "benign ventricular tachycardia" that is often noted in coronary care units. Treatment should be rapid.

If the blood pressure seems adequate, testifying to a reasonable cardiac output, a bolus of lidocaine (1 mg per kg) should be given. Additional lidocaine may be given—up to a total of 3 mg per kg or until the arrhythmia subsides. If the maximum permissible dose has been given and the VT persists, procainamide (Pronestyl) and/or bretylium can be tried next. If the arrhythmia still persists, cardioversion should be employed.

In the unstable patient with chest pain, dyspnea, or hypotension, synchronized cardioversion starting at 100 joules is the first treatment of choice. If time permits, some form of analgesia or sedation should be employed prior to the cardioversion. In the patient with pulseless VT and witnessed arrest, a precardial thump is delivered. If this is unsuccessful, defibrillation is started at 200 joules. More energy is given if needed—up to 360 joules if the initial shock is not successful. If the arrhythmia persists, cardiopulmonary resuscitation is begun, followed by intravenous epinephrine (1 mg), intubation, and repeated attempts at defibrillation at 360 joules. If unsuccessful, lidocaine is given, followed by defibrillation. If this is unsuccessful, the standard ACLS algorithms should be followed, but the odds for long term survival are not great.

In this case, the patient converted spontaneously after a brief run of five ventricular beats. One could question whether five beats make a ventricular tachycardia, but a more important question is whether this was indeed VT or just aberration of conduction through the ventricles from a supraventricular tachycardia. Normally, one can tell a supraventricular tachycardia from VT simply by the width of the QRS. In some cases, when there is aberrant conduction through the ventricle of the supraventricular beat, the QRS is widened. Even a cardiologist with plenty of time to study the tracing may have trouble differentiating a VT from a supraventricular tachycardia with aberrancy. In this case, the absence of a written record to study makes things even more difficult, and it is not wise to observe a patient too long in order to secure evidence. Too long of a delay may be diagnostic for the physician but lethal for the patient. This patient presented with faintness, and lidocaine should be given intravenously in a 100-mg bolus and followed by a lidocaine drip at 2 to 4 mg per minute.

Patients with myocardial infarctions may or may not have serious arrhythmias. On the other hand, a patient with life-threatening arrhythmias may not have had an infarction even though he has atherosclerotic coronary artery disease. Coronary artery disease may present with sudden death, myocardial infarction, self-limiting or benign arrhythmias, congestive heart failure, or angina pectoris. These may occur in combination or singly. With no clear history of pain or an ECG diagnostic of infarction, we cannot yet say whether this patient had a myocardial infarction. However, he surely should be hospitalized. His atrial fibrillation may be a recent change and may be responsible for his faintness. He may have had a brief but more serious arrhythmia at the bowling alley. His blood pressure is probably low and may be related to the arrhythmia or to the cause of the arrhythmia. Pulmonary embolism should be searched for as a cause of the atrial fibrillation. If this patient has been on digitalis, "dig" toxicity should be considered as another possible cause of his various arrhythmias.

Transportation to another hospital should not be done at this time because of the inherent instability of the patient's situation. The emergency physician caring for the patient is responsible for making sure the patient is stable for transport. The Comprehensive Omnibus Budget Reconciliation Act of 1988 (COBRA) requires that all patients presenting to an ED undergo a proper medical screening examination before being transfered, discharged, or triaged out of the ED. If deemed stable enough to transfer, the patient (or a representative) must, by law, be informed of the risks involved and sign a consent form. The emergency physician is responsible for care delivered (or not delivered) en route and until the patient is seen by the physician at the receiving facility.

The fact that this patient diagnosed his own ventricular tachycardia should not lessen its serious import for us. We should be doing the monitoring and should not have to rely on the patient to do this. At no time should the patient's monitoring be unattended—from arrival in the ED to the coronary care unit. A cardiac monitor with built-in rate alarms should be used.

REFERENCES

Review Article
Stapczynski, J. S., and Podrid, P. J. Coping with the vagaries of ventricular ectopy. *Emerg. Med. Rep.* 1989;10:(3)17–24.

Additional References

Cummins, R. O. CPR and ventricular fibrillation: Lasts longer, ends better. *Ann. Emerg. Med.* 1995;25:833–836.

Baerman, J. M., et al. Differentiation of ventricular tachycardia from supraventricular tachycardia with aberration: Value of the clinical history. *Ann. Emerg. Med.* 1987;16:40–43.

Levitt, M. A. Supraventricular tachycardia with aberrant conduction vs. ventricular tachycardia: Differentiation and diagnosis. *Am. J. Emerg. Med.* 1988;6:273–277.

Case records of the Massachusetts General Hospital. Weekly clinicopathological exercises. Case 9-1992. Wide-complex tachycardia in a 65-year-old woman without previous evidence of cardiac disease. *N. Engl. J. Med.* 1992;326:624–633.

McCabe, J. L., et al. Intravenous adenosine in the prehospital treatment of paroxysmal supraventricular tachycardia. *Ann. Emerg. Med.* 1992;22:358–361.

Lee, K. L., and Tai, Y. T. Adenosine in wide complex tachycardia: Potential pitfalls in diagnostic value. *Ann. Emerg. Med.* 1994;24:741–747.

CASE 43 FALLING DOWN STAIRS

A 44-year-old man came to the emergency department complaining of chest pain after a fall down stairs four hours earlier. He had begun to hurt then, and the pain was worst at the right lower rib cage. He also hurt over the right buttock, where he had bounced down several steps. He noted pain in his chest on breathing deeply. He had smoked about one pack of cigarettes daily for about thirty years and always had a morning cough. Alcohol intake was not commented on.

On physical examination, the patient had marked tenderness over the right fifth through tenth ribs, maximal in the midaxillary line. His chest was clear to auscultation. He was afebrile, and otherwise normal.

X-ray pictures were taken, and no hip fracture or pulmonary infiltrates were seen. The patient had several lateral rib fractures. After his chest was painted with benzoin, 3-inch adhesive tape was applied from past the anterior midline around the painful hemithorax to a point past the vertebrae posteriorly. The tape was applied in overlapping strips to cover the hemithorax from the fourth to the eleventh ribs. The patient was given 20 tablets of acetaminophen with ½ grain of codeine and told to take 1 tablet every 4 hours as needed for pain. He felt much better after the taping and thanked the physician.

Two days later the patient returned with more pain and a fever. Examination showed decreased breath sounds, rales, and wheezes at the right lung base. His temperature was 38.0°C orally. A chest x-ray showed an extensive right lower lobe pneumonia. He was admitted to the hospital for therapy.

Was the pneumonia an obligatory complication of the rib fractures?

What should have been done differently?

DISCUSSION

Rib fracture should be suspected if sharp pain that increases with cough or deep breathing develops after trauma or a heavy cough. The diagnosis can be made clinically, and, in simple cases, confirmation by rib x-rays is unnecessary because rib bruises and rib fractures are treated similarly. We do recommend taking a standard PA and lateral chest x-ray to rule out hemothorax, pneumothorax, pulmonary contusion, or pathologic fracture from metastatic disease. Most rib fractures will be seen on these films. If no fracture is seen, we tell patients that we believe they may have a fractured rib and treat them for it. We explain that if the injury is only a contusion, they will be better sooner. Older patients (over age 65) with multiple medical problems or in whom you suspect three or more rib fractures may need rib films, because if there are more than three fractured ribs they will most likely require admission.

An effective cough, an effective mucociliary apparatus, and adequate local ventilation all help to maintain the health of the lung. When these three mechanisms or other resistance phenomena are subverted, pneumonia is more likely. Smokers have considerable suppression of the ciliary activity in their bronchi and may not clear bacteria and debris from the lungs in the usual fashion. A cough may be essential. Codeine suppresses cough easily and, in this case, may have been instrumental in pneumonia development. The splinting induced by pain may be considerable, but taping adds to this and decreases local ventilation. This patient should have been urged to stop smoking and instructed in deep-breathing exercises. Patient compliance will not be good unless adequate analgesia is prescribed. A simple nonsteroidal anti-inflammatory (NSAID) will not be sufficient.

The pneumonia rate is high in smokers who have fractured ribs, and the pain problem is difficult to deal with. This patient's alcohol intake was not discussed with him. Alcohol suppresses host defenses in several ways, including suppression of the bone marrow resulting in leukopenia and suppression of the pulmonary mucociliary apparatus. If he was indeed a drinker, he should have been urged to abstain after his rib fractures. Finally, the actual fall down stairs was not defined clearly enough. Why and how did he fall down stairs? Had he been faint? Dizzy? Drunk? The event before the event bringing him to the ED (the fall) may be the most important part of his illness, and patients like this should be questioned about syncope, vertigo, dizziness, or light-headedness. This may prompt further workup.

"Prophylactic" antibiotic therapy may be used in this sort of case to treat the bronchitis and avoid the development of pneumonia.

References

Review Article

Lee, B. B., et al. Three or more rib fractures as an indicator for transfer to a Level I trauma center. *J. Trauma* 1990;30:689–694.

Additional References

Thompson, B. N., et al. Rib radiographs for trauma: Useful or wasteful? *Ann. Emerg. Med.* 1986;15:261–265.

LaBan, M. M., et al. Occult radiographic fractures of the chest wall identified by nuclear scan imaging. *Arch. Phys. Med. Rehabil.* 1994;75:353–354.

Jackimczyk, K. Blunt chest trauma. *Emerg. Med. Clin. North Am.* 1993;11:81–96.

Case 44 PROBABLY DRUNK

A 30-year-old man was brought to the emergency department by ambulance. He was described by the EMT as confused and probably drunk. He was noted to be absent without leave from a local private psychiatric hospital where he had been treated for alcoholism and had been on disulfiram (Antabuse) for one week. Today he had left the hospital and had drunk 1 quart of wine. Feeling ill, he went to a nearby police car and asked for assistance.

On arrival at the ED, the patient was observed to be uncooperative and lobster-red in color. He had a tachycardia of 140 beats per minute with a systolic blood pressure of 70 mm Hg. His chest was clear. His heart seemed normal except for the tachycardia. He appeared to be otherwise normal. Rectal exam revealed brown stool that was negative when tested for occult blood. There was no obvious evidence of trauma. His jugular venous pressure seemed normal (i.e., low). His skin was warm and dry.

He was given 2000 ml of normal saline solution intravenously over 60 minutes. A chest x-ray and an ECG were done; they were normal. One gram of ascorbic acid (vitamin C) was given intravenously, and the patient lost his flush. The blood pressure moved up to 110 systolic by the end of his first liter of intravenous fluids. He left the ED four hours later feeling much better.

What causes hypotension in the alcohol-Antabuse reaction?

How should it be treated?

What did the vitamin C do?

DISCUSSION

Hypotension is a cardinal sign of a serious disease state and should be attacked vigorously. In order to do so, one needs certain parameters, and some of these were not obtained in this case. Most important are blood pressure, temperature, pulse, an estimate of the central venous pressure, weight, hematocrit, BUN, urine output, and serum sodium levels. With these, one can attempt to distinguish among the three main mechanisms of hypotension and can monitor treatment. Cardiogenic shock usually is accompanied by an elevation of the venous pressure. Of course hypotension from any cause may lead to insufficient coronary artery perfusion and secondary pump failure. Hypovolemia resulting from bleeding (from cuts, or into fracture sites, the gastrointestinal tract, the peritoneum, the retroperitoneum, or the chest cavity) will lead to hypotension when about 30% of the blood volume is lost. In hypovolemia, water and salt may be lost externally or internally or simply moved out of the vascular compartment (as is thought to be the case in alcohol-Antabuse reactions). Finally, vascular collapse due to adrenal insufficiency, sepsis, hypoxia, or drugs may lead to hypotension. Treatment of vascular collapse or hypovolemia is similar—rapid infusions of large amounts of crystalloids, colloid, or blood. A solution of 5% dextrose in water is a poor fluid for this purpose, and we usually start with normal saline solution or lactated Ringer's solution.

Antabuse interferes with the metabolism of alcohol in the same way that metronidazole (Flagyl) does. It causes a pile-up of acetaldehyde, presumably by blocking the enzyme acetaldehyde dehydrogenase. Acetaldehyde can mimic some of the features of the alcohol-Antabuse reaction but *not* the hypotension; it is not in itself enough to explain the reaction. The additional effect may be caused by a breakdown product of Antabuse that interferes with catecholamine metabolism. The profound shock that results from these combined effects may be resistant to all catechols except intravenous norepinephrine. As little as 7 ml of alcohol can produce the syndrome.

The reasons for use of vitamin C are obscure, but it does seem to lessen the symptoms of the alcohol-Antabuse reaction. Some alcoholics even take oral vitamin C to "counteract the Antabuse" before drinking.

Drug reactions should always be considered in the differential diagnosis of patients who are on any medications. Many mild reactions result from common medications (such as aspirin or NSAIDs leading to asymptomatic gastrointestinal bleeding, or diuretics leading to generalized mild weakness). There are also a number of rare but potentially lethal reactions, such as mixing Demerol (meperidine) and a MAO inhibitor, or Antabuse and ethanol.

REFERENCES

Review Article

Barrera, S. E., et al. The use of antabuse in chronic alcoholics. *Am. J. Psychiatry* 1994;151(suppl. 6):263–267.

Additional References

Saxe, T. G. Drug-alcohol interactions. *Am. Fam. Phys.* 1986;33:159–162.

Motte, S., et al. Refractory hyperdynamic shock associated with alcohol and disulfiram. *Am. J. Emerg. Med.* 1986;4:323–325.

Antabuse. Proceedings of the Elsinore Antabuse Conference. Elsinore, Denmark. November 7–8, 1991. *Acta Psychiatr. Scand. Suppl.* 1992;369:1–72.

Gallant, D. M., et al. Antabuse and AIDS. *Alcohol Clin. Exp. Res.* 1991;15:900–901.

Case 45 PAIN ON URINATION

A 54-year-old woman came to the emergency department complaining of pain on urination over a period of several hours. She was urinating almost every thirty minutes and noted that her urine had become red. She had experienced many past episodes of similar suprapubic and low back pain with passage of urine. A total abdominal hysterectomy had been done ten years earlier for "pelvic relaxation." Cystoscopy had been done five years earlier with a diagnosis of trigonitis but no evidence of obstruction. Several intravenous pyelograms (IVPs) had been done in the past and were normal.

On physical examination the patient was observed to be obese, had a blood pressure of 174/110, and had a temperature of 37.5°C orally. There was no costovertebral angle tenderness, and her abdomen was normal. No rectal or pelvic examination was done.

A urinalysis showed 2+ protein—over 50 RBCs, and over 50 WBCs—per high-power field of spun sediment. A urine culture was done and later showed over 100,000 colonies of *E. coli* per milliliter. All antibiotics tested were effective against the organism in vitro. The diagnosis then considered was hemorrhagic cystitis. She was placed on ampicillin (500 mg orally qid for 10 days) and pyridium (100 mg tid for 3 days). Another IVP was scheduled and was performed the next day. It was normal. The patient was referred to the urology clinic. Despite her referral, she returned to the ED ten days after her first visit, now complaining of back pain and chills. She admitted to not taking her ampicillin regularly. She was afebrile but now had left flank tenderness. Her repeat urinalysis showed about 4 RBCs and WBCs per high-power field; there was no more proteinuria. She was given more ampicillin and urged to take it as directed.

What is the most common reason for failure of drug therapy?

How should follow-up care be arranged for patients with urinary tract infections?

When should an IVP be done in patients with urinary tract symptoms?

What is a significant white blood cell count in a urinalysis?

DISCUSSION

It should not be surprising that the primary reason drug therapy fails is the patient's failure to take the drug. Many patients will follow directions poorly even when given only one drug, and the failure rate goes up as the number of prescriptions given increases. In general, one should try to limit therapy to a single drug. If several drugs or procedures are being advised, one should clearly define expectations and plans for the patient. The patient should understand why the drug was prescribed, how it is to be taken, its significant side effects, and when to expect resolution of symptoms. The patient must understand the plan, and that is best achieved by providing the patient with a legible discharge instruction sheet, written in plain English, in addition to an oral communication. You know that your message has been communicated if the patient can recite it back to you.

Most patients who present with urinary tract symptoms at the ED have disease limited to the urethra or bladder. The question of which patients with urinary tract infection (UTI) need a urine culture remains controversial. Some physicians think that cultures need not be done in a woman with an apparently benign case of cystitis. Others, however, believe that all patients with suspected UTI deserve a urine culture because of the confusion that results when a patient's symptoms fail to resolve on therapy and the patient had no culture initially. Symptomatic UTIs often fail to produce more than 100,000 organisms per ml on culture, and, if a woman is symptomatic with pyuria, we consider a clean-catch culture to be positive if there are more than 10,000 per ml, especially if there is only one organism. The standard treatment for cystitis used to be a 10-day course of sulfa, tetracycline, or ampicillin. Clinical research over the past several years has demonstrated that seven-, five-, or three-day courses or even a single dose with any of a variety of antibiotics may be effective. The most effective of the single-dose regimens is trimethoprim/sulfamethoxazole (two double-strength tablets). Cranberry juice has been proven to be a helpful dietary adjunct to antibiotic therapy.

If the antibiotic is appropriate, the pyuria or hematuria should be nearly cleared in 2 days, and the dysuria should be gone in 24 hours.

Repeat urinalysis should be done 2 to 3 days after conclusion of antibiotic therapy.

Any evidence of renal involvement in a UTI (such as flank pain, high fever, or costovertebral angle tenderness) suggests acute pyelonephritis, a form of acute interstitial nephritis from infection that produces a septic picture with fever, chills, flank pain, nausea, tachycardia, and malaise. Signs of cystitis, leukocyte casts, and bacteria in unspun clean-catch urine samples may also be seen. As with most clinical syndromes, not all these signs and symptoms need be present in any one patient. Patients who are toxic should be placed on parenteral antibiotics and admitted. Any patient who is less sick, is able to keep down fluids, is not pregnant, and has no underlying disease such as HIV disease or diabetes may be treated as an outpatient if close follow-up and home support are available. Any evidence of obstruction warrants an emergency IVP.

An IVP with postvoiding films should also be done as part of a urologic workup in cases of repeated UTI. We usually work up a male with his second infection and a female with her fifth. Cystoscopy is appropriate at this stage, so a referral to a urologist is needed. If gross hematuria is present (as opposed to pink or reddish urine) referral is best, even with a "first infection."

It is not clear what amount of leukocytosis in the urine constitutes pyuria. Women may have several WBCs per high-power field with no infection, but in men even a few WBCs may be significant. A surprising number of women have some pyuria but no bactiuria and recover with or without antibiotics in 3 to 7 days.

Recurrent urethritis or cystitis in *postmenopausal* women may be associated with atrophic vaginal mucosa caused by estrogen lack. Treatment with estrogens improves the status of vaginal and urethral mucosa and decreases the incidence of infections. The full effects of this treatment in terms of possibly inducing some types of cancer and protecting against others are still being looked into.

REFERENCES

Review Article
Hooton, T. M., and Stam, W. F. Management of acute uncomplicated urinary tract infection in adults. *Med. Clin. North Am.* 1991;75: 339–357.

Additional References

Shea, D. G. Pyelonephritis and female urinary tract infection. *Emerg. Med. Clin. North Am.* 1988;6:403–417.

Werman, H. A., and Brown, C. G. Utility of the urine cultures in the emergency department. *Ann. Emerg. Med.* 1986;15:302–307.

Patton, J. P., et al. Urinary tract infection: Economic considerations. *Med. Clin. North Am.* 1991;75:495–513.

Hooton, T. M. A simplified approach to urinary tract infection. *Hosp. Pract. (Off. Ed.)* 1995;30:23–30.

Hooton, T. M., et al. Randomized comparative trial and cost analysis of 3-day antimicrobial regimens for treatment of acute cystitis in women. *J.A.M.A.* 1995;273:41–45.

Case 46 MENTAL STATUS: CONFUSED

A 50-year-old woman was brought to the emergency department by paramedics. On arrival, they stated that she had been found by her landlady lethargic and confused. The landlady had been concerned about the patient after not seeing her in the previous two days—an unusual occurrence.

The EMTs said that at the scene they found one hypertensive medication, although they "did not have time to look real well" for other pill bottles.

Her initial blood pressure at the scene was 230/140. The patient was described at that time as incoherent and generally lethargic with periods of combativeness.

On preliminary exam the ED physician found the mildly obese woman to be making "nonsense statements" but moving all extremities. She had periods of thrashing about on the stretcher. She was breathing at a rate of 20 without apparent difficulty. Her pulse was 70, her temperature 96.5 rectally, and her blood pressure in the ED was 250/140.

The heart and lung exam revealed fine rales at the bases and an S3 gallop. She had blurred optic disc margins with anteriolar narrowing and bilateral hemorrhages and exudate.

The neurologic exam revealed bilateral extensor response of the great toes. No other focal abnormality was noted.

When dealing with hypertensive disease syndromes, how does one gauge the relative severity of the initial presentation?

What initial treatment regimens would have been appropriate in this case?

Discussion

Much confusion exists concerning the treatment of patients with acute elevation of blood pressure. When treating such patients, it is crucial to be neither overly cautious nor overly aggressive. Too little therapy can result in life-threatening end-organ dysfunction of the central nervous system, heart, or kidneys; too much therapy can also threaten those same organs by diminishing their blood flow.

One useful method of categorizing acute hypertensive syndromes is to define them as being either a hypertensive emergency or a hypertensive urgency.

In cases of *hypertensive emergencies,* the diastolic blood pressure is usually 135 or greater, and evidence exists of significant dysfunction of the central nervous system, heart, or kidneys. Obviously, the physical exam, a mental status exam, a serum BUN level, and a routine urine analysis are critically important in making this categorization. Funduscopic and neurologic exams may reveal papilledema or focal deficits, or the heart and lung exams may show signs of congestive heart failure. The patient's mental status exam is always abnormal in cases of hypertensive emergency. To quickly assess the patient's mental status, one should determine if he or she is alert and oriented to person, place, and time. If not, does the patient respond appropriately to verbal or painful stimuli, or is he or she unresponsive?

Patients may present with less severe manifestations of hypertensive disease, often termed *hypertensive urgency,* in which the diastolic blood pressure is generally less than 130 and end-organ dysfunction, particularly of the central nervous system, is absent or very mild. In these cases, emergency therapy (i.e., therapy within the first hour) is generally not critical.

Clearly this patient's clinical presentation is that of an hypertensive emergency given her alteration in mental status, retinopathy, and evidence of congestive heart failure. In addition, her diastolic blood pressure is 140. Therefore, it is very important in this particular patient to initiate therapy quickly but cautiously to limit morbidity and mortality. Current standards suggest that the diastolic blood pressure should not be lowered below 105 in the initial treatment phase. The fear of lowering the blood pressure too much with subsequent underperfusion of vital organs is a real one, and careful monitoring of blood pressure at all times is mandatory.

Many pharmacologic agents are available to treat patients with hypertensive emergencies. Sodium nitroprusside is presently the single best agent, but it must be used with great caution and careful monitoring. Labetalol (an alpha- and beta-blocking agent), nifedipine (a calcium channel blocker), and loop diuretics are second-line agents that may also be useful in treating these emergencies. A useful method of gently lowering elevated pressure in a patient without altered mental status or congestive heart failure is giving a single sublingual dose of 10 mg of nifedipine. This is a common, although not currently an FDA approved, use of this drug, and its use is controversial.

REFERENCES

Review Article

Just, V. L., et al. Evaluation of drug therapy for treatment of hypertensive urgencies in the emergency department. *Am. J. Emerg. Med.* 1991;9:107–111.

Additional References

Catapno, M. S., and Marx, J. A. Management of urgent hypertension: A comparison of oral treatment regimens in the emergency department. *J. Emerg. Med.* 1986;4:361–368.

Gonzalez-Carmona, V. M., et al. Single-dose sublingual nifedipine as the only treatment in hypertensive urgencies and emergencies. *Angiology* 1991;42:908–913.

Heller, M. B., et al. Prehospital use of nifedipine in severe hypertension. *Am. J. Emerg. Med.* 1990;8:282–284.

Fagan, T. C. Calcium antagonists and mortality: Another case of the need for clinical judgment. *Arch. Intern. Med.* 1995;155:2145.

CASE 47 SEEING ZEBRAS

A 38-year-old woman was taken to another hospital's emergency department by concerned relatives. She stated that she awoke in the morning and saw two strange men in her house. She called the police, but the men mysteriously disappeared. Later there were "several zebras walking across the wall." Her son stated that she was a heavy drinker and that she drank to keep from being nervous.

On physical examination the patient was noted to have a tachycardia (120) but to be afebrile. Her blood pressure was 114/90. She was anxious and tachypneic but well oriented. Reflexes were brisk and pupils dilated but reactive. She complained of thirst and a dry mouth. The ED doctor at the time, a retired surgeon, gave her 100 mg of Librium intramuscularly and then called a medical resident to see her. The second doctor noted that she had a peripheral neuropathy. His diagnoses were (1) delirium tremens, (2) alcoholic myopathy and neuropathy, and (3) depression. She was referred to our ED for admission to the alcohol detoxification unit.

On arrival at our ED the woman denied much recent drinking. Her blood pressure was 100/70 supine and 80/65 sitting, and her pulse was 120 sitting. A hematocrit was 42% and stool hematest negative. She said she really did not want to go to the detoxification ward—she did not consider herself to be an alcoholic. The staff physician seeing her pointed out that not everyone in the ED that day was hallucinating and the sooner she realized she was an alcoholic the sooner she might be able to do something about it.

Samples were drawn for complete blood count, electrolytes, BUN, sugar, biochemical survey, VDRL, and blood alcohol analyses. Urinalysis and chest x-rays were done. The patient was admitted to the alcohol detoxification unit, and ten minutes later the electrolytes were reported to be Na 118, Cl 83, HCO_3 9, and K 2.8 mEq/L. Alcohol level was only 27 mg per 100 milliliters. A phone call to the woman's relatives uncovered the fact that she had indeed been depressed and probably had taken an overdose of aspirin and an over-the-counter sedative containing scopolamine. Serum salicylate level was 47 mg per 100 milliliters, several times the normal therapeutic level.

47. SEEING ZEBRAS 151

Did the patient have DTs?

Why was she hallucinating?

How do you treat overdoses of acetylsalicylic acid (aspirin)?

Discussion

Although this patient is indeed an alcoholic, she probably was not hallucinating because of alcohol withdrawal. She clearly does not have DTs; she is neither delirious nor tremulous. Scopolamine is a hallucinogen. In the past it was available in over-the-counter sedatives, but now requires a prescription. Other drugs such as bromides, lysergic acid (LSD), mescaline, and psilocybin may also cause hallucinations.

This patient's thirst, dry mouth, tachycardia, mental status changes, and dilated pupils are characteristic of an anticholinergic toxidrome. Some of the more common responsible drugs include scopolamine, tricyclic antidepressants, antipsychotics, and antihistamines. This patient also had an anion-gap metabolic acidosis. Normally the anion gap $(Na^+) + (K^+) - (Cl^-) - (HCO_3^-)$ is 8 ± 4 mEq/L. This patient was acidotic (HCO_3 9) with an anion gap of 28.8 mEq/L. We use the mnemonic *A MUD PILES* to remind us of the differential diagnosis of metabolic acidosis with an elevated anion gap.

A   Alcohol

M   Methanol
U   Uremia
D   Diabetic ketoacidosis

P   Paraldehyde
I   Iron/INH
L   Lactic acid
E   Ethylene glycol
S   Salicylates

Salicylate toxicity is often underestimated because the patient is usually awake and alert. The serum salicylate level decreases over time as it is metabolized, so one should always check the "Done Nomogram" (a graphic representation of how fast the serum level drops) to see if the patient's serum level is in the toxic range from an ingestion hours earlier. If we do treat, it usually is with forced alkaline diuresis. We use a solution of 1000 ml 5% dextrose/0.45 normal saline plus 88 mEq $NaHCO_3$ plus 10 mEq KCl, and infuse it at 1000 ml per hour for the first hour. After the patient is fully hydrated, we use the same solution to keep urine output at around 3 to 6 ml/kg per hour (approximately 200 to 300 ml per hour in a normal-sized adult). This can produce pulmonary edema, so the patient must be watched carefully with chest x-rays, intake and output records, and chest auscultation. Because this can derange sodium or potassium levels and can produce dangerous levels of alkalosis, these parameters must be carefully monitored. Most of these patients need admission, especially if the salicylate level is over 80 mg per 100 milliliters.

In the end, alcoholism will be the patient's major problem. However, correction of her present metabolic abnormalities must precede any significant psychiatric therapy. She should not be obliged to admit to being an alcoholic to get such therapy. Alcoholism does not limit the patient's susceptibility to other drugs or diseases, but it often leads the physician away from a careful consideration of other diagnoses.

REFERENCES

Review Article
Yip, L., Dart, R. C., and Gabon, P. A. Concepts and controversies in salicylate toxicity. *Emerg. Med. Clin. North Am.* 1994;12:351–364.

Additional References
Snodgrass, W. R. Salicylate toxicity. *Pediatr. Clin. North Am.* 1986;33: 381–391.

Hillman, R. J., and Prescott, L. F. Treatment of salicylate poisoning with repeated oral charcoal. *Br. Med. J.* 1985;291:1472.

Chan, T. Y., et al. The clinical value of screening for salicylates in acute poisoning. *Vet. Hum. Toxicol.* 1995;37:37–38.

Case 48 OD

A 45-year-old man was brought to the emergency department by ambulance. He was said to have ingested several drugs. On arrival he was drowsy but arousable. Although he refused to communicate, he could walk and had a good gag reflex. He was given syrup of ipecac (30 ml orally) and 300 ml of warm tap water. This resulted in copious vomiting over the next thirty minutes. The patient was kept in the ED and observed. After three hours he seemed more alert and was walking about and asking the staff for cigarettes. He was referred to the emergency psychiatry team for further evaluation. Perusal of his old chart revealed that he had long carried the diagnosis of paranoid schizophrenia and had been on phenothiazines in the past.

The nurse on the psychiatry team saw the patient in the fifth hour of his ED stay and reported to the referring physician that he was too sleepy to be interviewed. On rechecking, the patient was found to be comatose and unresponsive to pain but breathing well and with a normal blood pressure. His pockets were emptied and found to contain prescription bottles for Thorazine, Seconal, and Kemadrin. A nasotracheal tube was easily inserted, his stomach was lavaged with 2 liters of tap water via an Ewald tube, and he was admitted to the medical intensive care unit.

Why do overdose patients have fluctuating levels of consciousness?

What is "observation" in the ED?

Discussion

The patient probably took more of his drugs covertly after entering the ED. He was a "double overdose." We occasionally observe an alcoholic becoming more drunk while in the ED (more ataxic, sleepier, thicker speech) and find a half-full bottle of wine in his or her clothing. Usually overdose patients are stripped and searched and thus relieved of any drugs.

Varying depth of coma may be due to:

1. On and off gastrointestinal absorption. This is true for any drug but classic for meprobamate, which forms concretions in the gut. Duodenal storage may have been the problem in this case, and a cathartic should have been given.
2. Enterohepatic circulation.
3. Secondary effect of hypoxia on consciousness.
4. Brief action of narcotic antagonists versus long action of opiates.
5. Brief action of glucose versus long-acting hypoglycemic agents.
6. Subdural hematomas (especially worrisome in an alcoholic who is not properly waking up).
7. Repeated ingestion, as in this case.

This patient ingested three drugs with multiple side effects. They are all sedative-hypnotic drugs and may produce a decreasing level of consciousness and respiratory depression. Thorazine and Kemadrin (a drug used to treat extrapyramidal side effects of Thorazine) possess anticholinergic properties, and the patient should be monitored for cardiac arrhythmias, hypotension, seizures, and agitation.

Certain words have awesome implications in our ED that are not conveyed by their literal meaning. *Observed* should mean closely watched, yet often it is used to mean neglected, booth curtain closed, and no further evaluation. *Stable* is another such term. It should be used to describe a patient who is the same for at least two successive observations with time intervening. It should not be used in reference to one set of normal vital signs.

Finally, we don't usually give ipecac anymore in the acute treatment of overdoses, even when we suspect a serious OD. First, it causes prolonged patient discomfort and occasional injury from prolonged vomiting. Additionally, "gut decontamination," when really needed, is faster with gastric lavage.

REFERENCES

Review Articles

Henneman, P. L., et al. Prospective evaluation of E.D. medical clearance. *Ann. Emerg. Med.* 1994;24:672–677.

Perrone, J., Hoffman, R. S., and Goldfrank, L. R. Special considerations in gastrointestinal decontamination. *Emerg. Med. Clin. North Am.* 1994;12:285–300.

Additional References

Cann, H. M., and Verhulst, H. L. Accidental ingestion and overdosage involving psychopharmacologic drugs. *N. Engl. J. Med.* 1960;263: 719–724.

Davis, J. M., et al. Overdosage of psychotropic drugs: A review. *Dis. Nerv. Sys.* 1968;29:157–164.

Riba, M., and Hale, M. Medical clearance: Fact or fiction in the hospital emergency room. *Psychosomatics* 1990;31:400–404.

American College of Emergency Physicians: Management of observation units. *Ann. Emerg. Med.* 1995;25:783–830.

Case 49 WALKING AWAY FROM A CAR ACCIDENT

A 20-year-old man walked into the emergency department. He told the interviewing nurse that he had been in an auto accident three hours earlier but had felt more-or-less all right and had gone home. Then his shoulders, arms, and neck had begun to hurt, so his mother told him to go to the hospital. When he arrived, he was placed in an exam room, where he was interviewed by one of the more junior physicians available.

A full examination was done, including full range of movement of the neck. Then a complete set of cervical spine films was obtained, including flexion, extension, and odontoid views. The radiologist was not available, so the physician viewed the films alone. He mentioned to a staff physician that he had an interesting case of cervical spondylolisthesis. The second physician immediately placed sandbags on either side of the patient's head and a cervical collar on his neck. He told the patient not to move his head. A review of the films indeed disclosed an unstable cervical fracture-dislocation of C5-6. Skull tongs were placed, and the patient was admitted to the hospital for constant traction.

What is the usual presentation of a broken neck?

Is there anything unusual about this case?

What is the danger to the patient of further neck movement?

DISCUSSION

This patient had no apparent neurologic defect. By amazing luck his injury had not yet impinged on his cervical cord or nerve roots.

The most common spinal fracture site is at the C6-7 vertebral level, an area which is not easily seen on x-rays because the patient's shoulders may get in the way. A patient with a cord injury at that level is brought in by stretcher with arms flexed at the elbow and hands together on the chest because the elbow flexors (C5-6) are no longer opposed. This patient has flaccid paralysis elsewhere and may have hypotension from loss of sympathetic innervation. It is not actually rare, however, for a patient with a cervical fracture to walk into our department unassisted and neurologically intact.

Accident victims brought in by ambulance should always be fully immobilized. This includes a hard cervical collar around the neck, sand bags or rigid foam on either side of the neck, and the patient strapped to a long spine board. Some patients will be immobilized this way even though they have no spine injury. In our ED, a patient that has *no* neck pain, has a normal mental status (not psychotic, somnolent, overly anxious, distracted by severe pain elsewhere, or under the influence of alcohol or drugs), *and* who has no neck tenderness on palpation and no pain on gentle, slow, self-applied movement of the neck can have the neck "clinically cleared." All others must have their cervical spine x-rayed. Patients who present without full immobilization should be immobilized when they are first seen in the ED.

One should sandbag the patient's head straight. If it is turned, we usually try to straighten it *gently* with traction. If the patient is alert, he or she must be told to hold his or her head perfectly still, and, if not, someone must constantly hold it in place. The patient cannot be left alone. A cross-table lateral x-ray of the cervical spine should be done first. The arms should be pulled slowly down toward the feet before the x-ray—otherwise spasm of the shoulders may obscure much of the film below C5. Seven full cervical vertebrae must be seen for the film to be technically adequate. The x-ray should be carefully inspected for misalignment of the anterior and posterior border of the vertebral bodies with the anterior border of the spinous processes. The soft tissues anterior to the vertebral bodies should be examined for widening and the area of the odontoid (C2) closely looked at. The vertebral bodies themselves should be intact. If a fracture is present, only an A-P (anterior-posterior) film should then be taken. The patient should be immobilized by skeletal traction on the same stretcher and moved only once more—onto a circle bed or rigid frame. If no fracture is seen on the lateral view, a full cervical spine x-ray series is obtained. In our institution, this consists of A-P, odontoid view, and right and left oblique films. Flexion and extension views are occasionally used when the initial films are negative and the patient still has severe pain. They evaluate the degree of ligamentous laxity but can be dangerous and should always be done under the guidance of an experienced physician.

Any movement may render the patient paraplegic or quadraplegic (depending on the injury level). If quadraplegia develops and is still present after 24 hours of traction, there is little chance of full recovery.

The three common types of incomplete cord injuries are:

1. Central cord syndrome—the patient may have weakness or flaccid paralysis of the arms and fairly normal legs. Note that this is the opposite of what would usually be expected with a spinal injury. The prognosis is usually good, and recovery usually takes place within hours.
2. Anterior spinal cord injury—loss of all but position and vibratory senses. The injury occurs (as do most spine injuries) with the neck flexed. Probably the anterior spinal artery is damaged. These cases may recover well if incomplete injury occurs.
3. Brown-Séquard syndrome—hemisection of the cord usually caused by a knife wound. There is a loss of position and vibratory sense on the side of the injury, with loss of pain and temperature sense on the other side. Recovery is rarely complete.

Incomplete cord syndromes may also present as combinations of all three types. Look for sparing of light touch sensation around the anus (sacral sparing) as a sign of incomplete damage. These cases have a better prognosis than a complete spinal cord transection.

A 1990 report by the National Acute Spinal Cord Injury Study demonstrated that methylprednisolone is surprisingly effective in treating both complete and incomplete spinal cord injury. If the drug was given in high dose and within 8 hours of the injury, significant improvement (motor and sensory) was seen in acutely injured patients.

REFERENCES

Review Article
Rizzolo, S. J., et al. Cervical spine trauma. *Spine* 1994;19:2288–2298.

Additional References
Baker, J. S. The awake, alert patient can deceive (letter). *JACEP* 1978;7:289.

Freemyer, B., et al. Comparison of five-view and three-view cervical spine series in the evaluation of patients with cervical trauma. *Ann. Emerg. Med.* 1989;18:818–821.

Macdonald, R. L., et al. Diagnosis of cervical spine injury in motor vehicle crash victims: How many x-rays are enough? *J. Trauma* 1990;30:392–397.

Bracken, M. B., et al. A randomized, controlled trial of methylprednisolone or naloxone in the treatment of acute spinal-cord injury. *N. Engl. J. Med.* 1990;322:1405–1411.

el Khoury, G. Y., et al. Imaging of acute injuries of the cervical spine: Value of plain radiography, CT, and MR imaging. *AJR Am. J. Roentgenol.* 1995;164:43–50.

Case 50 HAND LACERATION

An 18-year-old man came to the emergency department after lacerating his left palm. He stated the accident occurred when he "broke a glass" while washing dishes. He was alert, well-mannered, and denied any other complaint. Though the ED was busy at the time he arrived, the patient's wound was bleeding briskly, and he was quickly brought to a treatment booth. A physician who was attending several other patients at the time was summoned to see the patient. He quickly examined the wound and had the patient "make a fist," which he did easily. The sensory exam was normal as well. The laceration was 2 cm in length, transversely placed just proximal to the fourth and fifth metacarpal phalangeal joints. The physician probed the wound and found no glass or bleeding arterial vessels. At that point, he anesthetized the wound with 5 ml of 2% plain Xylocaine solution and closed it with six 4-0 synthetic, nonabsorbable sutures. The wound was covered with an antimicrobial ointment, and a bulky dressing was applied. Prior to discharge the patient was given a diphtheria/tetanus toxoid booster because his last "tetanus shot" had been given ten years ago. He was instructed to return for suture removal in ten days and subsequently discharged. Five days later he returned to the ED because of increasing pain in the area of the wound and because he had noticed the wound had become red and tender. An x-ray of the hand was ordered at this time and revealed a 5 x 5 mm foreign body present deep in the soft tissues. Careful examination of tendon function revealed extreme pain on even 1 cm of passive motion of the fifth and fourth digits, as well as a diminished ability to flex the fourth finger at the distal interphalangeal (DIP) joint.

What are the complications from the initial injury that this patient is experiencing?

Was his initial treatment appropriate?

What should be done at this point?

Discussion

Patients with hand lacerations involving the palm must be carefully examined. It is not by coincidence that hand wounds are among the most common types of cases ED physicians are successfully sued over. It is very easy to miss a partial flexor tendon injury unless each superficialis and each profundus flexor tendon is examined! The profundus tendons each attach on the palmar surface of the digit's distal phalanx and are tested by asking the patient to bend the DIP joint with the rest of the finger immobilized. The superficialis tendons each insert on the palmar surface of the digit's middle phalanx and are tested by immobilizing the entire hand on a flat surface with the palm facing up and with only the finger in question free to move. If the patient can bend the finger in question at the proximal interphalangeal joint, that flexor superficialis tendon is intact.

In this case, an injury to the profundus component of the flexor tendon was missed on the initial exam. Whenever there is a laceration in the soft tissues involving an object made of glass, particularly when that object shatters, suspicion must be high that a retained foreign body is present in the wound. Careful examination and exploration of the wound may not always reveal the foreign body. We do not know the true incidence of unsuspected retained glass fragments, but we sometimes recommend obtaining a "soft tissue density" x-ray in these situations because 95% of commercial glass is radiopaque. In general, it is always a good idea to copiously irrigate such a wound using strict sterile technique.

On return, the patient also had evidence of wound infection that had extended into the flexor tendon sheath—a so-called flexor tenosynovitis. This is a dreaded complication of any penetrating wound to the palm area because permanently disabling adhesions may develop. The initial treatment of this particular patient should have included a careful flexor tendon exam. Had the foreign body and the flexor tendon injury been discovered on the initial visit, an appropriate consultation with a hand surgeon could have been obtained at that time, and the complications might well have been avoided.

This patient will now require hospitalization and intravenous antibiotics, as well as surgical intervention to remove the foreign body. Whether or not the tendon sheath will require incision and drainage will be determined by the response to antibiotic therapy.

REFERENCES

Review Article

Overton, D. T., and Uehara, D. T. Evaluation of the injured hand. *Emerg. Med. Clin. North Am.* 1993;11:585–599.

Additional References

Altman, R. S., et al. Initial management of hand injuries in the emergency patient. *Am. J. Emerg. Med.* 1987;5:400–404.

Hart, R. G., and Kutz, J. E. Flexor tendon injuries of the hand. *Emerg. Med. Clin. North Am.* 1993;11:621–636.

Lampe, E. W., and Netter, F. Surgical anatomy of the hand. *Ciba Clin. Symp.* 1969;21:1–46.

Sach, R. The injured hand. *Aust. Fam. Physician* 1992;21:920–924, 927–930.

Sood, R., et al. Extremity replantation. *Surg. Clin. North Am.* 1991;71:317–329.

Case 51 THE WEEKEND TOOTHACHE

A 26-year-old woman walked into the emergency department complaining of severe pain where one of her teeth had been removed four days previously. She said her dentist had warned her she might have some difficulty with unresolved infection and advised her to see an oral surgeon if any problems arose. He had then left town for the weekend. She was taking 1 acetaminophen with codeine every 4 hours for pain and 250 mg of penicillin every 6 hours.

She appeared to be in pain. Her vital signs included a pulse of 72, respiratory rate of 18, blood pressure of 140/90, and oral temperature of 99°F. Her mouth opened easily to reveal silk sutures in the empty socket with underlying clot, edema, and tenderness. No sign of gingivitis was seen around the other teeth. The gingival-buccal sulcus was unremarkable to inspection and palpation. The right maxillary sinus was tender to percussion. Sinus x-rays were obtained and showed mucosal thickening but no air-fluid level or opacification. The emergency physician changed her antibiotic to cefaclor and her pain medication to oxycodone and referred her to an otorhinolaryngologist the same day with a diagnosis of early maxillary sinusitis.

Two days later she returned to the ED saying she was in worse pain than before. Her vital signs were the same and her examination was the same except for increased tenderness. An oral surgeon was called in. He removed the sutures, probed the socket with a clamp, and released several milliliters of pus, causing immediate improvement of the patient's pain.

What are the appropriate pain medications and antibiotics for dental infection?

What are common pathways of extension of dental infection?

When is it appropriate for the emergency physician to incise and drain a dental infection?

Discussion

Oral and pharyngeal infections are appropriately treated with penicillin or a second-generation cephalosporin. Erythromycin is used in penicillin-sensitive individuals.

Both the dentist and the emergency physician used appropriate medications. The two problems in this case were insufficient surgical drainage of the infection and insufficient referral instructions.

Mandibular dental infection may spread through the soft tissue of the lower face and neck. Maxillary dental infection tends to spread through the upper half of the face and into the maxillary sinus. Advanced infections, especially in compromised hosts, may extend into any of the fascial planes of the neck and to the mediastinum.

If this patient's dentist had given her the specific name and phone number of an oral surgeon, she could have saved money and two days of pain by seeing him or her directly. The original emergency physician could have done her a similar favor by referring her directly to an oral surgeon the same day or by removing the sutures, or both.

If her abscess had presented with fluctuance in the gingiva facing the buccal mucosa or in the gingival-buccal sulcus, the emergency physician could have anesthetized the gingiva superficially with topical benzocaine and then 2% lidocaine with epinephrine (1:100,000), incised the fluctuant area until pus was obtained, probed with a mosquito clamp, irrigated, and packed the abscess cavity with a small amount of iodoform gauze.

References

Review Article

Klokkevold, P. Common dental emergencies: Evaluation and management for the emergency physician. *Emerg. Med. Clin. North Am.* 1989;7:29–64.

Additional References

Camp, J. H., and Stewart, C. Dental trauma: Diagnostic considerations, emergency procedures, and definitive management. *Emerg. Med. Rep.* 1995;16:79–86.

Krasner, P. R. Treatment of tooth avulsion in the emergency department: Appropriate storage and transport media. *Am. J. Emerg. Med.* 1990;8:351–355.

Medford, H. M. Temporary stabilization of avulsed or luxated teeth. *Ann. Emerg. Med.* 1982;11:490–492.

Case 52 "NO FRACTURE"

An 80-year-old man was brought to the emergency department by ambulance. He had fallen in his boarding home and could no longer walk because of right hip pain. He was in good general health but almost totally blind as a result of macular degeneration. He took no medicines, did not smoke, and drank no alcohol. On initial examination no remarkable abnormalities were noted except for his very poor vision and slight pain on rotation of his hip. An x-ray of the hip was obtained, but the emergency doctor could not find a fracture. He called in an orthopedist who agreed with the physical findings and the x-ray interpretation. "No fracture," he said. "This man can go home."

Accordingly, the patient was discharged home; that is, the medical record was filled out, signed, and "Home" checked in the disposition column. When a nurse went to escort the patient out, however, she found that he could not stand. The patient insisted that he had excruciating pain. He also explained to her that he lived two floors up in a boarding home without an elevator and that he had to come down to the dining room for meals. "How," he wondered, "can I get up and down for meals if I can't stand up?" The original physician had gone home by then, so the nurse went in search of his successor. The new physician was puzzled. The orthopedist had discharged the patient, yet he could not go back to his boarding home. What was to be done? The emergency physician called the orthopedist and, after much conversation and some argument, managed to have the patient admitted to the inpatient service. The patient spent twelve hours in the ED, during which time he was not fed because no one thought of it and because he was officially discharged for the greater part of the time.

What pathology might have caused this man's hip pain?

What does this orthopedist need to know?

Discussion

Hip pain after falls may be severe and incapacitating, even in the absence of a fracture. This case was no exception to the rule that patients who acutely cannot walk, for any reason, should not be sent home.

Fractures of the hip or pelvis are often hard to find and may easily escape detection until several days after the initial injury. It was not clear whether the films taken in this case included adequate views of the entire pelvis to rule out a small pelvic fracture. Sometimes a fracture that is invisible on x-ray may be found with the aid of a bone scan, although even the bone scan may be negative until 48 hours after the injury.

The first emergency doctor and the orthopedist probably suffer from a common confusion that they are caring just for fractures rather than for people. Even though the pathology was unclear in this case, the initial ED physician and the orthopedist should have realized that this elderly man could neither stand nor walk, could not return to his boarding house, and was relying on them for help. Physicians need to understand that they must care for people in distress, some of whom will have easily understandable medical problems and some of whom will not. In any case, medical staff members need to make great efforts to help all patients. Until the arrival of the second ED physician, the ED staff was letting this patient fall through the cracks.

References

Review Article
Miller, M. D. Commonly missed orthopedic problems. *Emerg. Med. Clin. North Am.* 1992;10:151–162.

Additional References
Lundberg, E. J., Marcias, D., and Gipe, B. T. Clinically occult presentation of comminuted intertrochanteric hip fracture. *Ann. Emerg. Med.* 1992;21:1511–1514.

Alba, E., and Youngberg, R. Occult fractures of the femoral neck. *Am. J. Emerg. Med.* 1992;10:64–68.

Freed, H. A., and Sheilds, N. N. Most frequently overlooked radiographically apparent fractures in a teaching hospital emergency department. *Ann. Emerg. Med.* 1984;13:900–904.

Frank, J. Physical diagnosis and the doctor–patient relation (letter). *N. Engl. J. Med.* 1976;294:1464.

Platt, F. W., and McMath, J. C. Clinical hypocompetence: The interview. *Ann. Intern. Med.* 1979;91:898–902.

CASE 53 A SHOOTER WITH VOMITING

A 26-year-old man came to the hospital because he was vomiting and had lost his appetite. He reported that his illness had begun about three weeks earlier when he noted malaise and anorexia with slight nausea. He was able to take only fluids. Two days previously he had begun vomiting everything he ate. He had night sweats but no fever. He also admitted to having some diarrhea, and his urine was darker than usual.

On examination, his temperature was 99.5°F, pulse 120, blood pressure 122/86, and respirations 26. He was not icteric. His skin showed multiple scars along the path of his arm veins. When confronted with these, he admitted that he had been an intravenous drug user for many years and was still actively shooting about $150 of heroin daily. He also admitted that he frequently shared needles. Further examination showed shotty cervical lymphadenopathy and liver enlargement and tenderness. There were no bruises or spider angiomata. He felt light-headed when he sat up, and his pulse in the upright position was 136, with a blood pressure of 118/86.

Blood was sent for CBC, liver enzymes, coagulation studies, BUN, glucose, and electrolytes. Tests for hepatitis A antibodies and hepatitis B surface antigen were also done. The staff nurse drawing the blood took extra care to prevent accidental needlesticks. An intravenous line of lactated Ringer's solution was begun, and he was given 2 liters over the next hour.

He could not keep any oral fluids down, so he was admitted for intravenous hydration. An immediate consult was placed to the infectious disease service.

What is the emergency department treatment of the patient with acute viral hepatitis?

What are "universal precautions" against contact with the AIDS virus?

Discussion

This patient probably has hepatitis and probably has the long-incubation or serum hepatitis type. He is not clinically icteric but may still have an elevated serum bilirubin. Most observers cannot detect jaundice until the total bilirubin is over 2 mg per 100 milliliters. Nevertheless, the urine may contain enough conjugated bilirubin ("direct-reacting bilirubin") to display yellow foam if shaken or to produce a positive dipstick reaction to bilirubin.

Hepatitis, when seen in our ED, is usually of viral or toxic etiology. The virus may be short-incubation "infectious hepatitis" with an incubation period of 2 to 6 weeks and hepatitis A antibody present. It may be parenterally transmitted long-incubation (6 to 24 weeks) "serum hepatitis" with hepatitis B antigen present throughout the course. Hepatitis may be caused by a variety of "non-A, non-B" viral causes, including mononucleosis (indicated by a positive Monospot test). Viral hepatitis usually presents with a prodrome of several weeks of malaise, anorexia, and miscellaneous, functional-sounding symptoms, although a rash or arthralgias may begin the illness.

Toxins producing hepatitis include many chemicals and drugs. Antituberculosis therapy, halothane anesthesia, and others have been incriminated. In our ED, by far the most common hepatotoxin is ethyl alcohol.

We usually obtain a weight on any presumed hepatitis patient. Anorexia or vomiting severe enough to cause continual weight loss may lead to hospitalization. In this case, the patient's symptoms were so severe that he became dehydrated. The signs of increased thirst, dry lips, and light-headedness all suggest dehydration. Orthostatic vital signs are useful in demonstrating the presence of significant fluid losses. In our ED, a pulse increase of 20 points on standing up from a lying position is considered a significant orthostatic change. This requires intravenous hydration, and if the patient is still unable to keep down fluids he must be hospitalized. We draw biochemical survey, CBC, prothrombin time, hepatitis screen, and bilirubin (direct and indirect), and we obtain a urinalysis.

Close contacts of patients with hepatitis A should receive gamma globulin as soon as possible to lessen the severity of the disease if they contract it. Any patient with presumed hepatitis A should be reported to the state health department by filling out the appropriate form. Contacts of hepatitis B patients, on the other hand, have far less chance of contracting hepatitis by an oral route, but sexual partners and persons who have had contact with the patient's blood need to be tested and treated. They should be tested for the presence of hepatitis B antigen and antibody, and if these are absent they should be given the hepatitis B vaccine and hepatitis B immune globulin. All ED personnel should be immunized against hepatitis B infection.

AIDS is also spread primarily by the sharing of contaminated needles and through sexual contact with an AIDS virus carrier. Universal precautions should be followed in all EDs. These include the use of gloves for all procedures involving possible contact with a patient's blood, wearing goggles when a likelihood of splattering exists (such as during intubation or irrigation of wounds), and assuming that *every* patient can have an infectious disease transmissible in their blood or secretions. Needles should never be recapped, and all soiled sharps should be disposed of in puncture-proof containers kept near the bedside.

HIV infection is a diagnosis that is usually not made in the ED. Patients will frequently come to be tested for the "AIDS virus." We refer them to a site where appropriate counseling is given before and after the test is performed.

AIDS patients will also present to the ED not previously diagnosed but complaining of what turns out to be the initial serious presentation of their disease. Most commonly this is a *Pneumocystis carinii* pneumonia, a diarrheal illness, or oral thrush. Many of these patients will require hospitalization because of poor follow-up in the community.

Because of recent animal studies, we have now begun offering immediate treatment with AZT to anyone who has just had a high risk exposure to the AIDS virus in the hope that immediate AZT treatment may prevent the virus from infecting the exposed individual. Anyone who has potentially infectious contact with blood from an HIV-positive patient should be tested at that time and again 3 and 6 months later. Failure to seroconvert after 6 months suggests that the person exposed did not acquire the virus, which luckily is much less contagious than hepatitis B.

REFERENCES

Review Articles

Marco, C. A. Presentations and emergency department evaluation of HIV infection, *Emerg. Med. Clin. North Am.* 1995;13:365–399.

The entire volume 13 issue 1 is devoted to HIV and the Emergency Department.

Balistreri, W. F. Viral hepatitis. *Emerg. Med. Clin. North Am.* 1991;9: 365–399.

Additional References

Go, G. W., Baraff, L. J., and Schriger, D. L. Management guidelines for health care workers exposed to blood and body fluids. *Ann. Emerg. Med.* 1991;20:1341–1350.

Varghese, G. K., and Crane, L. R. Evaluation and treatment of HIV-related illnesses in the emergency department. *Ann. Emerg. Med.* 1994;24:503–511.

Baker, J. L. What is the occupational risk of emergency care providers from the human immunodeficiency virus? *Ann. Emerg. Med.* 1988;17:700–703.

Trott, A. Hepatitis B exposure and the emergency physician: Risk assessment and hepatitis vaccine update. *Am. J. Emerg. Med.* 1987;5:54–59.

CASE 54 WOMAN WITH ABDOMINAL PAIN

A 20-year-old woman came to the emergency department complaining of abdominal pain. She had been well until two days previously, when she noted the onset of bilateral abdominal pain, most severely in the right lower abdomen. This pain was accompanied by nausea and vomiting. She had had no bowel movements for the past two days. She had noted no fever or chills and specifically denied any recent venereal disease or vaginal discharge. She was having sexual contacts and was on birth control pills. There was no prior history of abdominal or pelvic disease, and she had not had an appendectomy. Her last menstrual period had terminated three days earlier.

On physical examination, the patient appeared healthy but would pull away from an examining hand. Her blood pressure was 140/80, pulse 100, respiration 18, and temperature 38.0°C orally. The findings were normal except for her abdomen and pelvis. The abdomen was slightly distended, and she guarded throughout, especially the lower quadrants. Bowel sounds were present and unremarkable. The cervix was very tender, as were the uterus and adnexa. Because of this tenderness, the adnexa could not be clearly palpated. A rectal examination demonstrated the tenderness to be largely anterior to the examining finger. The stool was brown and negative for occult blood. Her pregnancy test was negative.

What is the diagnosis?

How should the patient be treated?

What are the most common misdiagnoses made in a case such as this?

DISCUSSION

Acute pelvic inflammatory disease (PID) is a common cause of lower abdominal pain in young, sexually active women. It affects 1% of women annually. The tubal scarring resulting from PID is a leading cause of infertility and is probably responsible for the recent increase in the rate of ectopic pregnancies in the United States. The most common agents that cause PID are *Neisseria gonorrhoeae, Chlamydia trachomatis, Myocoplasma hominis, Ureaplasma urealyticum,* and anaerobic organisms. The relative frequencies of occurrence of these agents are difficult to determine, as only *N. gonorrhoeae* and *Chlamydia* are routinely cultured.

Lower abdominal pain is almost universally present in PID. The onset of pain often follows a menstrual period, during which time the asymptomatic cervical infection ascends into the upper tract. Fever, guarding, and rebound tenderness are seen with advanced cases involving peritoneal irritation. Vaginal discharge and mucopurulent discharge from the cervical os are common. Marked cervical motion tenderness, a tender nonenlarged uterus, and adnexal pain without adnexal mass are typical and often clinch the diagnosis. Cultures should be obtained for gonorrhea and *Chlamydia* in every young, sexually active woman in whom a pelvic exam is performed, even if PID is not suspected. This is primarily for public health reasons and will identify women who are asymptomatic or have mild cervicitis.

In this woman, the other differential diagnostic considerations include appendicitis, ectopic pregnancy, ruptured ovarian cyst, and endometriosis. The evaluation of abdominal pain should always include a pregnancy test to help differentiate PID from ectopic pregnancy and septic or spontaneous abortion. Ectopic pregnancy can be fatal and typically presents with pelvic pain worse on one side than the other. A tender unilateral adnexal mass may be found. In our department we consider an ectopic pregnancy to be ruled out by a negative *serum* pregnancy test (BHCG). Unfortunately, we have seen patients with ectopic pregnancies who on presentation had a negative *urine* pregnancy test. Pelvic ultrasound is often done in cases of pelvic pain, when the pregnancy test is positive, to look for an ectopic. If no intrauterine pregnancy is seen on ultrasound in a patient with a positive pregnancy test, the patient should be admitted as a presumed ectopic pregnancy or, depending on local custom, followed up within 24 hours by a gynecologist. Early appendicitis may present with vague lower abdominal pain, fever, and leukocytosis mimicking PID. The progression of the symptoms, however, is usually different because the pain of appendicitis will localize in the right lower quadrant, whereas PID almost always remains bilateral. A ruptured ovarian cyst will also produce lateralizing lower abdominal pain and occasionally rebound tenderness. Fever and leukocytosis are typically absent in this condition. Laparoscopy is occasionally necessary to differentiate it from PID. Endometriosis may also cause pain and occasionally peritoneal signs that mimick PID. A history of recurrent pain at the time of menses or a prior history of endometriosis is helpful in making a diagnosis.

Treatment of PID varies somewhat between institutions. Because of tubal scarring and the possibility of infertility, some experts feel a nulliparous woman or a woman desiring a larger family should be hospitalized and intravenous therapy given. In our department, patients with first episodes of PID are admitted (to retain the patient's fertility), as are patients with fever, marked-rebound tenderness, and signs of systemic toxicity. Likewise, we admit patients who do not respond to outpatient regimens, patients whose compliance with therapy is in doubt, and those in whom other conditions cannot be ruled out.

Outpatient therapy with ceftriaxone (250 mg IM or IV) plus a 10- to 14-day course of oral doxycycline 100 mg bid is one recommended treatment, although other drugs and dosages are occasionally utilized. In addition to being given antibiotics, discharged patients should be rechecked in 3 days and told to avoid sexual intercourse for 7 days. Follow-up examination should always be done to ensure adequacy of treatment. Instructions should be given to the patient to return for fever, increased pain, or intolerance of the medications. The patient should receive HIV counseling and have a VDRL drawn to screen for incubating syphilis. In addition, all sexual partners should be treated.

REFERENCES
Review Article
Peterson, H. B., Galaid, E. I., and Cates, W. Pelvic inflammatory disease. *Emerg. Med. Clin. North Am.* 1991;9:437–449.

Additional References
Center for Disease Control and Prevention. 1993 Sexually Transmitted Disease Treatment Guidelines. *MMWR* 1993;42(RR-14):1–102.

Webster, D. P., et al. Differentiating acute appendicitis from pelvic inflammatory disease in women of childbearing age. *Am. J. Emerg. Med.* 1993;11:569–572.

Abbott, J. Pelvic pain: Lessons from anatomy and physiology. *J. Emerg. Med.* 1990;8:441–447.

Nuovo, J., et al. Cost-effectiveness analysis of five different antibiotic regimens for the treatment of uncomplicated Chlamydia trachomatis cervicitis. *J. Am. Board Fam. Pract.* 1995;8:7–16.

CASE 55 THE BLUE BRUISE

A 56-year-old man came to our emergency department complaining of pain in his right thigh. He had bumped it getting out of a car two days earlier, and it was getting more painful and swollen. Because his regular physician was out of town, he came to the ED. He had suffered a myocardial infarction six months earlier and was still on coumarin anticoagulant for this.

On examination, a large, blue bruise covering the anterior lower right thigh was observed. A sample was drawn to check prothrombin time, and the patient was sent for an x-ray of the thigh. The x-ray was normal. By the time the patient returned from the radiology department, the physician caring for him had finished his 12-hour shift and signed his cases over to another physician. The second physician noted that the x-ray pictures were normal and discharged the patient. The patient was unsatisfied and went to another ED, where he was hospitalized. We later noted the prothrombin time to be 45 seconds with a control of 11 seconds.

Was this an example of a physician's error, a patient's error, or a failure of the medical system?

How should the patient have been treated?

What instructions should patients be given when they are placed on anticoagulant therapy?

DISCUSSION

This patient was handled correctly initially, but there was a lapse in care in the change of physicians. Obviously, if a laboratory test is worth doing, the results should be obtained and acted on. Fairly frequently a patient is signed over to another physician at a shift change, and the new physician fails to review the course of events properly and take over management of the problems being presented. The time of sign-over is fraught with danger for both physicians and nurses. Serious errors have occurred more than once when the person taking over the patient's care did not perform his or her own evaluation of the patient's clinical status. Perhaps one factor is that patients seen at the end of a hard shift may not get the same level of diagnostic expertise applied to them as those seen earlier in the shift.

One must wonder why this patient did not question the second physician about the prothrombin time. He obviously was unsatisfied, but he did not communicate his dissatisfaction to the physician. Was this primarily a failure on the patient's part, a failure of the lab to provide data rapidly enough, or the physician's failure? Probably all three. Nonetheless, the physician must be assumed to have the ultimate responsibility. The nursing staff is responsible for actually discharging patients in most EDs. They are the "last line of defense" against obvious errors, such as missing lab tests. The nurse should always speak up in cases when, acting as a patient advocate, he or she feels the patient is not ready for discharge.

In any case, any bleeding while on coumarin must be recognized as a dangerous problem. The patient must know that he or she should discontinue use of the anticoagulant and see a physician. The patient should also know that many other drugs are dangerous when he or she is on coumarin and that over-the-counter preparations should not be taken without checking with a physician. Most important, the patient should remind his or her physician that he or she is on an anticoagulant. Patients usually assume their physicians remember everything, a dangerous assumption.

Proper therapy for this patient would include bed rest, withdrawal of the anticoagulant, and probably some vitamin K to allow synthesis of needed clotting factors by the liver. Vitamin K is fat soluble and needs bile salts for absorption. If there is any suggestion of obstructive liver disease (intrahepatic or extrahepatic), the vitamin K should be given parenterally. In order to avoid another hematoma, it is usually given subcutaneously rather than intramuscularly in a 5- to 10-mg dose. Oral therapy is often acceptable. "Rebound hypercoagulability," an often-stated danger, probably is not as hazardous as overanticoagulation. Because his prothrombin time was so high (more than three times control), this patient probably should also have been treated with fresh frozen plasma to reverse his anticoagulation status. This was an example of a potentially unstable patient being dealt with as a nonemergent

55. THE BLUE BRUISE

problem (even though he could have bled seriously with no warning at all).

Whether or not the patient is on anticoagulants, the evaluation of soft tissue trauma should include examination of the area of injury and the joints immediately above and below the injury. Marked point tenderness, a large hematoma, injury at a joint, and limitation of function are factors that prompt an x-ray. Older patients can have extensive hematomas from relatively minor trauma. The detection of an exceptionally large hematoma should be followed by a CBC, platelet count, prothrombin time, and partial thromboplastin time.

REFERENCES

Review Article
Wessler, S., and Gitel, S. N. Warfarin. *N. Engl. J. Med.* 1984;311:645–652.

Additional References
Scott, P. J. W. Anticoagulant drugs in the elderly: The risks usually outweigh the benefits. *Br. Med. J.* 1988;297:1261–1263.

Lowe, G. D. O. Anticoagulant drugs in the elderly: Valuable in selected patients. *Br. Med. J.* 1988;297:1260.

Sinert, R., and Scalea, T. Retropharangeal and bowel hematomas in an anticoagulated patient. *Acad. Emerg. Med.* 1994;1:67–72.

Hylek, E. M., and Singer, D. E. Risk factors for intracranial hemorrhage in outpatients taking warfarin. *Ann. Intern. Med.* 1994;120:897–902.

Case 56 MISTAKEN IDENTITY, SHOT IN THE HEAD

A 28-year-old policeman was brought to the emergency department by ambulance. He had made a call on a residence to investigate a prowler complaint. After an initial inspection, he knocked on the house door. The occupant reached around the partly opened door and fired a revolver at the policeman. Once the deed was done, he looked at his victim and called for an ambulance.

On arrival at the ED the patient was alive. He had a pulse and obtainable blood pressure of 140/80. His respirations were spontaneous at a rate of 14. He had an entrance wound between the eyebrows and an exit wound posteriorly, just to the right of the occiput. His pupils were midposition and reactive. He was comatose with no response to voice or painful stimuli.

An endotracheal tube was inserted, and the patient was hyperventilated with an Ambu bag at a rate of 30 per minute. Two intravenous routes were started and a solution of 5% dextrose in water was run very slowly at a keep-open rate. He was given 50 gm of mannitol. In the operating room an anterior craniotomy was done. The damaged right frontal lobe was debrided, the frontal sinus lining was curetted, and the craniotomy was closed. A similar procedure was done posteriorly. Two weeks later the patient left the hospital with a left hemiparesis.

How predictable is the outcome of head injury?

What is the reason for the hyperventilation and mannitol?

DISCUSSION

The priorities in treating this kind of trauma begin with the ABCs. An adequate airway with ventilation and oxygenation must be secured. If midfacial trauma is present, nasotracheal intubation is contraindicated because the tube may penetrate the cribiform plate and enter the brain. Massive oropharyngeal hemorrhage may preclude orotracheal intubation, and cricothyroidotomy may be necessary. Tracheostomy takes too long and is almost never indicated in the ED setting.

56. MISTAKEN IDENTITY, SHOT IN THE HEAD

Unless the patient is completely comatose, intubation should be done after the patient is sedated and paralyzed. Rapid sequence intubation (RSI) prevents increased intracranial pressure secondary to the gagging or coughing that may occur during normal intubation of a less than fully comatose patient. We begin by preoxygenating with an Ambu bag and mask, then premedicating with lidocaine (100 mg IV push—to blunt the cough reflex), vecuronium (1 mg IV push—to reduce muscle contraction) and midazolam hydrochloride (Versed) (2 mg IV push—for sedation). After this, the main paralyzing drug, succinylcholine (100 mg IV push) is given. The patient then becomes paralyzed (usually in about 1 minute) and intubation is carried out.

The results of head injuries are not always predictable. Physicians should not hesitate to treat patients with even disastrous-appearing injuries.

In general, an anteroposterior bullet course is more likely to be benign than a side-to-side wound. Nonetheless, many bullets take courses not defined by a straight line connecting entrance and exit wounds. A high-velocity bullet tends to take a straighter course than a low-velocity missile. Computed tomography can identify the extent of injury and bullet path and is always indicated if an attempt is going to be made to save the patient.

Initial therapy includes attempts at decreasing secondary injury by avoiding brain edema. Specific treatments include keeping intravenous fluids at a minimum, elevating the head of the patient's bed, and hyperventilation (which is probably the most effective maneuver).

There is a saying that every medical specialty is allowed one irrational use of steroids. Nevertheless, steroids (which lower intracranial pressure in some settings) are of no proven benefit in head trauma, and many centers have discontinued their use in these patients. Mannitol (at a dose of 1 to 2 gm per kg) lowers intracranial pressure, but its use is somewhat controversial unless herniation is present. No human efficacy studies exist regarding the use of mannitol in head injury. Neurosurgical therapy must be prompt even though the brain is partly decompressed by the bullet wound of the cranium.

REFERENCES

Review Article

Rosenwasser, R. H., Andrews, D. W., and Jimenez, D. F. Penetrating craniocerebral trauma. *Surg. Clin. North Am.* 1991;71:305–316.

Additional References

Ordog, G. J., Wasserberger, J., and Balasubramanium, S. Wound ballistics: Theory and practice. *Ann. Emerg. Med.* 1984;13:1113–1122.

Cushing, H. A study of a series of wounds involving the brain and its enveloping structures. *Br. J. Surg.* 1918;5:558–684.

Ordog, G. J., et al. Spent bullets and their injuries: The result of firing weapons into the sky. *J. Trauma* 1994;37:1003–1006.

Case 57 EMS RADIO CALL

One morning in the emergency department, the EMS radio was activated and the following conversation took place:

Paramedic: Be advised we're on the scene with a 68-year-old white male, approximate weight 180 pounds, who suddenly became dizzy and complained of testicular pain and passed out. We found him on the floor, semiconscious, extremely diaphoretic. He is on the following medications: Slow-K, Minipress, and Lozol. Patient has no known allergies. His vital signs are as follows: respirations 28, pulse 104, systolic blood pressure 50, palpated. The patient has a history of high blood pressure, no other significant history. At this time the patient has a waxing and waning level of consciousness. We have him in MAST[a] pants pumped up to 50.[b] We have an IV of lactated Ringer's running wide open in his left arm. We are attempting a second IV. We have a nonrebreathing mask, O_2 15 liters.[c] His ECG shows a sinus tach, his lungs are clear. Be advised the patient is complaining of some abdominal pain radiating to his back . . . [At this point the physician interrupted the paramedic.]

Physician: Peter, what's your ETA[d] here?

Paramedic: Eight to ten minutes.

Physician: All right, it sounds like he's blowing an aneurysm. Blow up the MAST pants all the way including the abdominal segment. We'll be ready for you. Thanks a lot.

Paramedic: Thank you very much. We'll be there in eight to ten.

The physician immediately contacted the surgical house staff, described the patient, and asked that an operating room be prepared. Several minutes later the paramedic returned to the radio.

[a]Military anti-shock trousers.
[b]50 mm Hg.
[c]Oxygen at 15 liters per minute.
[d]Estimated time of arrival.

Paramedic: Be advised the patient is awake now [audible patient groaning and ambulance siren in the background] and complaining. We're coming down the avenue, and we'll be there in about three minutes.

Physician: Did you get a blood pressure, Peter?

Paramedic: We're getting one as we speak. Stand by.

Physician: Standing by.

Paramedic: Be advised the blood pressure is now 82 palp, and he's had a liter-and-a-half of lactated Ringer's.

Physician: How many lines do you have in him?

Paramedic: We have two 14s.*

Physician: Stand by . . . [a brief pause] . . . You're going to booth six.

Paramedic: Thank you, Doc.

The patient was wheeled into the booth, and a blood pressure was immediately obtained at 100 by palpation. Blood was drawn for routine preoperative studies and for typing and crossmatching of 6 units of blood. The patient was taken to the operating room within five minutes of his arrival in the ED. At operation he had a large ruptured aneurysm and an abdomen full of blood. He was discharged home eight days later.

Does all this radio jargon help?

What is the usual presentation of a ruptured or leaking aortic aneurysm?

Discussion

This patient presented with classic signs and symptoms of a ruptured abdominal aortic aneurysm. It was probably because of the paramedic's clear communications and the physician's ability to use these findings quickly that the man survived.

---

*Two 14-gauge intravenous catheters.

57. EMS RADIO CALL

The radio serves as the link between the paramedic and the physician providing medical control. Because paramedics are an extension of the emergency physician—the physician's eyes, ears, and hands in the field—their communications must be precise. At the same time, in order to avoid delays in getting the patient treated in a timely manner, the communications must be brief and to the point. Some jargon allows shortcuts to be taken on the radio. The paramedics are trained in the "prehospital approach" to the patient. This follows a standard medical model involving history, primary survey, and secondary survey. The primary survey is ABC followed by level of consciousness and vital signs. The secondary survey is a quick head-to-toe physical assessment of the patient to look for abnormal physical findings or injuries. Paramedics are not trained to diagnose. They are trained to always give the information in the same manner. This facilitates communication. When the communications are good, as in this case, rapid, excellent, prehospital care and sometimes even diagnosis can occur.

Class I shock will present without any easily observable signs. (This is also called occult shock. It should be suspected when a mechanism of injury for shock is present and can sometimes be diagnosed by demonstrating a mild, otherwise unexplained metabolic acidosis.) Class II shock shows only tachycardia, tachypnea, and a decrease in pulse pressure. These changes occur when the patient has lost approximately 20% of circulating blood volume. Class III shock presents with hypotension, marked tachycardia, and cool skin. This patient was near class IV hemorrhage. He had shock with severe blood loss (over 2000 ml), hypotension, and evidence of end-organ failure (in this case central nervous system hypoperfusion). This degree of acute blood loss is immediately life-threatening.

The acute onset of testicular pain can also be caused by kidney stones, testicular torsion, or incarcerated hernia. When this patient was initially resuscitated with the MAST suit and intravenous therapy, he also complained of abdominal and back pain. These are common symptoms of acute aneurysmal rupture.

In older patients, a leaking aneurysm must always be considered in the differential diagnosis of abdominal or low back pain. Abdominal examination may show a pulsatile abdominal mass in the epigastrium (the bifurcation of the aorta is at the level of the umbilicus). Cross-table lateral and KUB films of the abdomen may show the aneurysm if its wall is calcified. If leaking, it is usually greater than 5 cm in diameter. Further workup may include an abdominal ultrasound or CT scan if the diagnosis cannot be made in the ED. Early surgical consultation with a vascular surgeon is mandatory. If time allows, an aortogram will help the vascular surgeon immensely.

REFERENCES

Review Article

Rothrock, S. G., and Green, S. M. Abdominal aortic aneurysms: Current clinical strategies for avoiding disaster. *Emerg. Med. Rep.* 1994;15:125–136.

Additional References

O'Keefe, K. P., and Skiendzielewski, J. J. Abdominal aortic aneurysm rupture presenting as testicular pain. *Ann. Emerg. Med.* 1989;18:1096–1098.

Nevitt, M. P., Ballard, D. J., and Hallett, J. W. Prognosis of abdominal aortic aneurysm: A population based study. *N. Engl. J. Med.* 1989;321:1009–1014.

Crawford, E. S., and Hess, K. R. Abdominal aortic aneurysm (editorial). *N. Engl. J. Med.* 1989;321:1040–1042.

CASE 58 CHRONIC SCHIZOPHRENIC ON DRUGS

A 48-year-old man was brought to the emergency department by police car. His wife had called the police because he seemed confused and disoriented. He had been sitting in the bathroom brandishing a butcher knife and worrying about someone "coming for him." A mental health hold was placed, and he was brought to the ED.

On initial evaluation, his vital signs were blood pressure 130/90, pulse 120, temperature 37.6°C (99.7°F). He was said to be "a chronic schizophrenic on drugs." A sheriff's deputy who knew him stated that he frequently stopped taking his prescribed drugs and then "became more crazy." A physical examination showed a thick green material coating his teeth. His chest was thought to be clear. The initial impression was acute schizophrenia.

A second examiner was then asked to see the patient. He noted that the patient's skin was very warm, and a repeat temperature was taken. Because the patient could not keep his mouth closed on the thermometer, a rectal temperature was obtained, and it was 39.9°C. The patient was noted to be tachypneic with a respiratory rate of 36. A more careful chest exam now showed rales, bronchial breath sounds, and dullness over the left lower lung field. The patient appeared terrified and kept looking over his shoulder "for the five men who were after him to gun him down like they had shot his three friends last week." The police were sure that such a mass murder had not taken place. Although this material was clearly delusional, the patient otherwise made sense and expressed his fears clearly.

A chest x-ray showed a left lower lobe pneumonia. Subsequent calls to the patient's wife revealed that he had been drinking heavily until three days earlier. The patient was admitted to the hospital and placed on high-dosage parenteral penicillin and sedation. He had a tumultuous early course, with delirium, and then slow partial clearing of his pneumonia. An effusion persisted, and eventually he required surgical decortication of the left lower lobe.

How can you differentiate an acute organic brain syndrome from schizophrenia?

What is the differential diagnosis in a "confused" patient?

Discussion

In this patient the temperature was the secret, and the first reading taken was erroneous. One must feel the patient and judge the approximate temperature. If the estimate is not close to the recorded value, retake the temperature and be careful to exclude artifactual errors such as mouth breathing or surreptitious heating of the thermometer by the patient. In the ED it is repeatedly made clear that the key to appreciation of the presence of severe disease lies in accurately reading vital signs. As one of our experienced clinicians likes to say, "They're not called *vital signs* for nothing."

This patient had an acute toxic delirium and needed admission for intensive medical therapy. Acute encephalopathy—usually metabolic rather than caused by a mass lesion—can mimic a functional psychotic state fairly closely. We have seen intoxications with alcohol, antihistamines, scopolamine, amphetamines, cocaine, LSD, and other medical problems confused with functional psychosis. Hypoxia, hypotension, or hypoglycemia may present with features suggesting schizophrenia. Subarachnoid hemorrhage, meningitis, and encephalitis have been misconstrued as nonorganic psychosis. Steroid psychosis and collagen disease vasculitis also may present in this way.

In general, the differential diagnosis of a "confused" patient includes three main groups: *confusion, dysphasia,* or *schizophrenia.*

The acute metabolic encephalopathy patient is confused and usually somewhat agitated. He or she may have hallucinations, but these are usually visual (as opposed to the auditory ones usually associated with schizophrenia). Paranoid ideation is common to any acute encephalopathy and in no way differentiates metabolic disorders from schizophrenia. The presence of a flap or ataxia, as well as the loss of orientation or the inability to do simple calculations, argues for metabolic brain disease.

Any abnormality of vital signs should lead to a search for metabolic or toxic causes of encephalopathy. A wide variety of tests are needed to screen for the many causes of acute confusion. These should include, at a minimum: CBC, BUN, glucose, electrolytes, calcium, liver function tests, blood alcohol, arterial blood gas, a urine analysis, and a chest x-ray. A CT scan of the head is also rapidly becoming part of the standard care for this type of patient workup.

The presence of perseveration, gibberish speech, or anger with the frustration of expressive difficulties may reveal the presence of dysphasia. Often such a patient can pick the right information from a list, even if he or she cannot spontaneously answer questions. The dysphasic or aphasic patient may be oriented, although this may not be initially apparent, and has no hallucinations or gross delusions. Other neurologic abnormalities may indicate the presence of an old or new cerebrovascular accident.

Infections presenting with an acute organic brain syndrome (encephalopathy) are immediately life-threatening illnesses. Meningitis, pneumonia, urosepsis, and intra-abdominal infections are commonly associated with this syndrome, especially in the elderly, alcoholic, or immunologically deficient patient. Pneumonia is usually caused by gram-positive organisms, but with increasing age and debility the number of gram-negative organisms and unusual organisms increases. Meningitis can be caused by *Neisseria meningitides, Listeria, E. coli,* or *Streptococcus.* Urinary tract infections leading to sepsis are usually caused by gram-negative rods, such as *E. coli, Pseudomonas,* or *Enterococci.* Anaerobes or mixed gram-negative infections are commonly the cause of intra-abdominal infections that lead to sepsis. Many of these patients are unable to give a good history, and specific clues to the location of the infection may be absent, especially in the elderly.

Other conditions that can present this way include hyponatremia, hypercalcemia, renal and hepatic failure, porphyria, and the postictal state. The ATO_2MIC^5 mnemonic will help you recall the differential diagnosis of the common causes of acute encephalopathy:

A   Alcohol
T   Trauma
O_2 Overdose, oxygen
M   Metabolic (hyponatremia, hypoglycemia, hypercalcemia, hepatic failure)

I Infection (meningitis/encephalitis, brain abscess, acute febrile illness)
C⁵ Cva, Cancer, Convulsion, Carbon monoxide, Cold (hypothermia)

REFERENCES

Review Article

Lipowski, Z. J. Update on delirium. *Psychiatr. Clin. North Am.* 1992; 15:335–346.

Additional References

Frame, D. S., and Kercher, E. E. Acute psychosis. Functional versus organic. *Emerg. Med. Clin. North Am.* 1991;10:123–136.

Kaufman, D. M., and Zun, L. A quantifiable, brief, mental status examination for emergency patients. *J. Emerg. Med.* 1995;13:449–456.

Erkinjuntti, T., et al. Short portable mental questionnaire as a screening test for dementia and delirium among the elderly. *J. Am. Geriatr. Soc.* 1987;35:412–416.

Case 59 ACUTE MYOCARDIAL INFARCTION

A 50-year-old man was sent to the outpatient lab by his family doctor for some routine blood work to monitor his hypertension and mild diabetes. While the phlebotomist was drawing his blood, the patient became weak and felt a slight pressure in his chest. The laboratory technician called an orderly, who found a wheeled stretcher and brought the patient to the emergency department. In the ED he was placed on a cardiac monitor, oxygen by nasal prongs was administered, and an intravenous line of 5% dextrose in water was begun. The monitor showed obvious ST-segment elevation.

A twelve-lead ECG was immediately done. It showed ST-segment elevations and T-wave inversions in leads II, III, and aVF, with reciprocal changes in I and aVL. The ED attending physician decided to begin treatment with tissue plasminogen activator (TPA) to attempt to dissolve what she assumed to be a coronary thrombosis.

Four intravenous lines were begun and heparin and TPA infusions were started. The patient's chest discomfort was treated with two nitroglycerin tablets sublingually, resulting in complete relief. Within ten minutes of the onset of the infusion, the elevated ST segments on the monitor were no longer present, and the patient felt much better. He had a few runs of ventricular tachycardia of four and five beats each. Lidocaine was given by bolus, and a constant infusion was begun. No further arrhythmias occurred. The patient was admitted to the coronary care unit as soon as a bed was available.

What is the standard treatment for an acute myocardial infarction?

When is TPA useful?

Can you diagnose an acute myocardial infarction from seeing ST-segment elevation on the cardiac monitor?

When should lidocaine be used prophylactically?

DISCUSSION

Two major problems face the emergency physician who deals with patients with chest pain or other symptoms possibly being caused by coronary artery disease.

The first problem is the task of identifying which patients are likely to die suddenly. This is not entirely possible with available methods and is not synonymous with identifying patients who are suffering myocardial infarctions. Even the diagnosis of an acute myocardial infarction is not always easy. Frequently, the patient does not present with a textbook description of crushing central chest pain associated with weakness, nausea, and diaphoresis. The patient may suffer a myocardial infarction, yet clearly deny chest pain. To approach this problem, we suggest the following steps:

1. The history is the best source of data. Above all, do not invest too much security in the ECG. A normal ECG in no way precludes sudden death.
2. If a history of pain is not forthcoming, listen more for the circumstances surrounding the patient's decision to call for help. What was the patient doing and how did he or she feel? Patients who deny much pain but say they felt that they were about to die probably should be admitted to the coronary care unit.
3. The physical examination must search for evidence of congestive heart failure, for an abdominal problem simulating myocardial ischemia, and for arrhythmias. The pulse should be carefully felt.

The next priority is the prevention of sudden death if possible. Any patient with chest pains that might conceivably be of cardiac origin needs three things right away: an intravenous line, oxygen, and a cardiac monitor. This should happen as early in the workup as is practical. The monitor is helpful in picking up arrhythmias but cannot diagnose an acute myocardial infarction because monitor ST-segment elevations may be artifactual. True ST-segment elevation is seen on a standard 12-lead ECG.

Patients who have acute myocardial ischemia are given nitroglycerin and morphine as needed for pain. This therapy will also improve coronary blood flow and decrease myocardial work and oxygen consumption. Because most cardiac arrests early in a myocardial infarction are caused by ventricular fibrillation, any arrhythmia should be quickly diagnosed and treated. New, multifocal, or frequent premature ventricular contractions, couplets (bigeminy) or trigeminy, or runs of premature ventricular contractions should be treated with lidocaine.

The next task is the initiation of treatment to limit the size of the infarction. Of the various therapies that have been tried for this, thrombolysis seems the most effective. If there is ST-segment elevation in contiguous leads and the patient has had pain for less than 4 hours, thrombolytic therapy should be started if possible. We usually use TPA to accomplish thrombus dissolution. Streptokinase is also widely used. TPA is contraindicated in any patient who has a bleeding disorder, recent surgery, bleeding ulcer, stroke, or prolonged cardiopulmonary resuscitation. Heparin, an oral aspirin tablet, and intravenous nitroglycerin are given at the same time. Reperfusion arrhythmias are a common sign of clot dissolution. We usually treat these with lidocaine.

The patient needs rapid evaluation and rapid decision-making. The national goal is that, when a thrombolytic is appropriate, it should take no longer than 30 minutes from the patient's arrival until the infusion of a thrombolytic is begun.

REFERENCES

Review Articles
Albrich, J. M. Acute myocardial infarction: Comprehensive guidelines for diagnosis, stabilization, and mortality reduction. *Emerg. Med. Rep.* 1994;15:51–62.

Eisenberg, M. S., et al. Thrombolytic therapy. *Ann. Emerg. Med.* 1993;22:417–427.

Additional References
Heesch, C. M., and Eichhorn, E. J. Magnesium in acute myocardial infarction. *Ann. Emerg. Med.* 1994;24:1154–1160.

Krone, R. J. The role of risk stratification in the early management of a myocardial infarction. *Ann. Intern. Med.* 1992;116:223–237.

Doorey, A. J., Michelson, E. L., and Topol, E. J. Thrombolytic therapy of acute myocardial infarction. Keeping the unfulfilled promises. *J.A.M.A.* 1992;268:3108–3114.

Ornato, J. P. Role of the emergency department in decreasing the time to thrombolytic therapy in acute myocardial infarction. *Clin. Cardiol.* 1990;Suppl. 5: V48–V52, V67–V72.

CASE 60 FACIAL TRAUMA

A 48-year-old woman came to the emergency department claiming that she had been in a fight with her husband. She smelled of alcohol, was disheveled, and lapsed into tears periodically. She had multiple puffy, bruised areas about her face, and her nose was obviously crooked. Both eyes were puffy, and one was almost shut. She was breathing easily and had normal vital signs. The resident radiologist recommended sinus views and a nasal view. The only abnormality of the bones was a fractured nose. She was sent home with an ice pack and told to return the next day to the ear-nose-throat (ENT) clinic to have her nose adjusted.

How do you determine what is broken in facial trauma?

What x-ray views may be helpful?

What about sending this woman home?

DISCUSSION

The first concerns in facial trauma have to do with airway, neck, and brain injuries. Laryngeal trauma can accompany facial trauma, and laryngeal edema may be progressive. Once these are dealt with, each of the bones of the face should be carefully palpated. Both sides should be compared at each step. Palpate the zygomatic arch, the orbital rim, the maxilla, and the jaw. Anesthesia of the infraorbital nerve suggests a fracture. The most important question to ask a patient with a suspected mandibular or maxillary fracture is whether his or her teeth fit together properly. The physical examination of the face should also include an examination of the nasal septum for signs of a septal hematoma, which should be evacuated if present. Visual acuity should be checked when there is any injury of or around the eyes. If the acuity is less than perfect, attempt correction by having the patient look through a pinhole or use his or her glasses. If the vision corrects, the problem is refractive only. If it does not correct, look for other results of eye trauma such as a hyphema, traumatic glaucoma, ruptured globe, or retinal detachment. A slit lamp examination is mandatory when there has been visual loss. If the extraocular movements are unequal or incomplete, suspect entrapment of one of the extraocular muscles in an orbital floor fracture.

Midface fractures may be maxillary—usually occurring in major traumas, such as those sustained in auto accidents. They may be blowout fractures of the orbit with an intact orbital rim and orbital floor collapse. They may be tripod fractures of the zygomatic arch, or they may be nasal fractures. There may be cerebrospinal rhinorrhea and associated basal skull fractures. Of all facial fractures, the nasal fracture is the most common and most benign. We usually do no emergency manipulation of a nasal fracture. We inspect the nasal septum for the presence of a septal hematoma, and, if none is found, we simply arrange for follow-up in 3 to 5 days.

Mandibular fractures may present with many loose foreign bodies (e.g., teeth) that can be aspirated by the patient if he or she is at all obtunded and lying on his or her back. There are often associated mouth wounds, making the fracture compound. In such cases we usually close all layers of the laceration and give the patient antibiotics. Ice packs should be applied to all facial contusions to decrease the swelling as rapidly as possible. The avulsed or loose teeth should be treated by a dentist or oral surgeon as soon as possible. Teeth may be reimplanted, but the success rate decreases rapidly as the time from the injury increases. If the tooth has fallen out of its socket, it should be rinsed off and replaced.

There are many possible x-rays for facial fractures. The best view is one that includes the bone that is fractured—the one with the greatest tenderness or swelling over it. Physicians should x-ray specific bones rather than order a general facial series. An upright Waters' view of the maxillary sinuses will frequently show fluid in the maxillary sinuses or a blowout of the floor of the orbit. Special dental films are often necessary to demonstrate tooth fractures. Maxillary and mandibular fractures may be best seen on a Panorex view of the mouth, and special "jughandle" views show the zygomatic arches most clearly.

Finally, all victims of domestic violence should be offered counseling and referred to a safe place to stay. Most cities have battered women's shelters where women who have been victims of domestic violence can go to be safe from further attacks. Returning this woman home with no effort to deal with the violence is shortsighted. The facial injuries are trivial compared to the marital disorder and its potential for even more disastrous results. The patient may need protection. Her husband may need help, too.

REFERENCES

Review Article

Colucciello, S. A. The treacherous and complex spectrum of maxillofacial trauma: Etiologies, evaluation, and emergency stabilization. *Emerg. Med. Rep.* 1995;16:59–70.

Additional References

O'Hare, T. H. Blow-out fractures: A review. *J. Emerg. Med.* 1991;9:253–263.

Center for Disease Control and Prevention. Emergency department response to domestic violence. *MMWR* 1993;42:617–620.

Dannenberg, A. L., Baker, S. P., and Li, G. Intentional and unintentional injuries in women. An overview. *Ann. Epidemiol.* 1994;4:133–139.

Loring, M. T., and Smith, R. W. Health care barriers and interventions for battered women. *Public Health Rep.* 1994;109:328–338.

Case 61 LACERATION

A 30-year-old man was brought to the emergency department by ambulance after his family called the city emergency number 911, reported that he was bleeding seriously from a cut, and requested an ambulance. The policeman who arrived minutes before the ambulance found a husky man with a tourniquet on his left upper arm and a 4-cm wound laterally on his forearm. The policeman replaced the tourniquet with a bath towel local-pressure bandage. The ambulance attendant removed this and found a no-longer-bleeding wound, which he bound with a sterile dressing.

Before leaving the scene, the ambulance attendant followed the trail of blood through the patient's house to the basement, where he noticed a small wooden table with a sharply broken leg. The table leg was splintered, and the attendant noted the possibility of splinters in the wound. He estimated there was about 500 ml of blood about the house.

On his arrival at the ED, the patient's wound was anesthetized, cleaned, and irrigated. A gloved finger could be inserted subcutaneously for about 8 centimeters.

How do lay persons generally try to stop bleeding?

How would you treat this wound?

Discussion

It is amazing how few people realize that steady pressure over a wound is appropriate to hold bleeding in check. We have people appearing at the ED who have tried to stop bleeding by applying anything from vitamin A to turpentine to the wound. Most people seem to be of the "dab and look" school—applying inadequate pressure for inadequate time and then checking to see if it is still bleeding. This patient probably lost a unit of blood, thanks in part to a tourniquet applied at too low a pressure. Fortunately, his family called 911 to access professional prehospital care for his wound; without it, he could have bled to death. EMTs usually attempt to stop bleeding by direct pressure and the application of a pressure bandage. If that fails, pressure on the artery proximal to the

61. LACERATION

wound is attempted in addition to direct pressure. Tourniquets are only applied as a last resort, lifesaving measure when other less potentially damaging maneuvers fail. The time a tourniquet is applied should be well documented on the patient's medical record. As a safety measure, we always write the time applied on the patient's skin, next to the tourniquet.

The cornerstone of wound care is careful closure after adequate cleaning. All wounds are contaminated. Problems that arise can almost always be traced to ineffective removal of this contamination during initial treatment. Wounds are contaminated by damaged or dead tissues and by ground-in dirt and bacteria. Removal of dead or damaged tissue and ground-in dirt or bacteria will leave a wound that heals primarily, leaving a minimal scar. Removal of dead or damaged tissue is accomplished by sharp excision of obvious necrotic material and ragged subcutaneous tissue, with "freshening up" of skin edges. This can be done with fine (Iris) scissors or with a scalpel. Removal of embedded dirt or bacteria can be accomplished by copiously irrigating the depths of the wound with a 20-ml syringe and a 20-gauge needle (or similar narrow lumen device), using at least 500 ml of saline solution for a moderate laceration (5 to 6 cm) and more for a larger laceration. This cannot be adequately done in a wound that has not been adequately anesthetized.

This patient's wound was opened with a scalpel to the full extent of the undermined tunnel. Several splinters of wood were removed. The rough skin edges were debrided and the opened wound rescrubbed and irrigated. As with all deep lacerations, this wound was closed in layers. Subcutaneous tissue may consist of fat, muscle, and fascia, but, because neither fat nor muscle holds sutures very well, we usually only sew fascial layers and the skin. Any buried (absorbable) suture material is acceptable, but we avoid both plain gut and "chromic" because they get sticky when wet and lack tensile strength. Similarly, many types and brands of skin (nonabsorbable) sutures are available, and it seems to make little difference which you use. Silk is popular because it is so strong and easy to use. Unfortunately, it is also quite inflammatory and tends to leave suture marks. Our common practice is to use 3–0 silk for scalp and intraoral wounds and 4–0 to 6–0 nylon or Prolene elsewhere. Tetanus prophylaxis for most clean wounds is given if ten years have passed since the last dose of tetanus toxoid. If no primary immunization has been given, or if it was inadequate, tetanus immunoglobin should be considered also. Sutured wounds are initially susceptible to infection by invasion from the outside, so after an initial cleaning in the ED we ask the patients to keep their wounds clean and dry for 48 to 72 hours. Antibiotic prophylaxis for most minor wounds will not prevent a secondary infection and generally should not be used. If the wound is especially dirty, involves a laceration into the tendon sheath, has nicked a joint, or involves some other special circumstance, a single dose of IV antibiotic (usually cefazolin sodium [Ancef]) is given and followed by a 3 to 5 day course of oral antibiotics.

Sutures are removed in 3 to 5 days for facial wounds, 7 to 10 days for most average wounds, and 10 to 14 days for slow-to-heal areas, such as the feet or over a joint. Because this patient's injury was deep and contaminated, he was told to return to the ED in 2 days to have his wound reexamined.

REFERENCES

Review Articles
Berk, W. A., Welch, R. D., and Bock, B. F. Controversial issues in clinical management of the simple wound. *Ann. Emerg. Med.* 1992;21:72–80.

Lammers, R. L., and Magill, T. Detection and management of foreign bodies in soft tissue. *Emerg. Med. Clin. North Am.* 1992;10:767–781.

Additional References
Bonadio, W. A., Carney, M., and Gustafson, D. Efficacy of nurses suturing pediatric dermal lacerations in the emergency department. *Ann. Emerg. Med.* 1994;24:1114–1116.

Cummings, P., and DelBeccaro, M. A. Antibiotics to prevent infections of simple wounds: A meta-analysis of randomized studies. *Am. J. Emerg. Med.* 1995;13:392–395.

Howell, J. M. Current and future trends in wound healing. *Emerg. Med. Clin. North Am.* 1992;10:655–663.

Bartfield, J. M., et al. Buffered versus plain lidocaine as a local anesthetic for simple laceration repair. *Ann. Emerg. Med.* 1990;19:1387–1389.

Case 62 CONSTIPATION

A 77-year-old woman was brought to the emergency department complaining of constipation. She had experienced trouble with bowel function for over ten years and had been diagnosed five years previously as having Parkinson's disease. At present she was on L-dopa and 1 teaspoonful of Metamucil daily. She complained of diffuse abdominal cramping pain, vomiting, and squirts of diarrhea despite a feeling of inability to pass a stool. On physical examination she had normal vital signs and a mildly tender abdomen. Her rectum was vastly distended by soft, brown stool that tested negative for occult blood.

The physician caring for her thought that she had obstipation resulting in a partial rectal obstruction.

Does Parkinson's disease lead to constipation?

How should the patient be treated?

When is constipation a sign of more serious disease?

Discussion

Most patients with Parkinson's disease are old, and colonic malfunction is common in the elderly. Probably the neurologic disease itself does not lead to constipation, but, of course, such patients are often treated with anticholinergics, and these drugs may induce more bowel dysfunction.

Therapy should begin with vigorous cleaning out of the distended rectum. This can usually be done with enemas. In this case enemas were unsuccessful, so the patient was given 10 mg of morphine subcutaneously. Nupercaine anesthetic ointment was placed in the anal canal, and the impaction was removed, bit by bit, digitally.

The woman was allowed to rest for an hour and then sent home with instructions to use a tap water enema once a day for 3 days; to drink at least 2 quarts of fluid daily; and to take 2 teaspoonfuls of Metamucil in water qid followed each time by a glass of hot water. She was encouraged to take a large glass of prune juice each morning; not to ignore any urge for a bowel movement; to increase her intake of fiber and fluids; and to set aside a time each morning after breakfast to attempt a bowel movement. She was told that if she went 3 days with no evacuation she should use glycerine suppositories, and, if that was unsuccessful, a tap water enema.

Because the diarrhea is a sort of overflow incontinence as a result of obstipation, opiates would be antitherapeutic and should not be used.

Of course, people may mean a variety of different things when they cite "constipation," and the physician's first task is to translate the code. Then, at the very least, abdominal and rectal exams are needed in order to get a sense of the problem.

One good way to stay out of trouble in the practice of emergency medicine is for the physician to consider in each case the worst thing that could be accounting for the patient's current symptoms. Constipation may be a local problem involving rectal dysfunction, as in this case, or it can be a sign of severe underlying disease. Particularly in the elderly patient, it can be difficult to differentiate between simple constipation and the low-grade ileus that often is seen as the first sign of an impending bowel obstruction or acute abdomen.

REFERENCES

Review Article
Wrenn, K. Fecal impaction. *N. Engl. J. Med.* 1989;321:658–662.

Additional References
Tedesco, F. J., and DiPiro, J. T. Laxative use in constipation. *Am. J. Gastroenterol.* 1985;80:303.

Floch, M. H., and Wald, A. Clinical evaluation and treatment of constipation. *Gastroenterology* 1994;2:50–60.

Edwards, L. L., Quigley, E. M., and Pfeiffer, R. F. Gastrointestinal dysfunction in Parkinson's disease: Frequency and pathophysiology. *Neurology* 1992;42:726–732.

Case 63 DIFFICULTY SWALLOWING

A 66-year-old woman presented to the triage nurse stating that she had eaten some chicken a day before and swallowed a bone. She thought that it was stuck in her throat. When asked where she felt it, she pointed at her mid neck. She said she could swallow, but then regurgitated everything including her saliva. She was comfortable and able to speak normally and had normal vital signs. Initial examination disclosed discomfort on laryngeal palpation but no other abnormalities. Because of the localization of her symptoms, a soft tissue x-ray of the neck was ordered. This showed what appeared to be a chicken bone sticking out of the upper esophagus. After her palate and posterior larynx were anesthetized with Cetacaine spray, indirect laryngoscopy was performed using a lamp, a head mirror, and a heated dental mirror. No foreign body was seen. After the patient was successfully able to take a sip of water, she was discharged.

Before she left, however, a more senior resident working in the department called her back. He sent her back to x-ray for a barium swallow that revealed a filling defect in the esophagus at the gastroesophageal junction. She was promptly sent to the gastrointestinal lab for esophagogastroscopy.

What is the treatment of a nonemergent gastrointestinal foreign body?

How is a choking emergency treated?

What is a "café coronary"?

Discussion

Esophageal obstruction commonly presents in this way, and meat impaction is common even without the presence of organic disease of the distal esophagus. There is much discomfort and a serious potential for emesis with aspiration. The patient should be taken seriously and treated quickly. If the patient is seen after about one hour, he or she is usually drooling or spitting out copious quantities of saliva. The patient often sits quietly with head bowed over a towel or basin and can be diagnosed from across the room. Barium swallow is a valuable diagnostic tool, but you must be careful that the patient does not aspirate any barium.

We do not advise the use of enzymes or meat tenderizer. These agents are very irritating and destructive to an already damaged esophageal mucosa. One or two milligrams of glucagon given intravenously may result in passage of the foreign body. If not, the patient needs endoscopy, which is usually done with local anesthesia after sedation.

Most foreign bodies (even sharp objects) that pass into the stomach will pass harmlessly through the intestines. Though there is debate about the safety of waiting for the passage of a sharp object, we believe that, for the reliable patient, invasive action is required only when pain or obstruction develops.

A "café coronary" refers to the sudden death of a restaurant patron from choking on a large piece of food. This food is usually steak, and the patient usually has consumed several alcoholic beverages. The patient may have dentures or may be a loud talker while eating. The food lodges in the hypopharynx and pushes the trachea closed or obstructs in the glottis. Treatment must be immediate or all is lost. Café coronary patients do not make it to the ED. The Heimlich maneuver is life-saving in these patients. It consists of standing behind the patient and placing both arms around him or her, with your hands making one fist on the upper epigastrium just below the xiphoid. Pressure is exerted with a quick upward and inward movement of the fists. This should expel the obstructing mass. If four thrusts are unsuccessful, try to remove the food with a finger sweep of the posterior hypopharynx, being careful not to ram the bolus deeper. (If the equipment is available, use Magill forceps.) If none of this clears the airway, a stab wound cricothyroidotomy should be done. Despite the name, the coronary arteries are not implicated in this illness.

In this case, the "chicken bone" that was seen on x-ray of the neck was later reread by the radiologist as a calcified hyoid cartilage. The patient was taken to the operating room, where a large bolus of meat was pushed out of her esophagus and into the stomach by an endoscope.

REFERENCES

Review Article

Brady, P. G. Esophageal foreign bodies. *Gastroenterol. Clin. North Am.* 1991;20:691–701.

Additional References

Nandi, P. E., and Ong, G. B. Foreign body in the oesophagus: Review of 2,394 cases. *Br. J. Surg.* 1978;65:5.

Dokler, M. L., et al. Selective management of pediatric esophageal foreign bodies. *Am. Surg.* 1995;61:132–134.

Losek, J. D. Diagnostic difficulties of foreign body aspiration in children. *Am. J. Emerg. Med.* 1990;8:348–350.

Case 64 ALLERGIC TO SHRIMP

The fire department paramedics were called to a local restaurant, where a 43-year-old woman was complaining of having an allergic reaction. She stated that she was allergic to shellfish and that she had accidently eaten a salad containing some shrimp. She realized her error too late.

Within minutes, she began itching and was covered with hives. She also complained of having some difficulty breathing. The paramedics reported that her skin was indeed covered with hives but her lungs were clear. Her pulse was 110 and her blood pressure was 100/60. Her respiratory rate was 28 and slightly labored. The paramedics started a rapid intravenous infusion of lactated Ringer's solution and contacted the medical control physician by radio for further orders. The medical control physician on duty ordered epinephrine (0.3 mg) to be given subcutaneously. The MAST garment was to be applied but not inflated unless the patient's blood pressure went below 100 systolic. The paramedics' estimated time of arrival at the emergency department was ten minutes.

When the patient arrived in the ED, she felt somewhat better. Her vital signs had not changed. She was given diphenhydramine and methylprednisolone intravenously and was admitted to the hospital for an observation period.

What kinds of allergens predispose to anaphylaxis?

What are the priorities in the treatment of anaphylaxis?

How can non-physicians treat complex medical emergencies in the street?

Discussion

Anaphylaxis occurs immediately after reexposure to an allergen. Allergens commonly causing anaphylaxis include penicillin, peanuts, seafood, and insect venom. The antigen-antibody interaction usually causes hives, wheezing, and laryngeal edema (hoarseness) and occasionally causes shock. Shock is a state in which vital organs are inadequately profused. Anaphylactic shock is caused by sharply decreasing the vascular tone and increasing vascular permeability.

In the early stages of the anaphylactic syndrome, the patients may complain of thirst, light-headedness, shortness of breath, gastrointestinal symptoms, a marked warmth and flushing of the skin, and pruritus (typically, intense itching of the palms of the hands). Laryngeal edema, marked wheezing, and hypotension develop later. Most patients with anaphylaxis respond to epinephrine, but some require endotracheal intubation or cricothyrotomy. The epinephrine is usually given subcutaneously for mild to moderate cases and intravenously or endotracheally for severe anaphylactic shock. Intravenous epinephrine has two undesirable features: a high peak blood pressure and a very short duration of action. We only use it in the most severe cases.

Patients with anaphylactic shock or laryngeal edema should be admitted for an observation period. Anaphylactoid reactions without shock or severe airway obstruction may be observed in the ED for a few hours, and then the patient should be released on oral steroids and antihistamines.

Paramedics are allied health professionals trained to recognize and begin treatment of medical emergencies at the scene of the illness or injury. Many areas of the country allow paramedics to administer epinephrine and other potent medications on standing orders (previously agreed-on protocols), but a few require some sort of physician contact before any drugs can be administered. This "on-line" medical control occurs when the paramedic establishes radio or phone communications with a physician, presents the patient's history and physical findings, and requests orders for further treatment. The use of crystalloid infusions by large intravenous lines is usually allowed under standing orders, but after they are begun the medic generally must contact the medical control authority for further orders. Most prehospital care systems allow the use of diphenhydramine and steroids. Anaphylaxis is one of the serious medical emergencies that can be nearly cured prior to the patient's arrival at the hospital.

REFERENCES

Review Article

Hailpern, K. L. The treacherous clinical spectrum of allergic emergencies: Diagnosis, treatment, and prevention. *Emerg. Med. Rep.* 1994;15:211–222.

Additional References

American College of Emergency Physicians. Guidelines for emergency medical services. *Ann. Emerg. Med.* 1988;17:742–745.

Hutcheson, P. S., and Slavin, R. G. Lack of preventive measures given to patients with stinging insect anaphylaxis in hospital emergency rooms. *Ann. Allergy* 1990;64:306–307.

Case 65 PEDIATRIC HEAD INJURY

A 2-year-old boy was brought to the emergency department by his concerned parents because he seemed unduly sleepy and had vomited several times. Three hours earlier he had fallen off the top bunk of a double bunk bed, landing on his right side and hitting the right side of his head.

On arrival in the ED, he seemed alert and would cry vigorously if stimulated. He could walk well, move all extremities well, had equal and reactive pupils, and had no facial or head abnormalities. He had no evidence of other injuries and had made no prior visits to the ED for injuries. A skull series of x-rays was done; they were unremarkable. The young physician seemed disappointed by these findings when he told the parents they were normal. The parents became more worried but agreed to observe the child closely that night.

How should "negative findings," such as a normal skull x-ray, be presented to patients and families?

Should a head CT be done?

What are the usual features of a case of child battering?

Discussion

Normal findings are good news and should be announced as such. A patient should feel that the doctor is working towards his or her health, not for diseases. This physician should have approached the parents more appropriately, with a statement such as "I have good news for you. The x-rays are normal. Your boy does not have a skull fracture."

Although vomiting is a serious symptom in an adult with head injury, it is of less diagnostic significance in a child, because it is present in a high percentage of children with relatively trivial head injuries. This child, like all others with head injury, needs careful observation over the ensuing 24 hours, with or without a CAT scan. He should be watched for arousability and the development of gross focal neurologic defects. Because he has a responsible family, we would send him home with careful instructions. We would tell the parents to wake him every 1 to 2 hours and have him touch the parent's finger tip or follow some other simple command. If he can do these highly coordinated maneuvers with ease, he has been adequately observed and can go back to sleep. An alarm clock must be set at 2-hour intervals. Of course if he deteriorates, he must be returned to the ED and studied further. If the parents are deemed unreliable, then the child must be admitted for observation.

Computed tomography has replaced all other modes to identify acute intracranial injury. A consensus on exact indications for CT in head trauma is still evolving. We perform a thorough neurologic exam including a mental status exam. If these exams are entirely normal and there is no sign of depressed or penetrating injury, the CT can usually be deferred in our current opinion. Continued observation and the ability to act on deterioration are mandatory.

This case is probably not one of parental abuse. Only one feature, the story of a fall from the top bunk, even suggests it. It must be considered, however, because child abuse ("child battering" or "nonaccidental trauma") may account for up to 30% of fractures, burns, and head injuries in young children. The physician's suspicions should be aroused by the following signals: an injury that is inconsistent with the reported trauma, prior injuries to the child or a sibling, the child's failure to thrive, and unusual injuries (for example, in this case one must ask what a 2-year-old child was doing on a top bunk).

Parents of battered children usually have a history of beating for discipline, but they rarely use one medical facility regularly. There may be a family crisis, perhaps a very small one, and no source of help, so the parents take out their hostility on the child. Long-bone x-rays and skull films often reveal many new and old fractures. Bruises in different stages of healing, scald burns to the buttocks, and cigarette burns are also typical patterns of abuse. It is usually not a good idea for the emergency physician to accuse the family of child abuse. We urge early involvement of the pediatric staff physician and social workers. The child may need hospitalization for protection, even if this is not warranted by the severity of his or her injuries. Any suspicion of child abuse must always be reported to the appropriate agency, as mandated by law.

The physician may either feel contempt for the injured child's family or despair of effecting any change in their treatment of the child, but neither attitude is warranted. Child-battering parents were usually battered or neglected children themselves, and only through support and encouragement can agencies help them change their pattern of child-rearing. The physician's or nurse's hostility may drive them "underground" and thus away from sources of help.

REFERENCES

Review Articles

Yealy, D. M., and Hogan, D. E. Imaging after head trauma: Who needs what? *Emerg. Med. Clin. North Am.* 1991;9:707–717.

Wissow, L. S. Child abuse and neglect. *N. Engl. J. Med.* 1995;332:1425–1431.

Additional References

Ros, S. P., and Cetta, F. Are skull radiographs useful in the evaluation of asymptomatic infants following minor head injury? *Pediatr. Emerg. Care* 1992;8:328–330.

Freed, H. Post-traumatic skull films: Who needs them? *Ann. Emerg. Med.* 1986;15:233–235.

Davis, R. L., et al. Cranial computed tomography scans in children after minimal head injury with loss of consciousness. *Ann. Emerg. Med.* 1994;24:640–645.

Cushman, R., et al. Helmet promotion in the emergency room following a bicycle injury: A randomized trial. *Pediatrics* 1991;88:43–47.

Hyden, P. W., and Gallagher, T. A. Child abuse intervention in the emergency room. *Pediatr. Clin. North Am.* 1992;39:1053–1081.

Reece, R. M. Unusual manifestations of child abuse. *Pediatr. Clin. North Am.* 1990;37:905–921.

Case 66 PREGNANT AND BLEEDING

A 17-year-old woman came to the emergency department complaining of vaginal spotting that had been occurring since four hours earlier that morning. She was four months pregnant and had already been seen twice in the obstetrics clinic. This was her first pregnancy, and she very much wanted the baby. Early in the pregnancy she had suffered with nausea and vomiting; otherwise, she was well. Her past history was uneventful except for an allergy to penicillin. This day she had lost about 2 teaspoonfuls of blood vaginally and was quite concerned.

The examining physician found the patient in bed, holding tightly to her young husband's hand. Her vital signs included blood pressure 120/72 supine and 110/50 seated, pulse 80 supine or seated, and temperature 36.2°C orally. Head, eyes, and throat were normal. Her chest was clear. Her abdomen showed slight tenderness throughout and a uterus halfway between pubis and umbilicus. A pelvic exam by speculum was done and disclosed a blue cervix with a closed os. There was no inordinate tenderness.

How often does bleeding occur in pregnancy?

Is it ever dangerous to do a pelvic exam in such a setting?

What is wrong with this young woman, and what should be done?

Discussion

Bleeding is common in pregnancy, occurring in perhaps a third of pregnancies—even those that go on to a healthy, full-term delivery. The significance of the bleeding varies depending on the stage of pregnancy.

We see a fair number of women with incomplete abortions in the first trimester. Such patients will have significant bleeding (usually more than their usual quantity for a menstrual period) or will pass actual tissue other than blood. We examine such patients, and, if the cervical os is open and there is active bleeding from the os, we will order a pelvic ultrasound to look for retained products of conception. Ultrasound and possible dilatation and curettage may follow. If the os is closed and the bleeding is minimal an ultrasound can still be done, but it is less urgent and patients can be followed as outpatients by their attending obstetrician or the obstetrical clinic. We draw a baseline hematocrit, type and Rh, and a serum human chorionic gonadotropin level at the time of the visit and advise that the patient avoid sexual activity and strenuous exertion until follow-up. Cultures are also obtained for chlamydia and gonorrhea. In order to prevent sensitizing to Rh factor, RhoGAM should be given to all Rh negative mothers having an abortion after 12 weeks of pregnancy. If there is any evidence of hypotension or lateralizing pain, or if adnexal tenderness or a mass is palpated, a pelvic ultrasound is performed to verify that the pregnancy is in the uterus. If no intrauterine pregnancy is found on ultrasound, the patient is admitted to be worked up for an ectopic pregnancy because it is a life-threatening condition.

In the second trimester abortions are much less frequent. This patient probably has less than a 10% chance of completing an abortion. She is having a threatened abortion and should be reassured and sent home. She should be told to return if she begins to pass copious amounts of blood (more than enough for one sanitary pad per hour), or any tissue, or if she begins to have increasingly severe pain. She should rest and avoid intercourse and douching (there should never be douching during pregnancy). She should be seen again soon in follow-up.

If bleeding occurs in the last half of the pregnancy, we advise against doing a pelvic exam in the ED. A placenta previa or abruptio may be present, and examination might increase the chance of losing the fetus. Of course, copious bleeding may require us to start several intravenous lines, give quantities of fluid, and perhaps transfuse many units of blood.

If the patient is hemorrhaging vigorously, her life takes precedence and a pelvic exam must be done. This should preferably be done in the operating room in case emergency cesarean section is necessary. Sometimes the products of conception are found in the cervical os, and simple removal quiets down the bleeding. When the bleeding is so severe as to force a pelvic exam, it should, of course, begin with a careful speculum examination, which has less chance than a bimanual exam of disturbing a placenta previa. Ultrasound is also available, and it is useful in diagnosing such pathology as placenta previa. Ultrasound should be used when the bleeding is not life-threatening and there is time to review the situation more closely.

The thoroughness of the physician's examination and his or her explanation of the patient's symptoms and reassurance that the pregnancy is a normal one are most important here. It is not enough for the physician to be assured that nothing is wrong; he or she must convey this feeling to the patient also. Women who are miscarrying often have a lot of guilt. Because about one third of pregnancies end in spontaneous abortion, it is important to tell the woman that she has done nothing wrong that caused it to occur. Even when there is a problem, the physician should be reassuring.

REFERENCES

Review Article

Turner, L. M. Vaginal bleeding during pregnancy. *Emerg. Med. Clin. North Am.* 1993;12:45–54.

The entire volume 12, number 1 issue of the Emerg. Med. Clin. North Am. *is devoted to emergency problems of the pregnant patient.*

Additional References

Gilling-Smith, G., et al. Management of early pregnancy bleeding in the accident and emergency department. *Arch. Emerg. Med.* 1988;5: 133–138.

Wathen, P. I., Henderson, M. C., and Witz, C. A. Abnormal uterine bleeding. *Med. Clin. North Am.* 1995;79:329–344.

Case 67 TROUBLE BREATHING

A 52-year-old man came to the emergency department complaining of difficulty getting his breath. He had been troubled with shortness of breath for the previous two weeks, and it had become even worse today. He said that he had asthma.

The man had smoked two packs of cigarettes a day for many years and had a total smoking history of over 60 pack-years. He had quit smoking six months earlier upon his discharge from the state penitentiary, where he had been a prisoner for nine years. He did not wish to discuss the cause of his incarceration. His shortness of breath had become noticeable at about age 40 and was more and more frequently a problem during the past year. While in prison, he had been told that he had asthma and had been treated with a combination drug containing ephedrine, theophylline, and a barbiturate. At times he had been on corticosteroids and used a bronchodilator inhaler.

During the past two years the patient had been bothered by a cough that usually produced a few ounces of yellow sputum daily. In fact, when pressed, he admitted to a "cigarette cough" most mornings for the past ten years. The cough had grown worse in the past few days, and the sputum was becoming darker—a sort of grayish green in color. During the past six months he had never been free of cough and could never walk more than three blocks without having to stop to catch his breath. The preceding night he was kept awake by coughing and difficulty getting his breath.

On examination the patient was observed to be having difficulty breathing at rest. He appeared fatigued and could say no more than a few words at a time between breaths. His chest was hyperexpanded, and he took a long time with each breath. Vital signs included blood pressure 160/90, pulse 90, respiration 24, jugular venous pressure elevated in expiration but normal in inspiration, and temperature 37.0°C orally. His breath sounds were altered; one could not hear any normal alveolar breath sounds, and he had high-pitched wheezes bilaterally. His heart was best heard in the epigastrium, and the heart tones were normal. His liver was low, with an upper edge percussible at almost the costal margin but with a total height in the midclavicular line of only 11 centimeters.

There was no edema, and the rest of the examination showed no abnormalities.

Does this man have asthma?

What sort of problems lead to the appearance of such a patient at the ED?

What can be done for him?

DISCUSSION

Most middle-aged or older patients who arrive at the ED with the comment that their asthma is getting worse do not have asthma. A few of them have severe congestive heart failure or even pulmonary edema. These can often be diagnosed by the presence of leg edema, hepatomegaly, and, above all, an elevated venous pressure. Patients with pulmonary edema may have no rales but rather a chest full of musical wheezes—hence, the term *cardiac asthma*. The history may include episodes of paroxysmal nocturnal dyspnea occurring 2 to 4 hours after going to bed, aiding diagnosis.

More often, as in this case, the older patient who labels himself or herself as asthmatic has a chronic obstructive lung disease of the emphysema-bronchitis type. The patient may present with a history primarily of dyspnea for many years, may be oxygenated but wasted, and can be described as a "pink puffer." Such a patient usually can be kept out of the hospital until his or her ultimate decline and thus never accumulates a large inpatient chart. The patient suffering from relatively pure emphysema is less common than the bronchitic patient who describes years of cough before he or she developed significant dyspnea. He or she often looks cyanotic. This "blue bloater" arrives frequently at the ED with the complications of infection (worsening bronchitis, pneumonia, or bronchiolitis), heart failure, mechanical disasters (pneumothorax, enlarging bleb restricting the vital capacity, etc.), or pulmonary emboli. Such a patient has many hospital admissions and typically has several volumes to his or her medical record.

This patient has characteristics of both emphysema and bronchitis. He may also have some airway narrowing that will respond to bronchodilators and is therefore termed *reversible*. In the ED we would treat him with low-flow oxygen, an intravenous loading dose infusion of corticosteroids such as methylprednisolone (Solu-Medrol), and inhaled bronchodilators such as metaproterenol or albuterol. We obtain baseline lab data including CBC, chest x-ray, ECG, and arterial blood gases. We sometimes look at the sputum for WBC and bacteria. It is seldom helpful to culture sputum unless the chest x-ray shows a pneumonia. Occasionally we can discharge such a patient on antibiotics (we prefer sulfamethoxazole/trimethoprim or ampicillin), but usually we are obliged to admit the patient for further evaluation and therapy.

One of the most vexing problems that faces the ED physician in treating the patient with chronic obstructive pulmonary disease is the decision to initiate mechanical ventilation. Such a decision depends on the physician's judgement and also on the patient's wishes. Certain warning signs or signals should prompt the physician to think of mechanical ventilation with these patients. First and foremost is the patient's clinical presentation. If he or she is unable to speak more than one or two words without gasping, seems to have an altered mental status, or is moving very little air on lung exam, the chances that he or she will need mechanical ventilation are very good. In addition, if the patient's respiratory acidosis is worsening because of increasing retained carbon dioxide despite appropriate therapy, mechanical ventilation may be needed. Remember that it is difficult to judge the need for intubation based on the result of one arterial blood gas. Some patients with chronic obstructive pulmonary disease (COPD) are chronically hypoxemic with pO_2's between 40 and 50 and pCO_2's between 50 and 60, even during their compensated periods; however, these patients are generally not acidotic and will not show evidence of acute decompensation on initial examination. More important are serial results from blood gases, which give a very good indication as to whether the patient is improving or worsening.

We hesitate to intubate the COPD patient because it is often very difficult or impossible to wean him or her from the ventilator. Intubation of these patients should *not* be undertaken lightly. Nevertheless, mechanical ventilation may be needed temporarily and can be lifesaving—thus provoking a very difficult clinical decision. If the patient is tiring and desires intubation, it should be performed. A recent alternative tool is C-PAP (continuous positive airway pressure), a non-invasive form of airway pressure similar to blowing into a balloon, which can successfully prevent intubation in some of these patients.

REFERENCES

Review Article

Murata, G. H., et al. Treatment of decompensated chronic obstructive pulmonary disease in the emergency department—correlation between clinical features and prognosis. *Ann. Emerg. Med.* 1991;20:125–129.

Additional References

Nicotra, M. B., Reveria, M., and Awer, J. A. Antibiotic therapy of acute exacerbations of chronic bronchitis. *Ann. Intern. Med.* 1982;97:18–21.

Cydulka, R. K., and Emerman, C. L. Effects of combined treatment with glycopyrrolate and albuterol in acute exacerbation of chronic obstructive pulmonary disease. *Ann. Emerg. Med.* 1995;25:470–473.

Stehr, D. E., Klein, B. J., and Murata, G. H. Emergency department return visits in chronic obstructive pulmonary disease: The importance of psychosocial factors. *Ann. Emerg. Med.* 1991;20:1113–1116.

Emerman, C. L., Effron, D., and Lukens, T. W. Spirometric criteria for hospital admission of patients with acute exacerbation of COPD. *Chest* 1991;99:595–599.

Case 68: GUNSHOT WOUND

A 33-year-old man was brought to the emergency department by ambulance. He had been despondent and had attempted suicide by shooting himself with a 38-caliber revolver. The bullet entered at a point two intercostal spaces below the left nipple and exited at the left posterior axillary line in the tenth intercostal space.

On arrival at the ED the patient was conscious and breathing. He had a palpable systolic blood pressure of 60 mm Hg. His cardiac rate was 130 per minute. Three large intravenous infusions were begun with lactated Ringer's solution. A right internal jugular line and two antecubital fossa lines were placed with large-diameter short intracatheters. Within 5 minutes 500 ml of fluid had been given, and his blood pressure was palpable and audible at 100 mm Hg. A single chest tube was placed in the left midaxillary line in the fifth interspace. The pectoralis major muscle was grasped and the tube placed just posterior to it. The tube was connected to underwater drainage and then to continuous suction via a three-bottle system. Less than 100 ml of blood returned via the chest tube.

A Foley indwelling bladder catheter and a nasogastric tube were inserted. A portable chest x-ray was taken. It showed a normal chest and a metal fragment probably below the diaphragm. The patient was told he needed an operation, and within 30 minutes of his arrival at the ED he was moved into the operating room. At that time the central venous pressure (CVP) readings from his jugular vein catheter were about 14 centimeters. Eight units of blood were readied, he was intubated and anesthetized, and his abdomen was opened.

The laparotomy exposed about 1000 ml of free blood in the peritoneal cavity, a bisected spleen, and tears in the stomach and the jejunum. As the spleen was being removed, the patient's blood pressure became unobtainable despite a CVP of 18 centimeters. The chest was then opened, and a bulging pericardium was incised. A large amount of clot was easily evacuated, and a tangential crease wound of the apex of the heart was reinforced with sutures. The blood pressure rose on opening the pericardium, and the rest of the operation proceeded uneventfully.

When and how should chest tubes be inserted?

When should a traumatized patient have his chest opened in the ED?

In this type of situation, is there any value to stabilization of the patient by prehospital caregivers such as paramedics?

DISCUSSION

Penetrating thoracic trauma can produce the following life-threatening injuries: tension pneumothorax, heart or great vessel injury with exsanguination, pericardial tamponade, and intra-abdominal hemorrhage. Initial treatment of the patient centers, of course, on the ABCs. Endotracheal intubation should be undertaken early if there are signs of airway compromise. At least two large-bore intravenous lines should be established, even if the patient appears to be stable on initial assessment. If the patient is unstable on presentation, three or four peripheral intravenous lines and a large-bore central line should be placed, and blood for type, crossmatch, and initial hematocrit should be sent immediately. Patients who present in shock can be transfused with O-negative or type-specific, uncrossmatched blood.

Tension pneumothorax is a deadly cause of hypotension in penetrating thoracic trauma. It causes displacement of the mediastinal structures followed by decreased cardiac output and cardiovascular collapse. Treatment is immediate decompression of the chest with a large-bore intravenous catheter placed in the second intercostal space at the midclavicular line. This should always be followed by insertion of a thoracostomy tube, as needle decompression is only a temporizing measure. Because this entity can be rapidly fatal, immediate action is necessary when it is clinically suspected. An x-ray study of the chest may cause a disastrous delay in patient care. Sucking (open) chest wounds should be temporarily sealed with a petrolatum gauze (such as Xeroform) taped on three sides to let air escape if under pressure but not be drawn into the chest cavity.

We feel rather free to insert chest tubes. Any traumatized patient who is dyspneic, tachypneic, or in whom we clinically suspect a pneumothorax or hemothorax may get one or two chest tubes placed even before the five minutes it would take to obtain a portable x-ray of the chest. Physical findings of the chest may often be nonrevealing and easily confused because listening to breath sounds and percussion can be suboptimal in a busy trauma room. A serious hemothorax may be missed by relying on auscultation. Chest tubes are fairly benign, considering the tremendous potential danger of the patient's basic problems.

We prefer to insert one tube in the fourth or fifth intercostal space between the anterior axillary and midaxillary lines. If the patient is awake, we try to anesthetize the skin and perichondrium with about 10 ml of 1% lidocaine, make a 1-inch long incision in the skin, separate deeper layers down to and including the parietal pleura (with a large clamp or with spreading movements of a pair of scissors), and then probe the wound with a gloved finger. If the tip of your finger tells you that you are in the chest cavity, a large chest tube is placed by grasping its tip in a large curved surgical clamp and advancing it over your probing finger. Tubes have been mistakenly placed below the diaphragm. This may damage the liver or spleen, so we try to avoid it. Occasionally a chest tube is placed on the wrong side (appearing correct until it is observed that the bullet's trajectory was bizarre and led to contralateral damage). If in doubt or if the patient is not improving, we do not hesitate to place a tube on the other side.

Penetrating injuries to the chest that damage the great vessels can be rapidly fatal. The majority of patients sustaining such injuries do not reach the ED alive. Stab wounds are usually less serious than gunshot wounds. The patient with heart or great vessel injury usually presents in hemorrhagic shock. Fluid resuscitation and rapid diagnosis of cardiac or great vessel injury are necessary for salvage. Findings that indicate the possibility of cardiac or great vessel injury include persistent hypotension and evidence of pericardial tamponade. Even when tamponade is found to be present, needle pericardiocentesis may be of very little value. It frequently returns nothing, even when much blood has clotted in the pericardium and led to cardiac tamponade. Searching for a paradoxical pulse is useless. This sign, defined in a spontaneously breathing patient with resting respiration, is grossly distorted in a patient who is in respiratory distress and is totally obviated in one who is receiving positive pressure ventilation. The only useful signs are hypotension and a high or rising CVP.

It is possible to plug some myocardial injuries with a finger or with an intraventricular Foley catheter balloon pulled gently back against the hole as a holding maneuver until the operating room's greater resources can be reached. In this most dramatic situation, one who hesitates is lost. Life-threatening hypotension following penetrating chest trauma may be caused by cardiac tamponade, and, after a brief but vigorous search for other sources of blood loss, the heart should be attacked directly. Sometimes this must be done in the ED. Emergency thoracotomy in the operating room is indicated for patients who continue to have hypotension despite aggressive fluid resuscitation, have an initial chest tube output of greater than 1000 ml of blood, have more than 250 ml of blood output in two consecutive hours, or have other signs of cardiac or great vessel injury. ED thoracotomy is indicated in patients who are victims of penetrating chest or abdominal trauma and have a cardiac arrest en route to or while in the ED.

In this case, the initial approach failed to turn up an intrathoracic cause for the patient's hypotension. The surgeon knew that the diaphragm can rise to the fourth intercostal space during expiration. The next obvious place to look was his abdomen, and it was quickly opened. However, the more serious disturbance was intrathoracic, and it was treated appropriately. If the patient had not responded promptly in the ED, a thoracotomy could have been done there. Nevertheless, the best place for these maneuvers is still a well-equipped and well-lighted operating room.

Prehospital care of these patients should be aimed toward rapid transport to the nearest trauma center. This "scoop and run" approach should include as much stabilization with peripheral intravenous lines and airway control as the paramedics are able to accomplish en route to the hospital. The caveat on the streets is that field care should not delay transport to the hospital. The use of MAST pants in these cases has been shown to increase rather than decrease mortality, probably by shunting blood to the area that is hemorrhaging.

REFERENCES

Review Article
Jorden, R. C. Penetrating chest trauma. *Emerg. Med. Clin. North Am.* 1993;11:97–106.

Additional References

Ordog, D. J. Emergency thoracotomy. *Am. J. Emerg. Med.* 1987;5:312–316.

Swan, K. G., and Swan, R. C. Principles of ballistics applicable to the treatment of gunshot wounds. *Surg. Clin. North Am.* 1991;71:221–239.

Case 69 PLEURITIC PAIN

A 65-year-old man came to the emergency department complaining of chest pain. He said the pain in his right side had begun about 24 hours earlier and had been getting worse since then. It was constantly present and especially excruciating when he coughed or moved suddenly. He was most comfortable sitting quietly or lying on his right side. Although he denied smoking or drinking, he did admit to having a cough the preceding few days that produced a small amount of yellow sputum. Prior to this illness he had been quite well and active and denied any chronic cough, prior chest pains, or shortness of breath.

On physical examination the patient appeared well. His vital signs included blood pressure 150/80, pulse 100, respiration 20, temperature 38.3°C orally, and a normal jugular venous pressure. His head, eyes, ears, nose, and throat were unremarkable. His neck was carefully palpated, revealing no adenopathy or other pathology. His chest was slightly tender laterally on the right side, and there were a few crackling rales audible there. His cardiovascular examination was normal, he had no edema, and the rest of the exam showed nothing remarkable. A chest x-ray showed a right lower lobe infiltrate involving almost the entire lobe.

What is the diagnosis in this case?

What further studies should be done?

What should be done for this man?

Discussion

This man seems to have a pneumonia, and most pneumonias are pneumococcal. Alcoholics, postinfluenza patients, diabetics, and the like all usually have the pneumococcus as causative organism when they develop a bacterial pneumonia.

After pneumococcus, the next most likely cause of pneumonia acquired in the community is mycoplasma. Mycoplasma most commonly occurs in the 10- to 30-year-old age group. The illness it causes is usually more gradual than pneumococcus in onset. Symptoms include fatigue, headache, myalgias, and a nonproductive hacking cough. Pleuritic chest pain and fever greater than 102°F (38.9°C) are unusual. In contrast, pneumococcal pneumonia often produces pleuritic chest pain, a cough productive of purulent sputum, chills, and temperature elevations exceeding 102°F. If the patient is immunocompromised by HIV, the most common pneumonia is caused by *Pneumocystis carinii*. Previously a rare disorder, *P. carinii* pneumonia (PCP) has grown to an epidemic along with AIDS.

The two most important procedures in confirming the presence of pneumonia are the chest x-ray and sputum gram stain. We recommend obtaining one or two blood cultures prior to initiating therapy, because blood cultures are frequently positive in pneumococcal pneumonia and may confirm the diagnosis when sputum cultures are negative. The WBC count, erythrocyte sedimentation rate, and the c-reactive protein are usually elevated in patients with bacteremia, but these tests provide only minimal additional information. When a good sputum smear is examined, it will often show a preponderance of one organism. If this is indeed a gram-positive diplococcus, therapy should be begun with penicillin. Care must be taken to obtain sputum, not saliva. This patient (if not allergic to penicillin) could be given 2.4 million units of procaine penicillin G intramuscularly, followed by 500 mg of penicillin V orally qid. In part because of the increase in the incidence of penicillin-resistant pneumococci, initial treatment with a second generation cephalosporin, such as cefuroxime sodium (Zinacef), or with erythromycin is increasingly common for the initial treatment of community acquired pneumonia.

Because our bed capacity is limited, and in order to keep costs down, we often do not admit patients with pneumonia to the hospital. Many do well at home. These outpatients need careful monitoring. The patient must return in 2 or 3 days—sooner if he or she is worse. The patients who have lowered host resistance or appear very ill should be admitted to the hospital. Any alcoholic or diabetic with pneumonia needs hospitalization, as do pregnant or dehydrated patients and those for whom adequate follow-up cannot be assured. Most patients over age 60 should be admitted. The presence of a high fever, tachypnea, severe chest pain, or hypoxia argues for admission.

The differential diagnosis of this patient included all of the other conditions that commonly can present with the sudden onset of severe respiratory chest pain: spontaneous pneumothorax, pleurodynia (a "viral pleurisy"), pulmonary embolism, pericarditis, and bronchitis with chest wall injury from coughing.

This patient was treated at home, and he improved rapidly. When seen again in three days, he felt much better and was afebrile. In two weeks his chest x-ray was normal and he had returned to work.

REFERENCES

Review Article
Emerman, C. L. Outpatient management of community-acquired pneumonia: Identifying etiologic agents and optimizing antimicrobial therapy. *Emerg. Med. Rep.* 1994;15:159–170.

Additional Reference
Sims, R. V. Bacterial pneumonia in the elderly. *Emerg. Med. Clin. North Am.* 1990;8:207–220.

The choice of antibacterial drugs. *Med. Lett.* 1994;36:53–60.

Case 70 LOOKED "TOO DRUNK" TO THE POLICE

A 38-year-old man was brought to the emergency department by city police. He had been arrested for being drunk in a public place and taken to the city jail. After seven hours in jail he had appeared "too drunk" to his jailers and was brought to the ED. Because no ED beds were available, the man was placed in the locked ED jail cell. A physician saw him within one hour of his arrival in the ED but quickly turned away. The patient was disheveled, malodorous, uncooperative, unshaven, ataxic, and appeared quite drunk. No careful neurologic or mental status exam was done, and he was left in the cell to sober up. When next seen three hours later, he was stuporous and had one large pupil. He was quickly taken from the cell, undressed, examined, and rushed to the operating room, where an epidural hematoma was evacuated. Despite these vigorous efforts the patient died on the operating table.

How can you tell that a patient is drunk?

How can you tell that he is just drunk?

Is it surprising that this man had no obvious signs of trauma and yet had an acute epidural hematoma?

Does an acute subdural hematoma also present this way?

Discussion

Alcohol intoxication is a common pathologic state in most EDs. The features that should be looked for include slurred speech, a tendency to drift off to sleep, inappropriate behavior, and mild ataxia. A blood, breath, or saliva alcohol is helpful. A level of 100 mg per 100 ml is used in most states to define a person as too drunk to drive. This level is also known as "100 milligrams percent" and is also equivalent to 100 mg per deciliter. One is usually ataxic at 200 mg per 100 ml, and stupor appears at about 300 mg per 100 ml in the occasional drinker. A chronic alcoholic (the "chronic" is redundant) may not become sleepy until a higher level—400 or 500 mg per 100 ml—because of central nervous system (CNS) tolerance to the alcohol. In this patient, who had been off alcohol for at least eight hours when first seen in the ED, a blood alcohol probably would have been under 100 mg per 100 ml. Becoming aware of such a low level would have alerted the physician to the presence of another problem.

The big problem is ruling out the existence of other pathology accompanying alcohol intoxication as the real cause of the ataxia or stupor. This patient was still "drunk" after seven hours of sobering-up time, so the physician should have made a more careful search for other pathology. A patient with a blood alcohol of 400 mg per dl may also have a subdural hematoma, an epidural hematoma, cerebellar degeneration, or any other pathology. The examination should include vital signs (a wide pulse pressure or bradycardia may be the tip-off to rising intracranial pressure), gait, mentation, and a careful search for head trauma. It is very difficult to evaluate CNS disorders in a drunk patient. A careful search for any lateralizing sign is essential, as is a cervical spine x-ray series if trauma is being seriously considered. If any doubt remains about the possibility of an acute intracranial bleed, a CT scan should be done.

It is not surprising that there was no gross evidence of head trauma. Epidural hematomas often result from a relatively small trauma that hits at precisely the right spot to tear the middle meningeal artery. A baseball or hockey puck can do this. The patient with an acute subdural hematoma is more often the victim of more massive trauma; being hit by a car or a truck rather than a baseball. As a result, he or she often has multiple injuries, and, as focal neurologic signs may be scant, we sometimes spend valuable time elsewhere before evaluating the cause of confusion or unconsciousness. A chronic subdural hematoma often presents weeks after the trauma, and the patient may no longer give a history of any trauma. This disorder is replacing syphilis as "the great imitator" and should be thought of in any confused or sleepy patient. This is especially true in elderly or alcoholic patients, in whom chronic subdural hematomas occur more frequently. In this case, the physician's instinct to avoid a malodorous, socially undesirable, uncooperative patient worked to the detriment of the physician as well as the patient.

REFERENCES

Review Article

Olshaker, J. S., and DePriest, W. W., Jr. Head Trauma. *Emerg. Med. Clin. North Am.* 1993;11:165–186.

Additional References

Macewen, W. The diagnosis of alcoholic coma. *Glasgow Med. J.* 1879; 1(January):1–15.

Galbraith, S. Misdiagnosis and delayed diagnosis in traumatic intracranial hematoma. *Br. Med. J.* 1976;1:1438–1439.

Wrenn, K. D., and Slovis, C. M. Neurologic complications of alcoholism. *Emerg. Med. Clin. North Am.* 1990;8:835–858.

Case 71 HEARING AIDS

A 78-year-old man was the driver of a pickup truck in a motor vehicle accident. He complained of some neck pain but otherwise felt fine. His pickup truck had collided with a small sedan and the damage to both cars was relatively minor. The driver of the other vehicle was also relatively uninjured. The pickup truck driver was taken to a community hospital ED, where an examination disclosed only some tenderness of his neck. He had been immobilized in a hard cervical collar and on a spine board, then was sent for x-rays of his cervical spine. These x-rays were read as negative. The patient was sent home in the care of his wife.

The next day he had some trouble getting around during the day. He felt "icky all over." That evening his wife was assisting him to the bathroom when he suddenly felt severe pain in his neck and the right side of his head. The whole right side of his face became numb. He promptly called for the rescue squad and was taken back to the hospital for reevaluation.

An evaluation of the patient's x-rays taken the previous night disclosed that the cervical spine films were taken without having removed the patient's hearing aids. The hearing aids obscured the C1-C2 junction and the dens process of C2. This area did not appear completely normal and repeat films were requested. The repeat films suggested a fracture through the dens process. Based on these, the emergency physician requested a CT scan. Because it was late at night, the radiologist had to be called. He objected to having to do the CT scan and felt that the x-rays read as normal the day before should be adequate. The ED physician, being quite certain that the repeat x-rays were abnormal, insisted that the radiologist come in and read the repeat x-rays himself. The radiologist came in, noted that there was an abnormality, and immediately ordered a CT scan. This showed a comminuted fracture of the C2 through the dens and the lateral pillar. The patient was subsequently taken to the operating room for a fusion. Fortunately, he suffered no neurological deficit.

What is the normal presentation of cervical spine fractures?

Under what circumstances should a CT scan be used to image the cervical spine?

What is the appropriate action when there is a disagreement between physicians?

Discussion

This patient presented and had an inadequate cervical spine film taken. When his symptoms recurred and he returned 24 hours later, the emergency physician was alert to review the films themselves and not just the report. This allowed him to note the problem with the hearing aids and request better films.

Any patient involved in a motor vehicle accident who has neck pain or tenderness should be suspected of having a cervical spine injury. The cervical spine can be clinically cleared if the patient has *no* neck pain or tenderness, is alert and awake, has a normal mental status (including no drugs or alcohol on board), and has no seriously painful distracting injury (such as fractured pelvis, multiple rib fractures, a fractured femur, etc.). In order to "clinically clear" the cervical spine, the neck should be examined by telling the patient to gently move the neck, first in a side to side "turning no slowly" motion and then, cautiously, "nodding yes slowly." If there is neither pain nor tenderness, the neck can be considered clinically cleared. All multiple major trauma patients should probably have their cervical spines cleared radiographically, because there is usually altered mental status or enough distracting injuries to prevent adequate examination.

As in this case, CT scan is useful in imaging the cervical spine to see if a fracture is present and to determine the presence of encroachment on the spinal canal from bony fragments. However, the ordinary radiographs of the cervical spine should always be taken first. If these are normal, the spine is generally considered cleared. If, however, there is still significant pain, flexion-extension views are sometimes used to delineate a ligamentous injury, which can be potentially unstable. In any case, the patient should remain in a hard cervical collar until all needed films are completed and read as negative.

In this case the emergency physician and radiologist disagreed on the case management. Of course, the patient's care comes first, and the emergency physician was correct in insisting that the radiologist come in to read the films personally. In some cases x-rays are faxed or teleradiographed to the home of the radiologist. However, the quality of these films may not be adequate to show fine details, as was necessary on this film.

Similar principles apply to other patient contacts. The emergency physician is the physician responsible for the patient—at least until another attending level physician comes in to care for that patient. The emergency physician should stand his or her ground and request what in his or her judgment is best for the patient. Occasionally, this can lead to conflict. In this case, if the patient's attending refused to come in to see the patient, the best plan would have been to ask for a third physician to come in to do so.

REFERENCES

Review Article
Mace, S. E. The unstable occult cervical spine fracture: A review. *Am. J. Emerg. Med.* 1992;10:136–142.

Additional References
Renfrew, D. L., et al. Error in radiology. *Radiology* 1992;183:145–150.

Scott, W. W., et al. Interpretation of emergency department radiographs by radiologists and emergency medicine physicians: Teleradiology workstation versus radiograph readings. *Radiology* 1995;195:223–229.

Daffner, R. H. Cervical radiography in the emergency department: Who, when, how extensive? *J. Emerg. Med.* 1993;11:619–620.

Freed, H. A., et al. Radiographic misreads as a function of level of training. *Acad. Emerg. Med.* 1995;2:345–346. Abstract.

Holliman, C. J. The art of dealing with consultants. *J. Emerg. Med.* 1993;11:633–640.

CASE 72 NO PULSE

A 55-year-old man was brought to the emergency department by ambulance. He was complaining of abdominal pain. As he was wheeled into the ED, the ambulance attendant mentioned that he had been unable to feel a pulse. The patient was immediately surrounded by a group of physicians and nurses, who noted that he was apparently conscious and communicating but indeed had no obtainable blood pressure and no obtainable peripheral pulses. His carotid pulse was palpable and his heart rate 110. There were several long scars on his chest, abdomen, and legs. An ECG showed a broad QRS with a duration of 0.16 seconds and a regular rate of 110. No P waves were evident. A CVP (central venous pressure) line was placed, and it read 28 centimeters. The physician's initial impression was probably tempered by his just having been involved in a case of dissecting aortic aneurysm in which the diagnosis had initially been missed. It was difficult to avoid the same diagnosis in this case.

A call to the patient's regular physician revealed that this man had undergone extensive vascular surgery including myocardial revascularization in the past two years. He had shown no palpable pulses for many months. The ECG was then reviewed, and the diagnosis of hyperkalemia was made. Therapy was begun with glucose, insulin, and sodium bicarbonate. Serum potassium level was 6.8 mEq per liter.

What is the usual first therapy given to a pulseless patient?

What are the ECG findings of hyperkalemia?

What are the usual causes of hyperkalemia?

DISCUSSION

A pulseless patient usually is assumed to be in ventricular fibrillation and greeted immediately with a very quick evaluation of the ABCs followed by cardiopulmonary resuscitation and a direct current shock of 200 watt seconds. This is done even before a diagnostic ECG. Occasionally, such a patient will be in severe shock, and there is indeed a possibility that a defibrillation will result in fibrillation rather than cure it. Even more rarely, as in this case, the pulseless patient will show evidence of adequate cardiac output (such as retaining consciousness), leading us to defer electroshock.

Extensive peripheral vascular disease in combination with hypotension and vasoconstriction may lead to poorly palpable pulses. Severe shock of any cause or a dissection of the aorta with or without aneurysm formation may also lead to poor peripheral perfusion without palpable pulses. Of course, if the patient is not awake, management proceeds according to Advanced Cardiac Life Support (ACLS) protocols depending on the presenting rhythm (i.e., ventricular fibrillation, asystole, and so forth).

Any adult patient with lower back pain, abdominal pain radiating to the back or groin, a pulsatile mass (particularly in the epigastrium), or shock must be suspected of having an abdominal aortic aneurysm. Chest pain of a tearing nature radiating to the back is typical of a dissecting thoracic aortic aneurysm. Signs include unequal pulses, neurologic dysfunction, hemothorax, and ECG changes. In this patient population, severe atherosclerosis may also affect the mesenteric vessels producing intestinal ischemia or infarction. Intestinal angina, a syndrome of abdominal pain following meals, is a warning sign of an impending mesenteric artery obstruction. The pain of a bowel infarction is usually out of proportion to the amount of tenderness found. The patient will complain of great pain but have an "unimpressive" abdominal exam, thus often deceiving the physician and delaying the diagnosis until it is too late.

Hyperkalemia, which was the diagnosis in this patient, usually first leads to peaked T waves and lengthening of the PR interval. More severe hyperkalemia may cause loss of P wave, widening of the QRS, and eventually a sine wave pattern easily mistaken for ventricular flutter or tachycardia. Hyperkalemia has two main causes: acidosis or uremia. This patient had renal failure, which led to both acidosis and uremia. Potassium therapy can of course worsen either of these.

REFERENCES

Review Article
Zull, D. N. Disorders of potassium metabolism. *Emerg. Med. Clin. North Am.* 1989;7:771–794.

Additional References

Lee, K. S., Powell, B. L., and Adams, P. L. Focal neurologic signs associated with hyperkalemia. *South. Med. J.* 1984;77:792–793.

Quick, G., and Bastani, B. Prolonged asystolic hyperkalemic cardiac arrest with no neurologic sequelae. *Ann. Emerg. Med.* 1994;24:305–311.

Zimmers, T., Brady, W., and DeBehnke, D. J. Cases in electrocardiography. *Am. J. Emerg. Med.* 1993;11:81–83.
Two cases of hyperkalemia.

Case 73: THREE DAYS OF COUGH/CYANOTIC

A 34-year-old man collapsed just outside the emergency department. His friend told of a three-day course of progressive cough and fatigue. The patient had been well previously and was not on any medication. He was hypotensive, grossly cyanotic, and had a sinus tachycardia of 140 beats per minute. His breathing was shallow at about 30 respirations per minute, and he had bilateral rales and rhonchi. His venous pressure was not elevated, and he had no edema. Oxygen therapy was begun but held to 4 liters per minute because the attending physician was concerned about the possible danger of high-flow oxygen. An arterial blood sample showed a pO_2 of 40 mm Hg that produced a saturation of less than 70%. A chest film showed multiple large infiltrates thought to be pneumonia. Increasing the nasal oxygen flow to 12 liters per minute raised the oxygen saturation to 80%.

How much oxygen should a patient be given?

When should intubation be performed?

DISCUSSION

This patient was in an advanced stage of acute respiratory failure. The early stages are characterized by dyspnea and an increase in the pulse, respiratory rate, and blood pressure. As the respirations become more labored, the partial pressure of carbon dioxide increases and the patient begins to tire. Soon the ventilations become more shallow, and the patient's mental status changes. Respiratory failure will then progress to unconsciousness and death if not immediately treated.

Assisting the patient's ventilations with a bag-valve-mask will do more than applying nasal oxygen. At 4 liters per minute, a nasal cannula will increase the inspired oxygen fraction by about 12 to 16%. Increasing the oxygen level to 12 liters per minute will only increase the oxygen by

Case 73 was adapted from Platt, F. W., Enough is not too much. *Emerg. Med.* 1972;4:46.

about 20%. A nonrebreather mask with 10 to 15 liters per minute oxygen flow would be more appropriate in this patient. This level of flow provides almost 100% oxygen concentration.

The critical factor in oxygen therapy is to give enough oxygen. Even though some patients with chronic obstructive lung disease cannot tolerate it without potentially life-threatening side effects, they need high-flow oxygen, perhaps with the use of a ventilator.

In adults, the only contraindication to high-flow oxygen therapy is in the subset of COPD patients who are CO_2 retainers. We give oxygen when it is desperately needed. If we do not know whether or not the patient is a CO_2 retainer, we watch the patient very closely for signs of respiratory depression. In some cases, a Venturi mask can fine-tune the amount of oxygen flow and help give the needed therapy while avoiding intubation. Oxygen therapy should never be withheld or kept to a low flow when the patient is dangerously hypoxic simply because the physician is afraid of giving too much oxygen.

In many situations, we see similar reluctance to give enough of an appropriate therapy. Patients in shock are given inadequate volumes of intravenous fluids; agitated withdrawing alcoholics are given too little sedation; patients in pain are given too little analgesia. Too much of a good thing may be bad, but too little can be too.

Intubation should be considered in any patient who is in imminent respiratory failure. Signs of this include evidence of overwhelming fatigue, falling blood pressure and pulse, and alterations in mental status. If these are present, the patient should be intubated. When these patients stop responding to spoken voice, our experience is that cardiac arrest occurs in about 1 minute. Adequate ventilation is the only preventative measure. Intubation can be done through the nose if the patient has a gag reflex and an adequate tidal volume; otherwise, it should be done orally.

REFERENCES

Review Article
Carden, D. L., and Smith, J. K. Pneumonias. *Emerg. Med. Clin. North Am.* 1989;7:255–278.
The entire volume 7 number 2 issue is devoted to adult respiratory emergencies.

Additional References

Brooks, K. R., et al. Acute respiratory failure due to *Pneumocystis carinii* pneumonia. *Crit. Care Clin.* 1993;9:31–48.

Ring, J. C., and Stidham, G. L. Novel therapies for acute respiratory failure. *Pediatr. Clin. North Am.* 1994;41:1325–1363.

Bezzant, T. B., and Mortensen, J. D. Risks and hazards of mechanical ventilation: A collective review of published literature. *Dis. Mon.* 1994;40:581–638.

Case 74 SEIZURE

A 40-year-old man was brought to the emergency department because he had been found lying on the street unconscious. Shortly after his arrival, he had a five-minute major motor seizure. He was lying on a cart in the hall while a room was being readied for him when he had the fit. He was observed by several patients as well as their relatives and friends, two persons from housekeeping, two clerks, a policeman, and a nurse. The consternation was considerable among this group. The nurse found a physician and urged him to give the patient an injection of 10 mg of Valium, which she handed him. The injection went in as the seizure was ending, to the great relief of the many observers. The patient was then given a brief physical examination that disclosed only stupor with no focal neurologic findings. He then was given 120 mg of phenobarbital intramuscularly. One hour later he was awake and alert enough to tell his story. He told of a seizure disorder of many years' standing but said he had recently stopped taking his usual phenytoin (Dilantin) to see what would happen.

If a patient has a seizure in the ED, how many has he probably already had that day?

How do seizure patients present in the ED, and how should they be treated?

Discussion

Usually, a seizure patient who has a fit in the ED is having the second one for that day—the first one brought him to the ED. Thus, therapy is usually but not always appropriate. Adult seizure patients arriving at the ED can usually be classified in four groups: (1) known seizure disorder, (2) alcoholic—withdrawal or "rum fits," (3) status—by definition: repeated seizures without awakening in the interim, and (4) first seizure. A blood sugar sample should always be obtained, as close to ictus as possible. In a person on medication, it is helpful to know his or her anticonvulsant drug levels.

1. *Known seizure disorder.* A person with a known seizure disorder may have a breakthrough in his or her control. This may be spontaneous, associated with drug juggling, or associated with alcohol intake, phenothiazines, or sleep deprivation. The therapeutic Dilantin level is 10 to 20 μg per ml (20 to 30 μg is associated with nystagmus; 30 to 40 μg with dysarthria and ataxia, i.e., "drunk-like state"; above 40 μg with drowsiness). A patient who ran out of medications a few days ago should be given a loading dose of his or her proper medications, either orally or intravenously.
2. *Alcoholic.* Withdrawal seizure may be associated with early alcohol withdrawal signs and symptoms, such as tremulousness, anxiety, fever, sweating, tachycardia, focal hallucinations, etc. It may occur while the patient is still drinking but tapering off. The term *rum fit* actually refers to withdrawal seizures and so is a misnomer. Alcohol withdrawal seizures tend to cluster over several hours. Other than protecting the airway and keeping these patients from hurting themselves on the stretcher, we do not specifically treat withdrawal seizures. A careful neurologic exam looking for signs of head trauma and lateralizing signs is essential in avoiding the pitfall of labeling an intoxicated patient with an epidural hematoma as a patient with simple alcohol withdrawal.
3. *Status.* This is a life-threatening disorder. Someone in a seizure can be first treated with intravenous diazepam (Valium) in 5- to 10-mg increments, but diazepam's two disadvantages are respiratory depression and recurrence of seizures within 30 minutes. Lorazepam (Ativan) in 2- to 4-mg increments up to 8 mg is as effective as diazepam in initial seizure treatment, lasts longer, and may cause less respiratory depression in young adults; but be prepared to intubate if respiratory depression occurs. The benzodiazepine is followed by thiamine and glucose (if not already given). The patient whose seizure continues must be loaded with Dilantin. We give 13 to 18 mg per kg intravenously at a maximum rate of 50 mg per minute (but preferably at 40 mg per minute) in normal saline, using an infusion pump and microfilter. The heart rhythm should be monitored during such an infusion. If the patient is awake and can wait several hours for a therapeutic blood level, it is safer and often more efficient to give the loading amount in one or two oral doses, but this is not an option

74. SEIZURE

in a patient who is still in status. One can always stop status with general anesthesia, usually barbiturates. We try phenobarbital 120 mg intravenously before calling anesthesiology.

4. *First seizure.* This is usually a good reason for admission and a full neurologic workup to determine the cause (toxic, metabolic, tumor, cardiovascular, subarachnoid hemorrhage, infection, etc.). A history is needed from observer and patient, first regarding warnings (aura). These can include visual hallucinations, olfactory hallucinations (funny or unpleasant smells), feeling of familiarity or strangeness, and sensations or jerking in limbs. Second, the history should include aspects of the seizure itself, such as lip-smacking, verbalization, head and eyes turning, focal limb-jerking, tongue-biting, incontinence, and generalized seizure. A postictal exam should be done. The sooner it is done the more likely it will be to disclose a deficit. Look for focal limb weakness, reflex asymmetry, unilateral Babinski's sign, dysphasic speech—in other words, any focal signs. The ED workup should include analysis of blood sugar, electrolytes, BUN, calcium, magnesium, ECG, and may also include toxicologic studies for agents such as cocaine, propoxyphene, and tricyclic antidepressants. A CT scan of the head is indicated for any patient with a first seizure (or if there is any lateralizing neurologic sign or if the patient is having seizures of unknown etiology or out of proportion to their prior pattern).

Pseudoseizures are a fairly common phenomena and sometimes are seen in known seizure patients. In a typical pseudoseizure, the tonic-colonic movement is asymmetric and there is no postictal somnolence. Pseudoseizure should be suspected if the patient blinks during the seizure when the eyelid is lightly touched or if the patient protects himself or herself from threats such as a hand approaching the face. Metabolic acidosis and elevation of creatine phosphokinase (CPK) enzymes, found after true seizures, are absent in pseudoseizures.

Finally, it should be said that the Valium given to this patient was probably unnecessary and unhelpful. His seizure was due to end shortly, and he was not in status epilepticus. The drug probably treated the onlookers' anxiety more than the patient's seizure disorder.

REFERENCES

Review Article

Engel, J., Jr., and Starkman, S. Overview of seizures. *Emerg. Med. Clin. North Am.* 1994;12:895–923.

The entire volume 12 number 4 issue is devoted to management of seizures in the emergency department.

Additional References

Turnbull, T. L., et al. Utility of laboratory studies in the emergency department patient with a new-onset seizure. *Ann. Emerg. Med.* 1990;19:373–377.

Pellegrino, T. R. An emergency department approach to first-time seizures. *Emerg. Med. Clin. North Am.* 1994;12:925–939.

Henneman, P. L., DeRoss, F., and Lewis, R. J. Determining the need for admission in patients with new onset seizures. *Ann. Emerg. Med.* 1994;24:1108–1114.

Jagoda, A., and Riggio, S. Psychogenic convulsive seizures. *Am. J. Emerg. Med.* 1993;11:626–632.

Case 75 MONEY TROUBLES

A 27-year-old man came to a community hospital emergency room at 11 P.M. on a Saturday evening. He told the reception clerk that he was having trouble catching his breath, that he was a patient in a local health maintenance organization (HMO), and that his primary doctor was Dr. A. The clerk asked him to sit in the lobby until she could contact his primary doctor for permission to treat him. If permission could not be obtained, she added, the HMO would not pay for his visit, and he would have to pay for it himself. He agreed and settled in to read old magazines. The clerk called Dr. A, reaching his answering service operator who promised to contact him. Sure enough, in a few minutes the operator had found Dr. A at home asleep in bed, and he returned the call to the emergency department. The admission clerk explained her problem, and, when the doctor asked for an initial appraisal of the patient's condition, the clerk said that she was not allowed to give one and that there was no available triage nurse at that time of the day. "Would Dr. A like the staff ED doctor to see his patient?" Dr. A agreed and asked that the staff doctor call him at home when he or she had finished evaluating the patient.

Three hours later, Dr. A was awakened by the emergency physician, who told him that his patient seemed to have a case of bronchitis and was being sent home to use a bronchodilator and antibiotics. The patient's examination had shown normal vital signs and diffuse pulmonary rhonchi. The arterial blood gases, chest x-ray, cardiogram, CBC, and biochemical survey had been normal. A sputum culture and blood cultures were cooking in the lab. Dr. A groggily agreed with the therapy and suggested that his patient be instructed to check back with him in a few days—sooner if he did not feel better quickly.

Four days later, the patient called Dr. A's office to say that he felt fine and would finish his prescriptions.

Three weeks later, Dr. A received a letter from the HMO office asking him why he had authorized such an expensive emergency visit and included a copy of the hospital bill totaling $937.00. The HMO reminded Dr. A that his office visits, currently being reimbursed at a rate of 65% of his usual charges, would suffer further payment cuts because of his excessive utilization of expensive consultant and emergency services. Dr. A called the emergency department administrator and complained of the charges. The hospital administrator explained that Dr. A was free to come in to the emergency room to see his own patients whenever he wanted to; if he chose not to, he had to accept what seemed best in the mind of the ED doctor, who, of course, did not benefit from "a better prior knowledge of the patients." Dr. A was not appeased. He called the ED doctor and berated him for excessive testing.

Dr. A felt misused and misunderstood. He was angered and humiliated. The ED doctor felt unappreciated and misunderstood. He was angry and vowed to let Dr. A "do his own dirty work in the future." The hospital ED administrator's opinion that the staff doctors "found it easy to stay home in bed and let our ED people take care of their patients and then complain afterwards, no matter what we do" was reinforced. The HMO administrators, knowing that their plan was hovering on the brink of bankruptcy, worried and fretted. The patient was unaware of all the consternation his evening visit to the ED had led to.

What is to be done?

Do you know what your hospital charges for an ABG? For a chest x-ray?

How do you feel about this statement: "Emergency department physicians must be extra careful. Many of the tests and procedures they do are important to guard against later malpractice suits."

DISCUSSION

There may not be easy answers for this kind of puzzle. We like to think of medical care as being outside usual economic considerations; that is, we like to worry not about how much it will cost but about whether it will help our patient to do it. That view of medicine—that you do what is best for the patient, disregarding cost—is common to perhaps no other activity in our lives. Some think that "National Defense" (i.e., spending on weapon systems and military activities) is the only other area that seems to escape economic scrutiny to a similar extent. But even medicine is becoming an object of cost analysis, and surely it must be.

75. MONEY TROUBLES

Resources are not unlimited. We must decide, as a society, where we want to spend our money.

For an individual physician, the problem is even more difficult; however, it must be addressed. The ED doctor cannot take refuge behind beliefs such as, "I don't know this patient's background, so I have to do everything." In this case, he could have called the primary physician during his evaluative process, instead of waiting until the end of the event. Nor can he hide behind ignorance of his hospital charges. And the primary physician must be a bit more willing to get up and go into the hospital if he cannot depend on the ED team to be parsimonious as well as precise. Surely the HMO cannot continue to accept outrageous hospital charges. As this physician estimated, the patient would have been well served to come to his office for a $50 visit and a $10 gram stain with the same outcome. If his primary care internist had seen the patient in the ED, the fee for use of the examination room would have led to a bill of about $200. A doctor who purports to be expert at emergency medicine should not routinely have to rely on four times the normal testing process to make good clinical decisions.

Our emergency department currently charges $70 for a visit like the one in this case. The hospital charges $97 for an arterial blood gas determination and $158 for a chest x-ray, and the radiologists add $25 to read the films the next day. Our ED doctor charge, which is independent of the hospital charge, is $100 for this sort of examination. The actual collection rate averages 50% of the above amounts. Hospitals vary in charges, and you should learn your own hospital's fees.

Arterial blood gases are usually not necessary in the patient who is not in acute respiratory distress and in whom pulmonary embolism is not a consideration. Other lab tests are equally useless in evaluation of these patients in the ED. Non-invasive fingertip pulse oximetry is a good screening for occult hypoxia if one is needed.

Malpractice defense is said to be rooted in a good doctor-patient relationship. Unfortunately, the emergency department physician usually lacks prior relationship with the patient and may be more vulnerable. However, if the relationship is of the essence, there is no reason why the ED doctor should not perform in a way that truly tries to satisfy his or her new patient. The ED doctor should be polite, be courteous, listen well, and explain well. Patients often complain that their doctors do not listen to them, and, when the interactions are studied, that is, in fact, what is observed. Your best protection against future suits is a gentle and humane style in communicating with the patient. This, of course, will not make you invulnerable, but it is better than over-testing.

REFERENCES

Review Texts

Congressional Budget Office. *Economic Implications of Rising Health Care Costs*. Washington, D.C.: U.S. Government Printing Office, 1992.
Free copy available through your member of Congress.

Cantrill, S. V., and Karas, S. *Cost-Effective Diagnostic Testing in Emergency Medicine*. Dallas: American College of Emergency Physicians, 1994.

Additional References

Fletcher, C. Listening and talking to patients. *Br. Med. J.* 1980;281:845–847, 931–933, 994–996, 1056–1058.

Platt, F. W., and McMath, J. Clinical hypocompetence: The interview. *Ann. Intern. Med.* 1981;94:405–409.

Rosensweig, S. Emergency rapport. *J. Emerg. Med.* 1993;11:775–778.

Case 76 FLANK PAIN

A 27-year-old man was brought to the emergency department by a good friend of his who was a third-year medical student. The patient had been well until two hours previously, when he was suddenly seized by severe pain in his left flank. He said that the pain was the worst he had ever experienced, that it came and went, and that he felt weak and nauseated when the pain was present. On his arrival at the ED, the pain had been absent for over 30 minutes, and he felt a bit embarrassed at being there. His friend had already done a urinalysis and reported seeing many white blood cells and bacteria in the urine. The patient was afebrile, and his physical examination revealed nothing noteworthy. His friend thought that the diagnosis was pyelonephritis and that antibiotics were indicated. However, review of the urinalysis by a staff physician showed red blood cells instead of white blood cells.

What is the diagnosis in this case?

Why the confusion in doing the urinalysis?

What should be done for this patient?

Discussion

This patient probably had ureteral colic. The story of sudden, varying, severe flank pain associated with hematuria suggests the presence of a stone in the ureter. Otherwise well persons may have episodes of ureteral colic which usually involve severe pain. The pain may be flank, groin, scrotal, or a combination of these. A woman may complain of vulva or vaginal pain. There is usually vesicle irritability with dysuria and frequency of urination when the stone is entering the bladder. This patient probably has passed the stone into his bladder at this time. Occasionally a kidney or ureteral stone will present with abdominal or back pain, and the diagnosis may be hard to make in the 10 to 15% of cases in which RBCs are not present in the urine.

Mistaking red blood cells for white is not an uncommon error for a neophyte to make while examining an unstained urine sediment. The identification of bacteria is almost impossible in an unstained sediment. Dust, debris, and amorphous crystals commonly oscillate in Brownian movement and simulate bacteria. Only a gram stain, or better still a urine culture, will identify bacteriuria. Of course, obstructive urinary disease and infective urinary disease are closely associated. Significant bacteriuria may be present in both, and a urine culture would be appropriate.

If the patient is in severe pain, we start an intravenous line, give several hundred ml of fluids and intravenous morphine or ketorolac (Toradol) for pain. We obtain a BUN or creatinine, and, if that is normal, we often get an intravenous pyelogram (IVP). If the patient has fever or chills, extravasation of dye, a stone over 6 mm in diameter in the renal pelvis, or a nonfunctioning (totally obstructed) kidney, we usually admit him or her to the hospital. If pain control is adequate and the stone looks small enough to pass, the patient can be discharged. If the patient is sent home, we give him or her a strainer with instructions to strain the urine as we have been doing in the ED. Follow-up is usually with the primary doctor or a urologist and within a week.

It is often helpful to give patients the discharge instructions in the presence of the people who brought them in. Patients frequently forget much of what is told to them in the course of treatment. We always give patients a discharge instruction sheet written in plain English (not "Medicalese") that explains the medications to be taken, possible side effects, and a referral for follow-up care. We also list the danger signs that would signal worsening of their condition and require them to come to the ED—in this case, any fever, chills, or increasing pain not relieved by oral analgesics.

This patient had an IVP that was normal except for slight dilation of the collecting system on the left. His friend became very upset when he heard that no antibiotics were to be given. When they left, the patient was reassured and his friend very anxious.

REFERENCES

Review Article
Peterson, N. E. Common urologic emergencies: A logical and practical approach to rapid diagnosis and treatment. *Acad. Emerg. Med.* 1994;1:186–189.

Additional References

Zangerle, K. F., et al. Usefulness of abdominal flat plate radiographs in patients with suspected uretheral calculi. *Ann. Emerg. Med.* 1985; 14:316–319.

Yealy, D. Acute pain management. *Acad. Emerg. Med.* 1994;1:186–189.

Cordell, W. H., et al. Indomethacin suppositories versus intravenously titrated morphine sulfate for the treatment of ureteral colic. *Ann. Emerg. Med.* 1994;23:262–269.

Case 77 TRICYCLIC ANTIDEPRESSANT OVERDOSE

On a Tuesday, a 23-year-old woman was brought in by a local rescue squad because of an alleged tricyclic antidepressant (TCA) overdose. The patient had been treated with imipramine one year previously. The rescue squad said that on their last shift, which was on Monday, they were called to the same woman because of a possible overdose, but she was acting normally and had no signs of any problem. She told them that she had taken her normal dose of medication, did not feel depressed, and wanted no further treatment. In fact, she said she felt so good that she now could easily see how to "solve all of her problems." Her parents, who were on the scene, told the paramedic that she was looking and acting better than she had in years, and they supported their daughter in refusing treatment. At the Monday call, the paramedics allowed her to sign a form stating she was requesting to be discharged AMA. The next morning her parents found her very drowsy in bed. Her medications were all missing. The rescue squad was called in and initiated an intravenous line and gave her 30 ml of ipecac. She did not vomit en route to the hospital.

On admission to the emergency department, she could be easily aroused but spoke with slurred speech. Her blood pressure was 100/60, pulse 124, and respirations 14. Her pupils were large and reactive, lungs were clear, heart sounds normal, and abdomen benign. Her deep tendon reflexes were depressed. She stated that she had taken all her pills about an hour previously and wanted to die.

The patient was initially uncooperative with therapy. Immediate gastric lavage was begun using a 36 French orogastric tube. Lavage continued for 30 minutes until the fluid return was clear. Fifty grams of activated charcoal was then placed down the tube.

At this point, her blood pressure dropped to 80/60 and frequent premature ventricular contractions (PVCs) were seen on the monitor. A 12-lead ECG showed a widened QRS of 0.14 seconds. She was given 100 mEq of $NaHCO_3$ and a liter of 0.5 normal saline over 30 minutes. This corrected the hypotension and the PVCs, and her QRS complex duration dropped to 0.12 seconds.

77. TRICYCLIC ANTIDEPRESSANT OVERDOSE

On the way to the intensive care unit, the patient became agitated. She tried to jump off the stretcher and required physical restraints. Physostigmine (1 mg) was given very slowly, and within a minute she began to calm but then had a sudden grand mal seizure and became asystolic. Full resuscitative efforts were unable to reverse this, and she was pronounced dead one hour after her cardiac arrest.

Should a patient be tied down and treated despite his or her refusal to give consent for such therapy?

What is the best initial treatment to empty the stomach in cases of massive overdose?

What went wrong here?

Discussion

Reasonable therapeutic restraint is always proper in emergency medicine. This includes the prehospital care given to any patient. The EMTs on the scene cannot simply allow a patient to refuse medical treatment (sign out AMA). If a patient with any but the most minor illness or injury wishes to sign out AMA, the EMTs should contact a medical control authority for assistance.

An AMA form is a potentially dangerous thing in an ED. It often allows poor therapy to be excused. A patient who refuses care for minor problems should have the refusal noted on his or her chart with a clear statement of the patient's mental status and the explanation that was given to him or her. If the possibility of a true emergency exists, however, then a complete, formal refusal should be documented. Even when we strongly disagree with their decision, patients may refuse care if they have the capacity to understand the risks and benefits associated with the refusal. They must have a "normal mental status," and this requirement excludes anyone clearly under the influence of alcohol or other drugs. If the patient seems to have the capacity to understand, and yet they still refuse a potentially lifesaving procedure or a necessary admission, we ask how the refusal fits into his or her lifestyle. Unless a satisfactory answer is obtained, the patient cannot sign out AMA. In these cases a psychiatrist should be called to help assess the "capacity" of the patient. The psychiatrist cannot assess "competency," which is a legal term. If the patient is found to lack capacity, he or she should be restrained and treated. Most patients become cooperative when they realize that we will not take no for an answer. Alternatively, a family member or friend can often talk the patient into accepting at least some of the treatment.

This patient's refusal to accept treatment the first time she was seen by the paramedics suggests that she had formulated a plan to kill herself. Any depressed patients who suddenly state that they are fine and have no further problems should be considered a high suicide risk.

A major evolving issue in the treatment of the overdose patient is how to empty the stomach. Syrup of ipecac is commonly used to induce emesis but can be dangerous. It should not be used in ingestions of severe caustics (acid or alkali), low-viscosity hydrocarbons (like gasoline), or in any patient who may develop a significantly depressed mental status. Finally, it must not be used when *rapid* gastric emptying is essential, as in TCA overdose.

A large-bore Ewald-type stomach tube can be used for gastric lavage; although, if the patient has an inadequate gag reflex or is lethargic, the airway needs to be protected first (i.e., intubate the patient before placing the Ewald tube). At least 2000 ml of water should be used in the lavage attempt. We fill and empty the stomach repeatedly with 400-ml amounts of saline or tap water. A small-bore nasogastric tube is of very little value in lavage, as it will not easily return pill fragments.

Possibly even more valuable than lavage is the administration of a slurry of charcoal. If both ipecac and charcoal are used, the charcoal must be held until vomiting has stopped. Charcoal is often mixed with a cathartic in order to further decrease absorption of the ingested drug.

Some potentially severe overdoses will show an initial lack of worrisome symptoms. This is the case with acetaminophen overdoses, which can produce a fatal hepatotoxicity that will manifest itself days after the asymptomatic overdose. The other drug overdoses we most often see underappreciated in our ED are the TCA overdoses, which may well present with a conscious patient and yet lead to fatal arrhythmias an hour after ingestion.

TCA overdoses are common. These drugs have strong anticholinergic properties, have quinidine-like membrane stabilizing effects on cardiac cells, and block the reuptake of norepinephrine. Clinically, the patient with TCA overdose may present with altered mental status, seizures, coma, hypotension, impaired cardiac conduction, supraventricular and ventricular arrhythmias, and respiratory depression.

Physostigmine is an antidote for the anticholinergic toxicity, but it should not be used in TCA overdose. Its effects are very short-lived, and studies have shown asystole, ventricular arrhythmias, and seizures in patients given this agent. The two most useful agents in treating TCA overdoses are activated charcoal and sodium bicarbonate. Repeated doses of activated charcoal have been shown to be effective in removing many toxins from circulation, including TCAs.

Sodium bicarbonate is extremely important in treating these patients and should be given intravenously until the arterial pH is 7.5. At this point approximately 98% of the tricyclic is protein bound, making it unavailable to tissues and hence limiting its potential for toxicity.

The toxic drug ingested by this patient was fairly clear. When a patient with an overdose of unknown substances presents, he or she should be evaluated for the presence of a recognizable toxidrome. Some of the more common and characteristic ones are:

1. *Anticholinergic*—hot flushed skin, tachycardia, dry mucous membranes, mydriasis, and altered mental status ("hot as a pistol, red as a beet, dry as a bone, blind as a bat, and mad as a hatter").
2. *Cholinergic*—SLUDGE syndrome (Salivation, Lacrimation, Urination, Defecation, Gastrointestinal hypermotility, and Emesis), bradycardia, miosis, wheezing, and respiratory distress.
3. *Sympathomimetic*—hypertension, anxiety, tachycardia, and mydriasis.
4. *Narcotic*—miosis and central nervous system depression, including respiratory depression.
5. *Sedative/Hypnotic*—central nervous system depression, including respiratory depression, with variable pupillary size.

Other poisons may turn up on laboratory analysis. Arterial blood gases clarify the patient's state of oxygenation, and acid-base status. Metabolic acidosis is seen in carbon monoxide and cyanide poisoning, as well as in some alcohol poisonings. The serum osmolality will detect the presence of all of the alcohols. The electrolytes will detect an anion gap. Acetaminophen levels must be measured specifically, because this drug cannot be detected by clinical or other laboratory means.

Poison control centers are a vital resource and provide first-aid telephone advice to the general public and more detailed information to inquiring medical personnel. Ideally, the phones are staffed by pharmacists, doctors of pharmacology, and physicians, with a toxicologist available. As the initial reference, many EDs use the Poisindex system. It is an expensive but reliable microfiche system published by the Rocky Mountain Poison Center and updated quarterly.

REFERENCES

Review Articles
Pimentel, L., and Trommer, L. Cyclic antidepressant overdoses. A review. *Emerg. Med. Clin. North Am.* 1994;12:533–547.

Mayer, D. Refusal of care and discharging 'difficult' patients from the emergency department. *Ann. Emerg. Med.* 1990;19:1436–1446.

Additional References
Wolfe, T. R., Caravati, E. M., and Rollins, D. E. Terminal 40m sec frontal plane QRS axis as a marker for tricyclic antidepressant overdose. *Ann. Emerg. Med.* 1989;18:348–351.

Buzan, R. D., and Weissberg, M. P. Suicide: Risk factors and therapeutic considerations in the emergency department. *J. Emerg. Med.* 1992;10:335–343.

Newton, E. H., Shih, R. D., and Hoffman, R. S. Cyclic antidepressant overdose: A review of current management strategies. *Am. J. Emerg. Med.* 1994;12:376–379.

Poisindex System available through Micromedex, Inc., 6200 South Syracuse Way, Englewood, Colorado 80111-4740.

Thibalt, G. E. The landlady confirms the diagnosis. *N. Engl. J. Med.* 1992;326:1272–1275.

Young, W. F., and Blivens, H. G. Evaluation of gastric emptying using radionuclides: Gastric lavage versus ipecac-induced emesis. *Ann. Emerg. Med.* 1993;22:1423–1427.

Case 78 ACTING WEIRD

A distraught mother called her family physician because her 18-year-old daughter was acting strangely. She said that her daughter thought everything was funny and at the same time could not remember anything. At first the mother thought this was a part of an adolescent mood swing, but a few hours after the onset of this behavior she decided to have the young woman checked. Because it was after office hours, the family doctor asked her to bring the daughter to the emergency department and explained that he would examine her there.

On arrival at the ED, the girl was indeed acting unusually, even for an adolescent. She thought that everything was funny and laughed in response to being questioned. When asked how old she was, she stated it was summer. Her past history was unremarkable, but her mother remembered that the girl had complained of a "cold" several weeks before. Physical examination was completely normal except for the mental status examination. The girl was not oriented to time or place. She was unable or unwilling to count backward from 100 by sevens, to interpret proverbs, or to respond to questions about how she was feeling. A complete blood count, routine blood chemistries, and a toxicology screen were drawn and sent to the lab for analysis. A lumbar puncture was performed. All these tests were negative. A neurologic consultant called into the case suggested liver function studies be done in order to test for the presence of a hepatic encephalopathy. Liver enzymes were elevated, as was her serum ammonia level. The patient was transferred by helicopter to a tertiary care center, where a diagnosis of Reye's syndrome was made. She recovered with only a mild memory deficit.

What is Reye's syndrome?

What is the hallmark of an acute metabolic encephalopathy?

What is the role of the family doctor in the ED?

Discussion

Reye's syndrome is a form of hepatic encephalopathy associated with viral illnesses, most commonly varicella and influenza B. This syndrome is strongly associated with aspirin use during the viral illness. The syndrome is most common in young children but can also be seen in adolescents and young adults. The oldest reported case was 63 years old. The initial symptoms are usually vomiting and altered behavior progressing to stupor and coma. In severe cases there is increased intracranial pressure. Treatment is supportive, and, with good intensive care, the prognosis is usually good. Residual neurologic sequelae are common but mild. The diagnosis is made in patients with an acute encephalopathy who have elevated liver function tests and an otherwise negative workup.

This patient presented with an acute alteration of her mental status. A common pitfall in the assessment of these patients is the assumption that because the patient is alert and just acting "weird," he or she probably has an acute psychosis or is under the influence of drugs. Delirium, an agitated and confused state, is the hallmark of the patient with an acute organic brain syndrome. To assess brain function, the physician must make a careful neurologic and mental status examination. A few simple questions will elicit indications of the more urgent problems: Does the patient respond to me? Is the patient awake? Does the patient know where he or she is, how far he or she is from home, what day it is, and about what time of the day it is? Is the patient responding appropriately to my presence, or is he or she struggling with and hostile to someone who is here to help? If the patient is confused, hostile, or asleep and not easily roused to full alertness, then he or she may have a life-threatening emergency.

The immediate workup of a patient with acute organic brain syndrome includes a CBC, glucose, urea nitrogen, electrolytes, serum osmolarity, and arterial blood gases. These can be followed by chest x-ray, ECG, CT scan of the brain, and lumbar puncture. A toxicologic screen may be helpful later in the patient's course but is often not available in the immediate treatment phase. If all these are negative, one must look for even more unusual causes.

Physicians in the community will often bring their patients to the ED for an evaluation after hours. In some cases the patient evaluation will be done in the ED by the family physician. This is quite appropriate, because the family physician knows the patient well. The emergency physician may function as an informal consultant in this setting. More often, the patient is instructed to come to the ED for an evaluation by the ED staff. The family physician will usually call ahead, notify the ED physician of the patient's arrival, and discuss the patient's past medical history and current situation with the ED physician. In this setting, as in others, two heads are often better than one.

REFERENCES

Review Article
Lovejoy, F. H., et al. Clinical staging and Reye syndrome. *Am. J. Dis. Child.* 1974;128:36–41.

Additional References
Reye, R. D. K., Morgan, G., and Baral, J. Encephalopathy and fatty degeneration of the viscera: A disease entity in childhood. *Lancet* 1963;2:749–752.

Henretig, F. M. Special considerations in the poisoned pediatric patient. *Emerg. Med. Clin. North Am.* 1994;12:549–567.

Quam, D. A. Recognizing a case of Reye's syndrome. *Am. Fam. Physician* 1994;50(7):1491–1496.

Case 79 DIARRHEA

A 26-year-old man arrived in the emergency department complaining of diarrhea and crampy abdominal pain. The illness had begun suddenly three days previously and was accompanied by two episodes of vomiting, slight nausea, and anorexia. He complained of eight to ten watery, foul-smelling bowel movements a day and said that he had to get up several times at night. This day he felt a bit weak and light-headed, especially when he rose quickly. His girlfriend had similar complaints, and her symptoms, although not as severe, had been present for about ten days. His past medical history was unremarkable, he was taking no medications, and he had no allergies. There was an epidemic of giardiasis in his town.

On examination he appeared in no distress and was afebrile, with a supine blood pressure of 120/76, pulse of 84, and respiratory rate of 20. Abdominal examination showed slight tenderness in the periumbilical area and slightly increased bowel sounds. Rectal examination was nontender, but the stool was trace positive for occult blood. When the patient stood up his blood pressure dropped to 104/64 and his pulse went to 112.

He was given 2 liters of normal saline intravenously over the next 2 hours. He was also given an injection of dimenhydrinate (Dramamine). Following this he was drowsy but otherwise felt better. He no longer had a drop in blood pressure when he stood up. A spun hematocrit was 43 initially and dropped to 40 after hydration. A stool sample was obtained for ova and parasites, and the patient was discharged with a prescription for oral metronidazole and a warning to avoid alcohol while taking that medication. He was to take only clear liquids for the first 24 hours and was to take Kaopectate for the diarrhea. It was also recommended that his girlfriend have a stool sample sent for ova and parasites.

What are the common causes of acute diarrhea?

How should diarrhea be worked up in the ED?

How should dehydration be treated in the ED?

DISCUSSION

Giardiasis is not the most common cause of acute infectious diarrhea, but it appears in local epidemic outbreaks. The classic presentation of *Giardia lamblia* infection includes crampy abdominal pain with watery, foul-smelling diarrhea. Nausea and vomiting are occasionally found but are not the prominent symptoms. Diagnosis by stool examination for ova and parasites is fairly accurate in the acute phase but less accurate as the infection becomes chronic.

The most common causes of acute diarrhea in adults are food poisoning and viral gastroenteritis. Food poisoning, usually caused by staphylococcal toxin, occurs within 4 hours of ingestion of spoiled food. Abdominal pain, vomiting, and diarrhea are usually severe, but the illness is self-limiting, lasting from 8 to 12 hours. Viral gastroenteritis also presents with the triad of abdominal pain, vomiting, and diarrhea but lasts longer. Clustering of cases in the home is common in both diseases. The abdominal examination is variable and frequently changes over the course of a brief observation period in the ED. Acute bacterial enteritis and pseudomembranous enterocolitis are serious but less common causes that must be considered. Bacterial enteritis should be suspected in any patient who appears toxic. Unfortunately, many stool samples may have to be cultured before the physician gets a diagnostic answer, even for a very sick patient with *Shigella, Campylobacter,* or *Salmonella* enteritis. Pseudomembranous enterocolitis is suspected in any patient who was recently on antibiotics. The physician should look for *Clostridium difficile* toxin in the stool sample.

Most physicians are unsure of what laboratory tests to order in the workup on these patients. Too much testing is more common than too little. A complete blood count will not differentiate viral from bacterial causes of diarrhea. Electrolyte panels are seldom helpful in young, healthy persons. We only check electrolytes on patients who have had serious vomiting or diarrhea over several days, are infants or elderly, are taking diuretics, or who have remarkably abnormal vital signs. It may help to stain the stool for white cells, a sign of bacterial diarrhea which is rarely seen in food poisoning or viral gastroenteritis.

An important examination in any patient with severe diarrhea is to check the vital signs for orthostatic changes. No one is exactly sure what degree of pressure change on rising from supine to standing is "signifi-

79. DIARRHEA

cant." Some emergency medicine experts accept a drop of 20 mm Hg in the systolic pressure or a rise of 20 beats per minute in the pulse as suggestive of significant dehydration. We try to estimate the "mean" arterial pressure by adding one-third of the pulse pressure to the diastolic reading. We consider a drop of 10 mm Hg of the mean pressure to be a worrisome fall and one of 20 mm Hg as quite likely to cause serious symptoms.

When the dehydration is thought to be significant, we start to treat these patients with intravenous 5% dextrose/0.5 normal saline, and most of them feel better after a liter is given. Medications to stop the vomiting and decrease gastrointestinal hypermotility include dimenhydrinate and prochlorperazine (Compazine). The latter will rarely produce acute dystonic reactions but may worsen hypotension. Diarrhea should not be treated with opiates or other potent antidiarrheal agents because these can increase mucosal invasion in bacterial diarrhea. Antibiotics are usually reserved for cases of *Shigella* or *Campylobacter*.

Oral rehydration is begun with clear liquids (water, flat ginger ale or other clear sodas, Jello, and clear broth) and advanced gradually to a BRAT (Bananas, Rice or rice cereal, Applesauce, and dry Toast) diet when the vomiting has ceased. We recommend that no dairy products be consumed for a week after the diarrhea ceases, because there is frequently some residual lactose intolerance.

Infants and young children who dehydrate with diarrhea may do so more quickly than adults because of their smaller fluid reserves. Children who have dry mucous membranes and a somewhat less than usual volume of dark-colored urine are clinically judged to be 5% dehydrated and need volume replacement. Those with lethargy, shrunken fontanelles, tenting of the skin, parched mucous membranes, and little or no urine output are estimated to be 10% or more clinically dehydrated and require intravenous hydration. We usually begin with a bolus of 10 to 20 ml per kg of 5% dextrose/$\frac{1}{3}$ normal saline over the first hour while laboratory studies are pending.

REFERENCES

Review Article
Panosian, C. B. Parasitic diarrhea. *Emerg. Med. Clin. North Am.* 1991;9:337–356.

Additional References
Fairchild, P. G., and Blacklow, N. R. Viral diarrhea. *Emerg. Med. Clin. North Am.* 1991;9:357–364.

Goodman, L. Evaluation of an outbreak of food borne illness initiated in the emergency department. *Ann. Emerg. Med.* 1993;22:1291–1294.

Farmer, R. G. Infectious causes of diarrhea in the differential diagnosis of inflammatory bowel disease. *Med. Clin. North Am.* 1990;74:29–38.

American Academy of Pediatrics Committee on Nutrition. Use of oral fluid therapy and posttreatment feeding following enteritis in children in a developed country. *Pediatrics* 1985;75:358–360.

Case 80 SYNCOPE

A woman was brought to the emergency department by ambulance after she fainted at home. She had been standing at the sink and helping her daughter dry the dinner dishes, when she slumped to the floor and was unconscious for a minute or two. There were no seizure movements and no incontinence, and she was feeling much better when the paramedics arrived.

On arrival at the ED, she said that she was "as well as one could be for 76 years." She denied smoking or drinking and said that she took only the Aldomet and digoxin her physician prescribed. She had never fainted before and had been feeling well earlier in the day. The examining doctor found that she had a pulse of 74 and a blood pressure of 134/80. He found nothing remarkable in his examination of her heart, lungs, and abdomen and no lateralizing neurologic findings.

Because it was her first faint, the doctor obtained some laboratory studies. A chest x-ray showed slightly increased interstitial markings. A cardiogram showed sinus rhythm with normal intervals but demonstrated ST sagging and T-wave flattening across the precordium. Her electrolytes and BUN were normal as were her CBC and urinalysis. Because of the T-wave abnormalities, the doctor wondered about a pulmonary embolism and obtained an emergency perfusion-ventilation lung scan that was interpreted by the radiologist on call as "low probability of pulmonary embolism, although not entirely normal."

The patient insisted that she felt well and wanted to go home. Accordingly, she was discharged to be taken home by her daughter, who was much reassured by all the normal test results but a little worried about the T waves and the "not quite normal lung scan."

The next day, while getting dressed to go shopping, the patient fainted again. This time she awoke unattended on the floor. She called her daughter and asked to be taken to her usual doctor. He found her blood pressure acceptable in the supine or seated position but 80/50 when she stood up. He gave her a liter of saline intravenously in his office, recommended drinking more water and salting her food liberally for a few days and stopped her alpha-methyldopa. She did well with his therapy.

The following week she received a bill for $780 for the ED treatment.

What are the essentials of an ED evaluation for fainting?

What was left out in this case?

Discussion

Fainting is common. The physician's first task is to distinguish a seizure from a faint and then to look for causes of syncope. In an elderly woman, one must worry about causes for decreased brain blood flow, most of which are to be found in the heart and blood vessels rather than in the brain. Surely a careful cardiovascular examination is necessary, and nothing can replace a careful examination of vital signs including an observation of the effect of sitting up and then standing. This patient was examined entirely in the supine position. Even her history cried out for a standing evaluation since she was standing when she fainted.

Postural drops in blood pressure can be caused by many drugs but are usually caused by direct vasodilators (e.g., nitrates, calcium channel blockers, phenothiazines, narcotics, and hydralazine and other alpha blockers), diuretics, or those that prevent the usual cardiac response to hypotension (beta blockers.) Of course any drug used to decrease blood pressure may do its job too well and produce hypotension.

If you are unable to document postural hypotension, your attention should turn to cardiac arrhythmias as the next most common cause of syncope in the elderly. Bradycardias, heart block, and rapid tachycardias can all cause syncope. In fact, because the first visit to the ED failed to reveal a clear cause for this patient's syncope, it would have been reasonable to admit her to the hospital and place her on a cardiac monitor. An arrhythmia may have been missed.

It is embarrassing when a simple maneuver like taking the blood pressure is found to be more useful than all the technology we are so proud of. Postural blood pressure readings cost considerably less than this patient's visit to our ED. She had reason to be puzzled and even distressed about our failure to diagnose her problem.

REFERENCES

Review Article
Kapoor, W. N. Evaluation and management of the patient with syncope. *J.A.M.A.* 1992;268:2553–2560.

Additional References
Silverstein, M. D., et al. Patients with syncope admitted to medical intensive care units. *J.A.M.A.* 1982;248:1185–1189.

Witting, M. D., Wears, R. L., and Li, S. Defining the tilt test: A study of healthy adults with moderate blood loss. *Ann. Emerg. Med.* 1994;23:1320–1323.

Case 81 RESPIRATORY INFECTION

A 26-year-old man came to the emergency department complaining of a cold. He thought that a shot of penicillin would clear him up. He claimed to have a cough productive of about one shotglass (2 ounces) of green-yellow sputum a day for the past week. The cough was associated with a ripping substernal pain that made the patient feel like he was "coming apart with the cough." He smoked about one-and-a-half packs of cigarettes a day but commented that he seldom finished a cigarette and that his friends bummed many cigarettes from him, contributing to that total. In describing his smoking, he said that he smoked "not too much." He also complained of a stuffy head but denied earache, ear drainage, or severe headaches. He noted mild hoarseness. He thought that he did not have a problem with shortness of breath but that recently any activity was causing coughing spells that were hard to stop. Deep breathing also provoked these spells, and the coughing frequently led to retching. He denied any drug allergies.

On physical exam, the patient had a temperature of 37.5°C orally, a respiratory rate of 18, a pulse of 94, and a blood pressure of 130/84 in the right arm when seated. His pharynx was a bit red. His tympanic membranes were normal. He had no tenderness over the maxillary sinuses or under the supraorbital ridge. His voice was slightly rough, and he sniffled frequently. As he took a deep breath, a vibratory sensation was palpable bilaterally over the middle ribs laterally. With a stethoscope, coarse rhonchi were audible. When asked to cough, he produced a few milliliters of yellow sputum.

What is a "cold?"

What does this patient have?

How would you treat this patient?

Discussion

The popular term *cold* has no exact medical significance but usually is equated with a viral upper respiratory infection. "Upper respiratory" is usually taken to mean bronchi and above, leaving the bronchioles and lungs to the "lower respiratory" system. Thus, upper respiratory symptoms include headache, earache, ear drainage, tinnitus, rhinorrhea, stuffy head, sore throat, pain on swallowing, swollen cervical nodes, loss of voice, and cough. Lower respiratory symptoms are chiefly three: cough, shortness of breath, and lateralized, pleuritic chest pain. Upper respiratory infections are either viral or bacterial. In adults, penicillin generally is good therapy if a strep throat is diagnosed; otherwise, no antibiotic is needed unless a septic focus (e.g., otitis media or acute sinusitis) is found. We then use amoxicillin, because other organisms such as haemophilus and neisseria species are often seen as well.

Severe hoarseness to the point of aphonia, severe dysphagia, or both may be the presentation of acute epiglottitis in an adult. This is a rare bacterial upper respiratory infection and deserves hospitalization and immediate ENT consultation. Trying to visualize the posterior pharynx or epiglottis in an epiglottitis patient can be a fatal error if one is not prepared, with equipment at hand, to do an emergency intubation or cricothyrotomy.

In this patient a chest x-ray may reveal bronchopneumonia but will probably be normal. The diagnosis is bronchitis, and the etiology may be either viral or bacterial. With yellow or green sputum, we usually treat bronchitis with an antibiotic and currently pick ampicillin, amoxicillin, erythromycin, or trimethoprim/sulfamethoxazole as a first choice.

Along with this treatment, and at least as important, is instructing the patient to stop smoking during the illness (and preferably thereafter). He or she should be encouraged to drink copious amounts of nonalcoholic fluids and to obtain some means of inhaling a high-humidity atmosphere to aid in bringing up sputum. Many patients will request cough medicines, but a patient with a productive cough or a fever should not usually be given powerful cough suppressants such as codeine; these patients need the cough to drain the purulent secretions. If given at all, codeine should be limited to nighttime use to allow sleep or used only occasionally to minimize prolonged, painful coughing fits.

REFERENCES

Review Article

Smith, P. L., Britt, E. J., and Terry, P. B. Common Pulmonary Problems. In L. R. Barker, J. R. Burton, and P. D. Zieve (eds.), *Principles of Ambulatory Care* (4th ed.). Baltimore: Williams & Wilkins, 1995. Pp. 633–649.

Additional References

Dunway, J., and Reinhardt, R. Clinical features and treatments of acute bronchitis. *J. Fam. Pract.* 1984;18:719–722.

Hueston, W. J. A comparison of albuterol and erythromycin for the treatment of acute bronchitis. *J. Fam. Pract.* 1991;33:476–480.

Hueston, W. J. Albuterol delivered by metered-dose inhaler to treat acute bronchitis. *J. Fam. Pract.* 1994;39:437–440.

CASE 82 SUDDEN SHOULDER PAIN

A 34-year-old physician came to the emergency department by private car. He arrived walking bent over, with his left arm held before him flexed at the elbow. He said that he was having terrible pain in his left shoulder and that it had begun 15 minutes earlier, immediately after he had thrown a 50-pound bag of wood chips in his backyard. This was the sixth time he had suffered such an episode.

On examination (once the patient's shirt was removed), he seemed in much distress and was somewhat pale and sweaty. His right shoulder curvature was more rounded than his left, and there was a bulge anteriorly on the left side. He could not move his upper arm and complained much of pain.

What is the diagnosis in this case?

Should x-rays be taken?

What can you do to relieve this patient's pain?

DISCUSSION

This patient has a recurring anterior shoulder dislocation. He probably should have a shoulder capsule reconstruction to avoid further recurrences. At the present time, the primary goal is to reduce his dislocation. Although fractures are seldom true emergencies, dislocations more often are, because nerve and vascular supplies may be damaged. A distal neurovascular examination should be done before and after reduction, looking for decreased sensation, diminished pulses, or delayed capillary refill. (Capillary refill is considered delayed if it takes longer for the normal color to return than for the examiner to say "capillary refill.") Patients will thank you for being brisk in your examination. Their priority is for you to reduce the dislocation as soon as possible.

We commonly see dislocated fingers, toes, shoulders, patellas, and hips. Dislocations of the hip often are difficult to reduce, whereas dislocations of fingers and toes usually can be easily reduced in the ED. One very easily reduced subluxation is the "nursemaid's elbow"—the radial head subluxation of childhood. It typically occurs when a walking child's arm is forcibly pulled, often by the parent. Reduction can be performed by supination and flexion of the involved elbow and is often performed by the x-ray technician when positioning the child to have the elbow x-rayed. A palpable pop indicates reduction, and the child will begin to use the arm normally within a short observation time.

Although we always x-ray a dislocation when it is a first-time event, we sometimes do not wait to obtain x-rays on repeat cases. The likelihood of a fracture-dislocation being present is very low in these cases.

For anterior shoulder dislocations, such as this case, we generally use intravenous Valium with 5 to 10 mg of morphine for analgesia and then attempt to reduce the shoulder dislocation. This patient was given 10 mg of Valium intravenously. Then, a sheet about his torso was pulled to the right, a large towel about his upper arm was pulled to the left, and gentle manipulation of the arm flexed at the elbow led to relocation of the shoulder. A number of other methods achieve the same results.

Once a dislocation is reduced, the pain diminishes radically, and any analgesia present will have much more effect. The patient often goes to sleep, and we have to beware of a respiratory arrest if a large dose of analgesic was given.

Prior to discharge, the dislocated joint must be fully immobilized. In shoulder dislocations we use a "sling and swathe" (a sling strapped to the torso).

REFERENCES

Review Article
Riebel, G. D., and McCabe, J. B. Anterior shoulder dislocation: A review of reduction techniques. *Am. J. Emerg. Med.* 1991;9:180–188.

Additional References
McNamara, R. Reduction of anterior shoulder dislocations by scapular manipulation. *Ann. Emerg. Med.* 1993;22:1140–1145.

Matthews, D. E., et al. Intraarticular lidocaine versus intravenous analgesic for reduction of acute anterior shoulder dislocation: A prospective randomized study. *Am. J. Sports Med.* 1995;23:54–58.

CASE 83 HIT BY A CAR

A 48-year-old man was struck by a fast-moving automobile. Paramedics found him confused and with a blood pressure of only 90/50 mm Hg. He was rapidly immobilized on a long board and transported to the emergency department. On arrival he was diaphoretic and cool with a blood pressure of 70/50, pulse of 120, and respiratory rate of 40.

His breath sounds were equal and clear, and his abdomen was distended and mildly tender. His pelvis was tender on compression of both the iliac crests and pubic symphysis. Blood was present at the urethral meatus, and the rectal exam revealed a "high riding" prostate. His right thigh was swollen, and his left leg was deformed, with the foot rotated externally. His right upper arm was swollen and bruised, but there was no evidence of neurovascular compromise.

Intravenous access was obtained for fluid resuscitation, and x-ray examination was initiated. Cervical spine and chest x-rays were normal. The pelvic film showed a diastasis (separation) of the pubic symphysis. Extremity films showed a right femur fracture, comminuted left tibia and fibula fractures, and a right humerus fracture. Because of the possibility of urethral injury, a retrograde urethrogram was performed that showed a posterior urethral rupture. He was taken to the operating room for further fluid resuscitation, pelvic fracture stabilization, and repair of his urethral injury.

Where exactly should paramedics take patients like this?

What are priorities in pelvic fractures?

DISCUSSION

Pelvic fractures usually involve multiple disruptions of the pelvic ring. A single fracture of the pelvic ring, like a single crack in a Lifesavers candy, is almost impossible. Multiple or displaced fractures are often unstable. Massive and fatal hemorrhage can occur from pelvic veins, arterial disruption, and the fracture site itself, which has a generous blood supply. MAST pants, when used in this setting, help to stabilize the fractures as well as maintain the blood pressure. Be careful when deflating them, because too-rapid deflation can cause a precipitous drop in the blood pressure of an otherwise stable-appearing patient.

When the pelvis is fractured, rectal, ureteral, and bladder injuries may be found. Blood at the urethral meatus, an inability to void, and high-riding prostate on rectal exam are cardinal signs of urethral injury. Generally, a Foley catheter should not be placed in these patients until a retrograde urethrogram is performed. An IVP to rule out higher injury usually follows. The mortality rate for patients with open pelvic fractures is over 50% because of complications such as hemorrhage, infection, and associated injury.

As always, aggressive fluid resuscitation is required if shock is present. Additional venous access may be required. When the vital signs reveal shock, an initial fluid bolus of 20 ml per kg (or 10 ml per pound) is appropriate. The patient's blood pressure and pulse must be scrupulously monitored.

Patients with multiple trauma and hypotension, coma, or respiratory failure should be transferred to a regional trauma center as soon as possible. With long transport times, these patients may be stabilized at a nearby hospital and subsequently transferred to a designated trauma center. Studies have shown that bypassing general hospitals and taking such patients directly to a trauma center saves lives. Regional prehospital protocols usually define which patients require trauma center care.

REFERENCES

Review Article
Stewart, C. Trauma to the pelvis: A systematic approach to classification, assessment, and management of pelvic fractures and their complications. *Emerg. Med. Rep.* 1994;15:99–106.

Additional References
Schneider, P. A., Mitchell, J. M., and Allison, E. J. The use of military antishock trousers in trauma—a reevaluation. *J. Emerg. Med.* 1989;7:497–500.

Perry, M. O., and Husmann, D. A. Urethral injuries in female subjects following pelvic fractures. *J. Urol.* 1992;147:139–143.

Resnik, C. S., et al. Diagnosis of pelvic fractures in patients with acute pelvic trauma: Efficacy of plain radiographs. *AJR Am. J. Roentgenol.* 1992;158:109–112.

Ben-Menachem, Y., et al. Hemorrhage associated with pelvic fractures: Causes, diagnosis, and emergent management. *AJR Am. J. Roentgenol.* 1991;157:1005–1014.

Case 84 KICKED IN THE GROIN

A 15-year-old boy came to the emergency department complaining of abdominal pain and nausea that had begun suddenly four hours before. He said that his right testicle was swollen and that "something like this" had happened in the past but had gone away spontaneously. Today he had played football and been kicked in the groin. He had been sexually active for almost a year but never had any sexually transmitted diseases, urethral discharge, or pain on urinating.

On physical examination he was noted to be an athletic adolescent male in marked distress. His temperature was 100°F, pulse 120, respiratory rate 18, and blood pressure 110/80. His abdomen was normal, but his scrotum was red and warm, with a tender and swollen right testicle.

His WBC count was 10,000 per mm^3, and his urinalysis showed 5 white cells per high-power field.

What is the diagnosis?

What diagnostic studies might be helpful?

Why is a prompt diagnosis so important in this case?

Discussion

In this case the priority diagnosis is testicular torsion. It is not the most common cause of a swollen testicle, but it is the most urgent. Although the peak incidence is in adolescence, it can be seen in adults, premature infants, and the elderly as well. Undescended testes have a tenfold increased incidence of torsion.

With a "bell clapper" deformity, the tunica vaginalis is capacious and has no posterior attachment. This allows the testicle to twist, compressing vessels and causing ischemia. The degree of testicular atrophy that follows torsion is proportional to the degree and duration of the torsion, so early diagnosis is important. If the diagnosis is made within 6 hours of the onset of symptoms, the salvage rate approaches 100%. In another 6 hours, only 20% of testes can be saved.

The classic presentation consists of the sudden onset of severe unrelenting pain that may be referred to the inguinal or abdominal region. In the classic description, the twisted testicle sits high, and the epididymis is in an abnormal position. The scrotum is red and edematous, and often a reactive hydrocele has formed, obscuring the testicle. Because of severe pain, these patients rarely tolerate a careful examination. It was once thought that if elevation of the testicle gave pain relief, then epididymitis was more likely than torsion. This feature, Prehn's sign, is now known to be unreliable. About one-fifth of patients with torsion have fever and about one-third have pyuria.

In the differential diagnosis, one must consider acute epididymitis, orchitis, and torsion of the appendix testis. Testicular cancer, which also tends to occur in young patients, may present with a swollen, red scrotum, although *usually* it is a painless condition.

Doppler flow studies are a quick and easy bedside test. If flow is not detected on the tender side, then torsion is likely. Unfortunately, detection of flow does not rule out torsion, as increased scrotal flow may mimic testicular blood flow.

The diagnosis of testicular torsion is made correctly on clinical grounds in only 50% of cases. Radioactive technetium scanning is somewhat more accurate than Doppler and is often used in equivocal cases. Unfortunately, both Doppler and nuclear studies have false-positives and false-negatives. To obtain a definitive diagnosis of the swollen, tender testicle, surgical exploration is most reliable. In adolescent and prepubertal boys when there is significant doubt about the diagnosis, surgical exploration should be undertaken. While the operating room is being prepared, manual detorsion may be attempted. Even if this is successful, an operation including exploration and surgical fixation of both testes within the scrotum (orchiopexy) is still mandatory, because recurrence is common.

REFERENCES

Review Article
Rabinowicz, R., and Hulbert, W. C. Acute scrotal swelling. *Urol. Clin. North Am.* 1995;22:101–106.

Additional References

Lindsey, D., and Stanisic, T. H. Diagnosis and management of testicular torsion: Pitfalls and perils. *Am. J. Emerg. Med.* 1988;6:42–46.

Cattolica, A. V. Preoperative manual detorsion of the torsed spermatic cord. *J. Urol.* 1985;133:803–805.

Joyce, J. M., and Grossman, S. J. Scrotal scintigraphy in testicular torsion. *Emerg. Med. Clin. North Am.* 1992;10:93–102.

Case 85 CHILD WITH A BARKING COUGH

A 4-year-old boy was brought to the emergency department at midnight because of difficulty breathing. He had had a low-grade fever and nasal congestion all day and began having noisy breathing and a barking cough in the middle of the night. The parents described the noise on inspiration to their pediatrician over the phone, and he requested that they bring the child right to the ED for examination.

The child appeared to be in no acute distress and was breathing more comfortably than at home. His temperature was 103.6°F, and he had frequent bouts of a barking cough. Further examination showed no abnormalities except a slightly red throat, and his parents were told to give him acetaminophen and use a cool mist humidifier at his bedside at home.

Several hours later they returned to the ED because the child began having more trouble breathing and could not lie down. The boy was sitting on the stretcher and was noted by a nurse to be drooling. His temperature was then 104.2°F. The pediatric resident seemed annoyed over having been awakened from sleep to see the child again. He asked the child to open his mouth, and when the child opened it only a small amount the resident became angry, asked a nurse to restrain the child, and placed a tongue blade in the mouth to visualize the tonsils better.

The child had a sudden respiratory arrest. Attempts were made to intubate him, but a large, red, swollen epiglottis prevented this, and, after about five to six minutes (because there was a great deal of confusion, no one kept track of the time), a surgeon was called to perform an emergency tracheostomy. The airway was finally established, and a stable cardiac rhythm returned, but the child never regained consciousness and was pronounced brain dead several days later.

What is croup, and when should the suspicion of epiglottitis be raised?

What is the correct treatment of epiglottitis in a child?

DISCUSSION

Acute epiglottitis in a child is an immediately life-threatening emergency. This case occurred 20 years ago and, along with many other similar cases, has led to the use of strict protocols for the treatment of this disease. Whenever a child with a clinical picture of acute epiglottitis (high fever, inspiratory stridor, drooling, and sitting forward, unwilling to speak or move) presents to our ED, a predetermined plan is set in motion. The operating room is immediately readied and an anesthesiologist and otolaryngologist are called. A "double setup" is prepared and brought to the bedside so the staff has the equipment at hand to endotracheally intubate or, if necessary, perform a cricothyrotomy. The child is made as comfortable as possible and is given humidified oxygen. No blood is drawn or intravenous line established at this point, although an intravenous antibiotic for presumed *Haemophilus* epiglottitis will be begun once the airway is secured. If the patient begins to tire or obstruct before the team is assembled, ventilations may be assisted with a bag-valve-mask apparatus. Once the patient is in the operating room, orotracheal intubation is attempted under inhalational anesthesia. If this fails, an emergency cricothyrotomy or tracheostomy is performed. This protocol has reduced the mortality for this disease. Fortunately, we are seeing fewer cases of childhood epiglottitis since the introduction of *Haemophilus influenza* type b vaccine (Hib).

Croup is usually a viral infection causing swelling of the subglottic area and is not as life-threatening as epiglottitis. The child is usually between the ages of 6 months and 3 years—somewhat younger than the usual epiglottitis patient. There is so much overlap, however, that age alone is not a reliable way to differentiate one from the other. In croup, the "croupy" (honking, barking) cough is usually preceded by an upper respiratory infection. Typically, the illness progresses slowly over days, as opposed to the more rapid progression over a single day common to epiglottitis. The characteristic barking cough sound is unmistakable. Most children improve after they are taken into a steamy shower, or while being driven to the ED. If the child arrives in severe respiratory distress, immediate treatment with racemic epinephrine given by a small-volume nebulizer may be lifesaving. The relief, however, is short lived, and frequently a rebound phenomenon occurs that results in stridor as bad or worse than the original condition. Any child treated with epinephrine should be closely observed, and many feel that hospitalization is the safest course. Fortunately, most children need only humidified air for treatment and can be discharged to their home. If there is still a question of epiglottitis after the child has been clinically evaluated, a good-quality soft tissue lateral neck x-ray can differentiate croup from epiglottitis in most cases.

REFERENCES

Review Article
Banks, D. E., and Krug, S. E. New approaches to upper airway disease. *Emerg. Med. Clin. North Am.* 1995;13:473–488.

Additional References
Hodge, K. M., and Ganzel, T. M. Diagnostic and therapeutic efficiency in croup and epiglottitis. *Laryngoscope* 1987;97:621–625.

Gorelick, M. H., and Baker, M. D. Epiglottitis in children 1979 through 1992. *Arch. Pediatr. Adolesc. Med.* 1994;148:47–50.

Prendergast, M., et al. Racemic epinephrine in the treatment of laryngotracheitis: Can we identify children for outpatient treatment? *Am. J. Emerg. Med.* 1994;12:613–616.

Frantz, T. D., et al. Acute epiglottitis in adults: Analysis of 129 cases. *J.A.M.A.* 1994;272:1358–1360.

Case 86 HIV POSITIVE

A 27-year-old man came to the emergency department with a tale of woe. He had been ill for about two weeks with fevers, night sweats, anorexia, and weight loss. After about one week, he had developed a bothersome but largely unproductive cough. He was homosexual but had not been sexually active recently. One previous sexual partner had died of acquired immunodeficiency syndrome (AIDS), and the patient himself had tested positive on a Human Immunodeficiency Virus (HIV) antibody test about a year ago. He was taking no medicine other than vitamins, did not know his T4-helper cell count, and rarely smoked a cigarette.

On examination, his temperature was 99°F orally, his chest was clear, he had a white pasty discoloration on his tongue, and there was shotty lymphadenopathy throughout his neck. There were no other remarkable findings. A chest x-ray appeared to be normal. The examining doctor suspected that the patient did indeed have HIV infection but that the acute illness was a viral or perhaps a bacterial bronchitis. He prescribed cephalexin (Keflex) orally and suggested that the patient contact his usual primary physician.

The patient went home and took the antibiotic for the next 10 days. Then, because his fevers had not diminished and he still felt quite ill, even worse than before, he contacted his primary care internist, who hospitalized him. The patient was now producing a bit of sputum, and special stains showed *Pneumocystis carinii* in the sputum. An arterial blood gas showed a surprising degree of hypoxia. The patient's hospital course was stormy. He developed severe nausea and vomiting, which were attributed to the high-dosage intravenous trimethoprim/sulfamethoxazole that he was being given. He was switched to intravenous pentamidine and then developed a worrisome neutropenia. The pentamidine was then given by inhalation, and his white cell count ceased to decline, but his fevers returned. Finally, corticosteroids were added and he improved. Because his T4 cell count was about 120, below the cutoff level of 200, he was treated with azidothymidine (AZT), 200 mg qid. As he improved, so did his chest x-ray and it became "even more normal" than it had been on admission or in the ED prior to admission. Some of the markings that had been explained as "normal bronchovascular markings" melted away under the therapy with AZT, predisone, and pentamidine. He went home 29 days after admission.

What do you think about the therapy with Keflex?

Would you be equally censorious about empiric outpatient therapy with inhaled pentamidine?

Is this patient a serious health risk to the workers in the ED? If not, who is?

Discussion

If we are treating a bacterial bronchitis in a patient who has normal immune status and an antibiotic is indicated, we choose a drug that covers such common organisms as *Branhamella catarrhalis* and *H. influenzae*. Two such drugs are cefuroxime axetil (Ceftin) and trimethoprim/sulfamethoxazole (Bactrim or Septra). Because of cost, the *Medical Letter* recommends the latter. A first generation cephalosporin such as cephalexin is probably reasonable for pneumococcus coverage but not as a "broad spectrum" respiratory antibiotic.

Of course, in an immunosuppressed individual, the usual organisms are "unusual." The most common is PCP *(Pneumocystis carinii)*, and you should either make a definite effort to reach a precise diagnosis or at least consider treatment with one of the two drugs that are usually effective against that organism. Because we usually use large doses of trimethoprim/sulfamethoxazole in such treatment and there are often allergic and other toxic reactions, it seems that the best course is, as usual, to establish a firm diagnosis. Inhaled pentamidine, which is becoming a preferred therapy in many centers, is perhaps less toxic but quite expensive if given in a therapeutic daily dosage. Again, it is best to have the diagnosis first.

As we see more and more patients with pneumocystis lung infections, we realize that our usual diagnostic requirements for pneumonia are bound to prove inadequate. A "normal" chest x-ray cannot rule out PCP, and, as in this case, the range of radiographic normality is wide and sometimes overlaps with modestly abnormal x-rays. Only a prior film, which is often unavailable, would help. Even patients with normal films may have striking hypoxia from diffuse lung involvement. Sometimes the arterial blood gas determination or even pulse oximetry tells the tale. Of course patients with HIV infections can suffer from other lung diseases, infections, and malignancies, but the majority have PCP. With fever, cough, and evidence of HIV infection, you can bet on PCP and win most of your wagers.

This patient, identified from the start as a carrier of HIV, is of little risk to those in the ED. We try to always use universal precautions and are generally careful handling blood, but we are probably on guard and safest with this type of patient. We are at greater risk when dealing with a trauma patient who is actively bleeding and whom we do not know to be an HIV carrier. Emergency departments, especially those in the big cities, are seeing more and more such patients (often IV drug users) who either do not know or cannot or will not tell of their health status. We must be careful.

REFERENCES

Review Article
Marco, C. A. Presentations and emergency department evaluation of HIV infection. *Emerg. Med. Clin. North Am.* 1995;13:61–72.

Additional References
Montgomery, A. B., et al. Aerosolised pentamidine as sole therapy for Pneumocystis carinii pneumonia in patients with acquired immunodeficiency syndrome. *Lancet* 1987;2:480–482.

Baker, J. L., et al. Unsuspected human immunodeficiency virus in critically ill emergency patients. *J.A.M.A.* 1987;257:2609–2611.

Guss, D. A. The acquired immune deficiency syndrome: An overview for the emergency physician. *J. Emerg. Med.* 1994;12:375–384, 491–497.

87 CHILD WITH SMALL TOYS

A 3-year-old boy was brought in to the ED by his mother because of a fever and drainage from his nose. He had been seen two days before by his pediatrician because of the runny nose, was thought to have a viral upper respiratory infection, and was treated with a decongestant. His nasal drainage became worse and the fever developed. His past history was unremarkable.

When seen in the emergency department, he had a temperature of 102.6°F but was cheerful and played with his mother when not annoyed by our examination. His head and neck were normal except for congestion of the right naris with a large amount of purulent discharge. This was vigorously suctioned, and a small wooden bead was seen inside the nose. The bead was removed with difficulty by the ENT resident who was called to see the child.

The child was discharged after we instructed his mother to use saltwater nose drops and to keep him away from small toys.

Two weeks later the same child was back. The mother stated that he was playing when he had a sudden coughing spell and perhaps even turned blue for a few seconds. She reported seeing no small toys in the area. He now seemed fine, and his examination was completely normal. Because aspiration was suspected, a chest x-ray was taken. The x-ray was normal, so the child was sent home and the mother reassured.

The next day, the child awoke with a fever and was returned to the ED. He had been coughing all night, his appetite was poor, and he was not interested in playing.

His temperature then was 102.4°F, his pulse was 124 per minute, and his respirations were 36 per minute. Examination was normal except for his chest, which showed wheezes and rhonchi in the right lower lung field. A repeat chest x-ray showed a right middle lobe infiltrate with atelectasis. The child was admitted.

What types of respiratory foreign bodies can cause problems in children?

When should aspiration be suspected?

Discussion

Small children may place toys or other objects in any orifice of the body. This exploratory behavior is common and usually harmless. For this reason, pediatricians advise that children this age have no toy smaller than their fist. Small beads or beans are commonly placed in the nose or ears, and unilateral drainage from the nose or ear suggests the presence of a foreign body. Removal may be accomplished using an ear curette, suction, or fine forceps. Irrigation with water should not be used when beans or vegetable matter have been inserted, because this will cause the object to swell.

Aspirated foreign bodies should be considered a medical emergency. If the patient is old enough, he or she may show the universal signs of a choking victim, which are the inability to speak and a hand held to the throat. For a voiceless child who is turning blue, the Heimlich maneuver, rapid upward thrusts into the midepigastrium, may help. Any person who is "choking" and is still able to speak can also breathe and should be left alone until the object can be removed under direct visualization.

A more subtle and common presentation occurred in this child. The typical history of sudden choking or coughing while the child was playing should prompt the physician to suspect a foreign body aspiration. The child may have a new cough and occasionally some blood-tinged sputum, although there may be surprisingly few objective signs in the first day. A chest x-ray should be obtained in order to look for a radiopaque foreign body or evidence of air trapping. Initial hyperinflation on the affected side (because of a one-way valve effect) with a tracheal shift toward the other side but no pneumothorax should be taken as evidence of a retained foreign body. Treatment is bronchoscopy and removal of the foreign body. If the child is left untreated, complications may include recurrent pneumonias and atelectasis.

References

Review Article
Mofenson, H. C., and Greensher, J. Management of the choking child. *Pediatr. Clin. North Am.* 1985;32:183–192.

Additional References

Standards and guidelines for cardiopulmonary resuscitation and emergency cardiac care. *J.A.M.A.* 1986;255(Suppl.):2841–3044.

Heimlich, H. J. A life saving maneuver to prevent food-choking. *J.A.M.A.* 1975;234:398–401.

Imaizumi, H., et al. Definitive diagnosis and location of peanuts in the airway using magnetic resonance imaging techniques. *Ann. Emerg. Med.* 1994;23:1379–1382.

Losek, J. D. Diagnostic difficulties of foreign body aspiration in children. *Am. J. Emerg. Med.* 1990;8:348–350.

Case 88 CHILD AFTER A SEIZURE

A previously healthy 2-year-old boy was brought to the emergency department after a generalized tonic-clonic seizure that had lasted 10 minutes. Following a 5-minute postictal period, he appeared well. The child's past medical history, developmental history, and family history were unremarkable and included no history of seizures. The child's mother had noted that he had nasal congestion and diarrhea for two days prior to his ED visit. Examination revealed a happy, playful child in no distress and with the following vital signs: temperature 102°F rectally, pulse 120, blood pressure 85/50 mm Hg, and 28 respirations per minute. His pupils were equal and reactive. Both tympanic membranes were red and immobile. The pharynx was erythematous, without exudate. No adenopathy was noted, and his neck was supple. Further examination revealed clear lungs, a nontender abdomen, and a normal neurologic examination. The child was discharged with a diagnosis of bilateral otitis media and febrile seizure. Treatment was initiated with amoxicillin and acetaminophen.

Should the child have had a lumbar puncture to rule out meningitis?

Can you have bacterial meningitis without meningeal signs?

Discussion

Febrile seizures occur in 2 to 5% of children under 5 years of age. A simple febrile seizure lasts less than 15 minutes, is generalized, and occurs between 3 months and 5 years of age in an otherwise normal child who is left with no residual focal neurologic deficit. Atypical febrile seizures may last longer, manifest focal seizure activity, result in a focal neurologic deficit during the postictal period, or recur within 24 hours. Febrile seizures usually result from a focus of infection detected on physical exam (e.g., pharyngitis or otitis media), and the primary infection may be treated with antipyretics and appropriate antibiotics, if

88. CHILD AFTER A SEIZURE

indicated, in an otherwise well-appearing child. If the child appears ill or the febrile seizures are atypical, a more thorough evaluation must be performed to rule out sepsis and meningitis (blood cultures, lumbar puncture, and occasionally CT scanning).

Examination of a febrile child begins with a complete history, including respiratory complaints, gastrointestinal symptoms, rashes, and any changes in the child's appetite or level of activity. The physical exam should add additional information about the potential source of infection.

In a child younger than 2 years old, fever over 102°F may result from many causes, including pharyngitis, tracheobronchitis, otitis media, pneumonia, cellulitis, osteomyelitis, appendicitis, septic arthritis, or urinary tract infection. The absence of a specific source of infection despite physical examination, chest x-ray, and urinalysis should raise the index of suspicion for sepsis, bacteremia, and meningitis. Experts differ about what constitutes the appropriate workup for a febrile infant. Because of the risks of "occult bacteremia," we think that if no source of infection is found, a blood culture should be obtained in any child younger than 2 years old with a temperature over 104°F, a sedimentation rate greater than 30 mm per hour, or a white blood cell count over 15,000. Additionally, a lumbar puncture is indicated in these cases if the infant appears ill.

Meningitis is a devastating disease with high morbidity and mortality unless diagnosed and treated early. Gram-negative rods and group B streptococcus are the major pathogens in neonatal meningitis. After the first month of life, the major pathogens include pneumococcus, *H. influenzae,* and meningococcus. Meningitis must always be considered in the febrile child who appears ill or lacks a clear focus of infection. Younger children may present with lethargy, irritability, and decreased feeding as the only symptoms. In children under 6 months of age, and particularly in children under 3 months of age, signs of nuchal rigidity may be subtle or absent. Particularly in a child less than 3 months old, indications for lumbar puncture and the use of antibiotics when no source of fever can be found is an area of controversy.

Because this child was already 2 years old and had such a clear source of infection, a history consistent with a simple febrile seizure, and a happy, playful demeanor in the ED, we think deferring the lumbar puncture was appropriate.

REFERENCES

Review Article

Stenklyft, P. H., and Carmona, M. Febrile seizures. *Emerg. Med. Clin. North Am.* 1994;12:989–999.

Additional References

Singer, J. I., Vest, J., and Prints, A. Occult bacteremia and septicemia in the febrile child younger than two years. *Emerg. Med. Clin. North Am.* 1995;13:381–416.

Jaskiewicz, J. A., et al. Febrile infants at low risk for serious bacterial infection: An appraisal of the Rochester criteria. *Pediatrics* 1994; 94:390–396.

Baraff, L. J., et al. Practice guidelines for the management of infants and children 0 to 36 months of age with fever without source. Agency for Health Care Policy Research. *Ann. Emerg. Med.* 1993;22:1198–1210.

Case 89 ABSCESS

A 24-year-old muscular male presented to the triage desk complaining of a sore arm, fever, and chills. The patient said that he was an intravenous drug user and that several days earlier he had been attempting to "shoot" what he thought was a combination of heroin and cocaine. It had not worked, and he thought he had missed the vein with at least part of the solution. By the next day, his arm had become warm, sore, and swollen, and this had continued to progress rapidly until he decided to come to the hospital. When he started to get sick, he spoke with his friends, who suggested that perhaps the packet he had injected contained Ritalin and not cocaine. The examining physician found a huge fluctuant abscess extending down the lateral side of the patient's arm, from the deltoid muscle to the elbow. The abscess required an incision and drainage, and it took five full bottles of iodoform gauze packing to fill the cavity.

Is this a "boil?"

How is a boil treated?

Discussion

An abscess usually begins with a small break in the skin or a superficial skin infection. If caused by staphylococcus, the infection may spread deeper and cause a "boil," which is a subcutaneous collection of pus surrounded by an area of cellulitis. Although antibiotic therapy will reduce and control the cellulitis around the pus collection, the only effective treatment of an abscess is drainage.

Adequate anesthesia is usually difficult to obtain. One option is to use a field block around the abscess. Lidocaine is injected in a ring surrounding the abscess and then subcutaneously over the area where the incision is to be made. For large abscesses, a more humane approach is through the use of conscious sedation. We use midazolam (Versed), an ultra–short-acting benzodiazepine, and fentanyl, a short-acting and very potent narcotic analgesic. They are given intravenously while the patient is closely monitored. The incision can then be made into the abscess cavity, and the pus can be released. A common error in this procedure is not going deep enough into the abscess cavity. There are usually fibrous septae in the cavity when it is large, and these must be broken up, either with a clamp or the physician's finger. The cavity should then be packed open with gauze to prevent it from closing and the abscess from reforming. The packing should be removed every 2 days and replaced with a smaller amount of gauze until the abscess cavity fills in.

Systemic antibiotics are usually not appropriate in the treatment of superficial abscesses but should be used in immunocompromised patients and when there is a large area of cellulitis or ascending lymphangitis associated with the abscess. Cultures of the abscess contents are usually not necessary and should only be taken if the patient is to be placed on antibiotics.

Deep perirectal abscesses, tendon sheath abscesses, and intracavitary abscesses usually require hospitalization and parenteral antibiotics.

Abscesses in drug abusers arise from multiple causes. The needle may be contaminated with bacteria, or the drug itself may cause the abscess. This is especially true with sympathomimetics, such as cocaine and amphetamines ("speed"), which produce intense vasoconstriction and cell necrosis at the site of subcutaneous injection. Ritalin (methylphenidate hydrochloride) is a synthetic, amphetamine-like drug with similar properties when injected.

This abscess is unusual in size and shape. One must wonder about its extent and consider unusual bacteria that tend to produce spreading infections that dissect along tissue planes. *Clostridium* species, for example, may be present. Any unusual infection deserves the best help our microbiology lab can give us. We should culture aerobically and anaerobically, and this patient should be hospitalized for observation and intravenous antibiotics. He may be immunosuppressed.

REFERENCES

Review Article
Lindsey, D. Soft tissue infections. *Emerg. Med. Clin. North Am.* 1992;10:737–752.

Additional References

Meislin, H. W. Pathogenic identification of abscesses and cellulitus. *Ann. Emerg. Med.* 1986;15:329–332.

Bidernan, P., and Hiatt, J. R. Management of soft-tissue infections of the upper extremity in parenteral drug abusers. *Am. J. Surg.* 1987;154:526–528.

Vlahov, D., et al. Bacterial infections and skin cleaning prior to injection among intravenous drug users. *Public Health Rep.* 1992;107:595–598.

Summanen, P. H., et al. Bacteriology of skin and soft-tissue infections: Comparison of infections in intravenous drug users and individuals with no history of intravenous drug use. *Clin. Infect. Dis.* 1995;20(Suppl 2):5279–5282.

Case 90 CARDIAC ARREST

A 55-year-old man developed chest pain while walking to work. When he got to his office, his co-workers noted that he was pale and diaphoretic and called the paramedics through the fire department's emergency number. A basic life-support truck and an advanced life-support rescue squad arrived at the scene at about the same time. Only 12 minutes had elapsed since the initial call was placed.

The paramedics noted that the patient was in distress and suffering squeezing substernal chest pressure, a feeling of "light-headedness," and slight shortness of breath. They immediately placed a nonrebreathing face mask, giving him almost 100% oxygen. He was attached to a cardiac monitor, and an intravenous line was started with 5% dextrose in water at a keep-open rate. By that time, his pain had subsided slightly, and his vital signs included blood pressure 110/50, pulse 56, and respirations 22. His skin had dried and become warm. His lungs had some bibasilar rales. He reported that he had a history of hypertension and was taking some medication for it. He smoked and had a family history of heart attacks.

The paramedics then called the emergency department physician on duty for further orders (on-line medical control). They were told to administer one nitroglycerin tablet sublingually and repeat the vital signs. This produced further relief of the patient's pain, but his pressure dropped to 96/50, and he became more light-headed. They were then told to give a fluid challenge of 300 ml of normal saline and to place the patient in a shock position. His pressure came up to 124/64, and he felt better. He was transported to the hospital in the supine position and had no further pain until he was about to be unloaded from the ambulance.

At this time his pulse was noted to be 40, his skin was cool and clammy again, and his chest pain recurred. The ED physician was called out to the ambulance ramp to see the patient and immediately ordered a bolus of atropine given by intravenous push. This was done on the ambulance ramp while the patient was being wheeled into the ED. As he was being pushed from the entrance of the department to the cardiac booth, his cardiac rate increased to 100, and some premature ventricular

90. CARDIAC ARREST

contractions appeared. An intravenous bolus of lidocaine was given, and he was transferred to the stretcher.

When he was transferred to the stretcher, he complained of increasing chest pain again, and within minutes his rate had slowed again to 44 with a sinus rhythm. He was then given another dose of atropine, and his rate again increased to 110. His blood pressure was 120/62 at this point. He was given another nitroglycerin tablet, and morphine sulfate was ordered in case his pain continued. A 12-lead ECG was begun, but, before it could be completed, the patient slumped unconscious and was seen to be in ventricular fibrillation.

Two precordial chest thumps were administered while the defibrillator was charged, and the patient was ventilated with a bag-valve-mask on 100% oxygen. An initial shock was delivered at 200 joules, but the rhythm showed no change. A second shock delivered at 300 joules and a third at 360 joules produced no change in the rhythm. Cardiopulmonary resuscitation (CPR) was begun after the first shock, and the patient's trachea was intubated after the third shock. Epinephrine was given intravenously, and he was shocked again at 360 joules with no change in his rhythm. After each shock, it was observed that the fibrillatory waves were of lower amplitude. Lidocaine was given by intravenous bolus, and the patient was shocked again. His rhythm deteriorated to asystole.

He was given another dose of epinephrine and atropine, and CPR and ventilations were continued. Because there was no change and the patient was young, the staff doctor elected to attempt transthoracic cardiac pacing. While this was being set up, another dose of epinephrine was given. The pacer functioned, but the patient's heart did not capture the paced beats. Further attempts at treatment with intravenous epinephrine and atropine were unsuccessful, and the patient was pronounced dead about 75 minutes after arriving at the hospital.

Do paramedics waste time by treating patients "in the streets"?

What are the priorities in a cardiac arrest? (hint: ABC)

DISCUSSION

Most patients who suffer cardiac arrest are found to be in ventricular fibrillation when a rhythm can be determined. The chance of successfully defibrillating such a patient falls off rapidly as time passes. Early defibrillation is essential. There is indeed a hazard in shocking a patient who because of hypotension or supraventricular arrhythmias has no palpable pulse—the same ventricular fibrillation thought to be present initially may be brought about by the shock. In some EMS systems, the standing protocol is to shock the pulseless patient first and look at the rhythm later. New, automatic external defibrillators will automatically determine the rhythm and shock only ventricular fibrillation. Most EMS systems now train their basic level medics to use these devices. These medics are termed EMT-Ds (EMT-defibrillation). Several studies have shown increased survival from out-of-hospital cardiac arrest in communities that have gone to this level of provider.

An ambulance crew properly planned to handle emergency resuscitation would consist of at least three persons. Most cities use existing services, usually fire departments, to provide basic and advanced life support (ALS) services. Many cities have initiated citizen CPR programs that train a large portion of the population to perform one- and two-person CPR. Often, however, the first responder in these cases is the basic EMT on a fire truck. The second responder is the paramedic or advanced EMT on a specially equipped rescue vehicle. Paramedics are trained to recognize and initiate treatment of many life-threatening cardiac problems. Most paramedics have between 700 and 1500 hours of training, including arrhythmia interpretation and observation in the coronary care units. Treatment is often begun on the scene by paramedics, and they will frequently delay transport of a cardiac patient until the initial treatment is begun. Transport can be done by these units or by a simultaneously dispatched ambulance. The crew needs skills in ventilation with Ambu bag and oral airway. They need good cardiac massage technique and a van-type vehicle large enough to allow them to work over the patient on the trip. They need intravenous infusion capabilities, including sufficient height inside the vehicles to provide a pressure head for intravenous infusions. Drugs usually carried are $NaHCO_3$, atropine, lidocaine, epinephrine, bretylium, dopamine, isoproterenol, furosemide (Lasix), morphine, naloxone (Narcan), glucose, glucagon, calcium, adenosine, and verapamil. The present standard of prehospital care is very high, and in some cities over 40% of victims of ventricular fibrillation now survive to hospital discharge because of the rapid care delivered by paramedics. The prognosis for patients presenting in

90. CARDIAC ARREST

asystole or electromechanical dissociation remains dismal.

Once in the ED, a pulseless patient is resuscitated in a standardized fashion. Most importantly, one physician must take charge of the procedure. Seldom should any other voice be heard, and, ideally he or she should not be involved directly in carrying out the procedures but rather should observe and command the entire team.

Advanced Cardiac Life Support (ACLS) teaches the principles of cardiac resuscitation through intensive courses. The Megacode is a lifelike simulation of a cardiac arrest performed on a mannequin with simulated arrhythmias. This training allows all persons involved in the care of patients in cardiac arrest to function smoothly as a team and eliminates much of the confusion that accompanied cardiac arrests in the past.

The following steps outline the American Heart Association's ACLS approach to cardiac arrest:

A. Attempt to reestablish spontaneous cardiac activity.
   1. In monitored ventricular fibrillation, a blow to the chest (precordial thump) may restore spontaneous activity.
   2. Follow this with three successive shocks of 200, 300, and 360 joules if earlier treatment is not successful.
B. CPR (one physician assumes the role of resuscitation chief).
   1. Suction airway when needed, place oral airway, and ventilate with 100% oxygen using a mask and Ambu bag to preoxygenate before intubation.
   2. Cardiac compressions start at about 100 per minute while a second person ventilates at about 20 per minute. Basic CPR must continue throughout the resuscitation efforts, pausing only momentarily to allow electric shock delivery and rhythm determination.
   3. Intubate the trachea with an endotracheal tube.
   4. Evaluate effectiveness of ventilation and massage.
C. Establish access and data base.
   1. IV, large bore if possible.
   2. ECG monitor with defibrillator capabilities.
   3. Blood gas on a stat basis.
D. Team leader evaluates the data obtained and the effectiveness of therapy.

E. Attempt definitive therapy. Continue massage and ventilation.
   1. Ventricular fibrillation.
      a. Epinephrine, 1 to 1.5 mg (1:10,000) IV.
      b. Defibrillate at 360 joules.
      c. Lidocaine, 1 mg per kg IV.
      d. Defibrillate at 360 joules.
      e. Bretylium, 5 mg per kg IV.
      f. Defibrillate at 360 joules.
      g. Repeat lidocaine or bretylium.
      h. Magnesium, 1 to 2 g IV.
      i. Give bicarbonate only, based on the results of arterial blood gas measurements.
      j. Lidocaine or bretylium infusions should be started after the establishment of a supraventricular rhythm.
   2. Asystole.
      a. Epinephrine, 1 mg (1:10,000) IV every 3 to 5 minutes.
      b. Atropine, 1 mg IV repeated every 3 to 5 minutes, up to a total dose of 0.03 to 0.04 mg per kg.
      c. Consider external (transcutaneous) pacemaker.
   3. Pulseless Electrical Activity (PEA); that is, electrical rhythm but no pulse. (Also known as Electromechanical dissociation [EMD].)
      a. Epinephrine, 1 mg (1:10,000) IV every 3 to 5 minutes.
      b. Look and treat for treatable causes of EMD, such as pericardial tamponade, tension pneumothorax, severe hypovolemia, acidosis, hypoxemia, or pulmonary embolism.
   4. Bradycardia or AV block. If hypotensive, accompanied by chest pain, or with ventricular escape beats, treat the patient; otherwise, observe.
      a. Atropine, 0.5 to 1.0 mg IV every 3 to 5 minutes, up to a total dose of 0.03 to 0.04 mg per kg.
      b. External pacemaker or isoproterenol IV infusion.
      c. In an otherwise stable patient with third-degree or second-degree type II heart block, a transvenous pacemaker is the treatment of choice. The external pacemaker should be on standby while it is being arranged.

Unfortunately, as in this case, sometimes the best we can offer is still too late or too little. After a failed resuscitation effort involving a large team of people, we all may feel depressed. Then there is still a difficult task at hand. This man's family needs to be told the bad news; another painful challenge for the emergency physician and the nursing staff.

REFERENCES

Review Articles

Emergency Cardiac Care Committee and Subcommittees, American Heart Association. Guidelines for cardiopulmonary resuscitation and emergency cardiac care. *J.A.M.A.* 1992;268:2172–2302.

Rose, J. S., and Koenig, K. L. Code blue: What's new? *J. Emerg. Med.* 1994;12:187–191.

Additional References

Tucker, K. J., et al. Cardiopulmonary resuscitation. Historical perspectives, physiology, and future directions. *Arch. Intern. Med.* 1994;154:2141–2150.

Becker, L. B., and Pepe, P. E. Ensuring the effectiveness of community-wide emergency cardiac care. *Ann. Emerg. Med.* 1993;22:354–365.

Gonzalez, E. R. Pharmacologic controversies in CPR. *Ann. Emerg. Med.* 1993;22:317–323.

Schmidt, T. A., and Tolle, S. W. Emergency physicians' responses to families following patient death. *Ann. Emerg. Med.* 1990;19:125–128.

Case 91 BOUNCE BACK

A 28-year-old man was in a bar fight. The next day, he came to the ED complaining of neck pain and multiple extremity bruises.

He was recognized by the ED staff as one of their regular patients. He called the ED periodically, and because he had no family physician he tended to use the ED for that purpose. He was known to be on public assistance, and some hospital staff members frankly resented his frequent "abuse" of the ED.

He was appropriately evaluated by the physician on duty, and, after his C-spine x-rays were read as normal by the radiologist, the ED staff cleaned his wounds, made sure his tetanus immunization was up-to-date, and recommended over-the-counter symptomatic care for his contusions.

Two days later, he called the ED and angrily stated that the treatments the ED had suggested had done "no good." He was somewhat belligerent on the phone, and a nurse suspected he was intoxicated. She advised him to continue the treatments, instructed him to follow-up with an orthopedic surgeon if he was still not improving, and suggested to the patient that he might feel a little better if he wasn't drinking so much. The following day, the patient presented to the hospital for the second time. The ED was packed with patients at the time. He loudly complained of pain and insisted on being seen immediately. He was a large man, clearly bigger than anyone else in the ED at that moment, and when he got unusually close to one of the nurses and loudly repeated his demands she became fearful of his threatening manner. Nevertheless, she was able to quiet him somewhat and convinced him to register and wait his turn.

When re-examined by the ED physician, the patient demanded repeat x-rays, even though he was reassured they had been read as negative on the first visit. Repeat x-rays were obtained and showed a fracture of the second cervical vertebrae, the odontoid. In retrospect, the fracture was present on the initial films taken days earlier but had been overlooked. The patient was tranferred to the nearest hospital with a spine treatment center for surgical stabilization.

What is a "bounce back?"

Wasn't the staff's reaction to this patient understandable?

Discussion

In the terminology of emergency medicine, a "bounce back" is a patient who presents to the ED, is treated and released, and then returns with the same or similar complaints. There are many reasons for a patient's "bouncing back." Nevertheless, it is widely recognized that this subset of patients has a much higher incidence of problems, both medical and medico-legal, than ED patients as a whole. Patients with unscheduled returns have a higher incidence of clinical errors, misdiagnoses, and interpersonal problems with ED staff. Minimizing such patients' complaints or blowing them off and not investigating them fully is well recognized by experienced ED physicians as unnecessarily risky behavior.

The ED staff was not impartial and wholly professional in the care of this patient. They were prejudiced against him because he used the ED frequently, because he was a drinker, because he was on public assistance, because he acted belligerently towards them, and perhaps in other ways as well. Their prejudice was understandable but not acceptable. When the ED staff feels that a patient is abusing them by seeking medical care, trouble often follows.

References

Review Article
Platt, F. W. *Conversation Failure: Case Studies in Doctor-Patient Communication.* Tacoma, WA: Life Sciences, 1992.

Additional References
Kelly, A. M., et al. An analysis of unscheduled return visits to an urban emergency department. *N. Z. Med. J.* 1993;106(961):334–336.

Renfrew, D. L., et al. Error in radiology. *Radiology* 1992;183:145–150.

Freed, H. A., et al. Radiographic misreads as a function of level of training. *Acad. Emerg. Med.* 1995;2:345–346. Abstract.

Case 92 RECENT BYPASS SURGERY

A 59-year-old man was discharged home from the hospital after having a coronary artery bypass graft done several days earlier. Two hours after discharge, he arrived in the ED complaining of substernal chest pressure and a pounding in his chest. He denied shortness of breath. His only medication was Tylenol with codeine for incisional pain.

On examination, he appeared to be in no distress, but his face was pasty in color. He stated that the pain stopped when oxygen was applied via a nonrebreathing face mask. Vital signs were blood pressure 124/80, pulse 188, respirations 18, and temperature 98.6°F. The remainder of the physical examination was normal.

The patient was placed on a cardiac monitor, and the rhythm was interpreted as a narrow complex tachycardia with what appeared to be P waves preceding each beat. On this basis, he was given a 5-mg dose of intravenous verapamil. This had no effect on the rate. Carotid sinus massage likewise had no effect on the rate. A 12-lead ECG was done at this time and showed a wide complex tachycardia. The patient was then given 100 mg of intravenous lidocaine. Several minutes later, his heart rate slowed to 100 per minute. He was placed on a lidocaine drip and transferred to the coronary care unit.

How can you differentiate supraventricular tachycardia from ventricular tachycardia?

What are the complications of supraventricular tachycardia and its treatment?

Discussion

This patient presented with symptoms attributable to a tachyarrhythmia. This symptom complex may range from vague feelings of apprehensiveness and fear to mental status changes, seizure from lack of blood supply, and full cardiac arrest.

Patients with tachyarrhythmias who present to the ED and are hemodynamically unstable should undergo immediate synchronized cardioversion, usually starting at 50 to 100 joules of energy. The usual indications include hypotension (systolic blood pressure less than 80), unconsciousness or obtundation, pulmonary edema, or other signs associated with a poor cardiac output. Chest pain alone may be enough to prompt electrical cardioversion from a tachyarrhythmia. Synchronized cardioversion is the safest and most reliable way to terminate tachyarrhythmias in these patients.

In a more stable patient, the physician should proceed to define the arrhythmia by careful assessment of the ECG and physical exam. Most patients tolerate supraventricular tachycardias (SVTs) better than ventricular tachycardias. Usually our diagnostic problem involves a wide QRS tachycardia (initially missed in this case), and our challenge is to differentiate a supraventricular arrhythmia with aberrant ventricular conduction from ventricular tachycardia. (Aberrancy occurs when a supraventricular reentrant impulse arrives at the AV node while one or both bundle branches are refractory and results in a widened QRS complex.) The treatment of these two entities in the hemodynamically stable patient is quite different. Misdiagnosis and subsequent inappropriate treatment have resulted in patient deaths.

ECG evidence favoring a diagnosis of ventricular tachycardia includes the presence of atrioventricular disassociation, a QRS complex greater than 0.14 seconds, the appearance of fusion or capture beats, concordance (all QRS complexes upright or all inverted in the precordial leads), a marked left-axis deviation, and the presence of qR in lead V_1. Findings on physical exam suggesting the diagnosis of ventricular tachycardia include the presence of cannon a-waves in the neck, varying loudness of the first heart sound, and beat to beat variability in the systolic blood pressure. Advanced age and a history of underlying coronary artery disease favor a diagnosis of ventricular tachycardia.

Once the diagnosis of ventricular tachycardia has been made, appropriate initial management should include administration of intravenous lidocaine or procainamide.

In those cases where the diagnosis of SVT is likely, vagal maneuvers may be useful. Carotid sinus massage, Valsalva maneuver, and the diving reflex (immersion of the patient's face into ice-cold water) are procedures that increase vagal tone and thereby prolong refractoriness at the AV node. This may aid in differentiating the type of SVT (atrial fibrillation, atrial flutter, or paroxysmal) and in some cases will abruptly terminate the arrhythmia. Carotid massage may be hazardous in an elderly or atherosclerotic patient. If vagal maneuvers are unsuccessful, adenosine administered by rapid intravenous injection has been shown to be effective in terminating many SVTs. Calcium channel blockers (e.g., Verapamil or diltiazem) should be used cautiously in patients with a history of congestive heart failure, hypotension, or heart block. They have also been shown to accelerate conduction over accessory pathways in patients with the Wolff-Parkinson-White (WPW) syndrome accompanied by atrial fibrillation.

Procainamide has also been shown to be effective in terminating both ventricular tachycardias and atrial tachycardias with aberrancy. In cases of wide-complex tachycardia where the diagnosis remains unclear, it may be best to choose between intravenous procainamide (if the patient is stable) or cardioversion (if the patient is not). That is because the diagnosis could be WPW syndrome with uncontrolled rapid atrial fibrillation and aberrancy; lidocaine, digitalis, and calcium channel blockers can all lead to more rapid conduction through the accessory pathway and death in this setting.

REFERENCES

Review Article
Ganz, L. I., and Friedman, P. L. Supraventricular tachycardia. *N. Engl. J. Med.* 1995;332:162–173.

Additional References
Lowenstein, F. R., and Harken, A. H. A wide, complex look at cardiac dysrhythmias. *J. Emerg. Med.* 1987;5:519–531.

Moore, G. P., and Munter, D. W. Wolff-Parkinson-White syndrome: Illustrative case and brief review. *J. Emerg. Med.* 1989;7:47–54.

Furlong, R., et al. Intravenous adenosine as first line prehospital management of narrow complex tachycardia by EMS personnel without direct physician contact. *Am. J. Emerg. Med.* 1995;13:383–388.

Waldo, A. L., et al. Ventricular arrhythmias in perspective: A current view. *Am. Heart J.* 1992;123:1140–1147.

DeLorenzo, R. A. Prehospital misidentification of tachydysrhythmias. *J. Emerg. Med.* 1993;11:431–436.

CASE 93 PATIENT WHO BECAME LOUD AND ABUSIVE

A 34-year-old man presented himself to the triage nurse complaining of severe low back pain. He was moaning and groaning and appeared in such severe distress from his pain that the nurse immediately triaged him to a booth. He was promptly seen by a nurse and a senior emergency medicine resident.

He stated that the pain had begun a few days earlier and was the result of an exacerbation of an old injury. It started while he was lifting heavy packages at work. He had undergone numerous operations for slipped discs in the past. He had no neurologic deficit but told the staff that the pain felt exactly like his last slipped disc. He begged for some pain medication. He was taking no medication at the time but had used Percodan in the past. He said that he was allergic to codeine and requested a prescription for more Percodan.

Examination was difficult because of the patient's writhing and groaning, but the resident noticed that the patient could be distracted and showed no sign of pain when he sat up with his legs extended before him, a form of "straight leg raising." The physician suspected that his patient was seeking narcotics and told him that there was no indication of a disc herniation and narcotics were not needed. The patient was instead given a muscle relaxant and ibuprofen, at which point he became angry and demanded "proper treatment" from the resident. The patient threatened to sue the resident, the nurse, and the hospital if he was not given the medication of his choice.

Distressed by the deteriorating situation, the resident asked for assistance from the attending physician on duty. This physician was equally unable to define the patient's level of pain and reproduced the resident's inconsistent findings on examination. The patient was again told that the use of narcotics in his case was inappropriate and that the resident's prescriptions should help for muscle spasms of the lower back. The patient, now loudly abusive of the physicians, shouted that he was going to sue the hospital and that the care given in the ED was substandard. The patient was told that if he was unsatisfied with the care, he was free to go to another hospital and get a second opinion. He then got dressed and left the department.

Later, the triage nurse reported to the physicians that as soon as the patient was outside the department and thought that he could no longer be seen by anyone inside, he began walking normally and appeared to be in no distress. The attending physician notified the neighboring EDs to be on the alert for this man should he show up in their departments seeking narcotics.

What is the function of the triage nurse?

How do drug seekers usually present?

What is the likelihood that he will sue?

Discussion

By their nature, EDs must be available 24 hours a day to everyone who seeks care, and without regard to the patient's ability to pay. This makes them targets for persons seeking drugs for nonmedical or recreational purposes. Drug seekers often simulate low back pain, headache, or renal colic, and it is difficult to separate patients who are seeking drugs from those with legitimate pain. Some subtle clues to drug-seeking behavior include the lack of or contradictory objective findings, "allergies" to non-narcotic analgesics or to codeine, and "allergy" to contrast medium, which makes an intravenous pyelogram impossible. These patients often demand immediate relief of their pain, and they usually have no physician available with whom telephone consultation can be made. Patients feigning renal colic have been known to bite their tongues and spit the blood into their urine specimen to mimic hematuria.

Some patients will threaten to sue if their demands are not met. This is almost always an idle threat. If the diagnosis and treatment are appropriate, the patient has no grounds to sue for malpractice. Patients who appear to be in pain but have puzzling aspects to their story may be given a two-day supply of medication and instructed to seek follow-up care within those two days. If no narcotic medication is prescribed, the provider should explain that the desired medication is too strong for the problem and is not medically indicated but that another analgesic can be used. There is very little to be gained by confronting the patient in most ED encounters. In many cases the EDs will warn each other and the patient's physician when they suspect drug-seeking behavior. When they realize that access to these drugs has been limited, these patients have been known to move on to other cities.

When patients walk into our ED, they first give their complaint to a triage nurse. The nurse has guidelines by which to distribute patients to different areas of the department. Inside our department, a nursing assessment is performed and documented on every patient. The nurse often uncovers facts that the patient is hesitant to tell the doctor. A physician who fails to read the nursing notes on a patient does so at his own and his patient's peril.

REFERENCES

Review Articles

Dubin, W. R. Evaluating and managing the violent patient. *Ann. Emerg. Med.* 1981;10:481–484.

Wiens, D. A. Acute low back pain: Differential diagnosis, targeted assessment, and therapeutic controversies. *Emerg. Med. Rep.* 1995;16:129–140.

Additional References

Johnson, R., and Trimble, E. C. The (expletive deleted) shouter. *JACEP* 1975;4:333–335.

Grove, J. E. Taking care of the hateful patient. *N. Engl. J. Med.* 1978;298:883–887.

Schwenk, P. L., et al. Physician and patient determinants of difficult physician patient relationship. *J. Fam. Pract.* 1989;28:59–63.

Graber, M., et al. The use of unofficial "problem patient" files and interinstitutional information transfer in emergency medicine in Iowa. *Am. J. Emerg. Med.* 1995;13:509–511.

Finch, J. Prescription drug abuse. *Prim. Care* 1993;20:231–239.

Peteet, J. R. and Evans, K. R. Problematic behavior of drug-dependent patients in the general hospital: A clinical and administrative approach to management. *Gen. Hosp. Psychiatry* 1991;13:150–155.

Case 94   MULTIPLE SHOOTING VICTIMS

The EMS dispatcher called in on the ambulance radio, saying there was a multiple-casualty incident in progress. Multiple shootings had occurred in a poor section of the city. Her initial report stated that there were at least five casualties. She heard that one might be dead at the scene, that one had head, chest, and abdominal wounds, and that there were several others. The trauma teams and several additional residents were called to the department to help deal with the anticipated disaster.

The department staff attempted to contact a local police dispatcher to get more detailed information, but none was available at the time. About 20 minutes later, a city paramedic unit called in on the medical control radio with the condition of one of the victims. They reported a man in his twenties who had been shot once in the head and was now unconscious. They had intubated his trachea, placed a large-bore intravenous line of Ringer's lactate, and were transporting him to the emergency department, with an estimated time of arrival (ETA) of five minutes. Indeed, in five minutes the team arrived with their patient. They reported that there were other victims, but they had no idea of how many or the extent of their injuries.

Moments later, a second paramedic unit brought in another man in his twenties who had been shot once in the neck. He seemed to be breathing adequately. He had been treated in the field with two large-bore intravenous lines of lactated Ringer's and placed on oxygen with a nonrebreather mask.

The second paramedic unit reported that one person had been declared dead on the scene, but they did not know if there were any other victims. Further radio calls to the EMS dispatcher were made, but she had no further information about the incident.

When the police supervisor at the scene arrived about 15 minutes later, he informed the ED team that the two patients who had just been brought in were the only living victims of the shooting. Another victim was pronounced dead at the scene, and they were still searching for other victims. They also knew of another incident, unrelated to this one, in which a man jumped out of a second-story window to avoid being shot. He was being transported to our department and arrived shortly thereafter.

The first patient, with the head injury, was rushed off for a CT scan, which showed widespread intracranial damage. He was placed on a ventilator, hyperventilated, and admitted but was declared brain dead several hours later. He was hepatitis B positive and thus unsuitable for organ donation. The second victim's wounds were explored in the ED under local anesthesia, and the bullet track was found to have pierced the platysma muscle. He was admitted to the operating room for a neck exploration.

What is a multiple-casualty incident?

What are the elements of a disaster plan?

Was the neck wound treated correctly?

DISCUSSION

An *EMS disaster* is defined as a sudden, calamitous event, producing injury and death, that is beyond the capacity of the normal EMS response. It may be a natural event or it may be human-made. Building collapses, explosions, plane crashes, fires, and major motor vehicle accidents with multiple victims all qualify. The events are sudden and result in many casualties. Most natural disasters disrupt communications in the area, making notification of hospitals difficult. Weather-related disasters usually cause many moderate to minor injuries and a trickle of more serious ones. Persons with serious injuries usually are not found soon enough to be brought to medical attention. Human-made disasters lead to a bolus of many serious injuries arriving rapidly, because the area of the disaster is usually well defined and can be quickly reached by police, fire, and medical rescue units. Multiple-casualty incidents are "minidisasters," in that they may stress the facilities of any one hospital if all the victims of the incident are brought there.

The keys to successful disaster management are proper command structure at the scene and coordinated communications. The paramedics should recognize any multiple-casualty incident as a disaster, and a senior member of the first squad on the scene should be designated as

94. MULTIPLE SHOOTING VICTIMS

the incident commander. This person will designate the role for each of the subsequent rescuers to play in the rescue and transport and is in charge of all communications from the scene. One rescuer assumes the role of the triage officer. This person goes from one victim to the next and performs a primary assessment on each patient before determining the priority with which each will be managed. This person will also begin treatment of the ABCs for each patient in need of an open airway and ventilation. Of course, such a scenario assumes an adequate number of well-trained rescuers. In well organized systems working correctly, the triage officer at the scene tags patients with color codes to direct the next arriving rescue teams. Black tags are placed on anyone who is without vital signs or considered unsalvageable. Red tags are put on those with immediately life-threatening injuries and designate the highest priority for treatment and transport. Yellow and green tags are put on those with lesser injuries. Immediately life-threatening (red) injuries usually involve the respiratory and cardiovascular systems. Less serious (yellow) injuries include multiple fractures and head traumas that lack signs of increasing intracranial pressure. Green-tagged patients are the "walking wounded" and can help themselves to get to the ambulances.

Prompt notification of the hospital by the incident commander is essential in allowing the hospital to ready itself for the patients and to allocate resources for each patient. Notification should include the number of casualties in each category and the approximate time it will take to extricate and transport the first patient. The hospital should be updated frequently.

We encourage our prehospital providers to treat any multiple-casualty incident as a disaster so that they can practice the elements of the disaster plan. This includes any incident in which there are more than two victims. Through this kind of practice, they will be familiar with the practical aspects of the plan and will be able to execute it when a major disaster strikes. In addition, many municipalities stage a major disaster drill once a year. This usually includes a hypothetical scenario with "patients" moulaged (made up) to appear as real injuries and then transported to hospitals and "treated." The drill concludes with a critique by all the participants in order to find weaknesses in the plan and its operation.

The second patient in this "disaster" had a penetrating wound of the neck. These wounds are usually explored in the operating room if the track of the bullet or knife penetrates the platysma muscle. Even apparently superficial neck wounds demand close observation because of the threat of expanding hematoma and undetected great vessel, tracheal, and esophageal injuries.

REFERENCES

Review Article
Pepe, P. E., and Kvetan, V. Field management and critical care in mass disasters. *Crit. Care Clin.* 1991;7:401–420.
The entire volume 7 number 2 issue is devoted to disaster management.

Additional References
Fain, R. M., and Schreirer, R. A. Disaster, stress and the doctor. *Med. Educ.* 1989;23:91–96.

Haynes, B. E., et al. A pre-hospital approach to multiple victim incidents. *Ann. Emerg. Med.* 1986;15:458–462.

Selden, B. S. Adolescent epidemic hysteria presenting as a mass casualty, toxic exposure incident. *Ann. Emerg. Med.* 1989;18:892–895.

Noji, E. K. Progress in disaster management. *Lancet* 1994;343:1239–1240.

Vukmir, R. B., and Paris, P. M. The Three Rivers regatta accident: An EMS perspective. *Am. J. Emerg. Med.* 1991;9:64–71.

Case 95 REFUSING TREATMENT

Paramedics were called to the home of a 69-year-old woman. Her daughter had noticed a change in her behavior over the past several days and tried to get her to the doctor. The day before, the daughter had called the ambulance twice, but it left both times after the mother refused transport to the hospital.

The paramedics attempted to get vital signs, but the patient refused; the only one they were able to obtain was a respiratory rate of 24 per minute. The patient was agitated and appeared upset at the presence of the paramedics in her home. She was answering their questions appropriately and still refusing to go to the hospital even for a "check up." The medics contacted their hospital base station for medical control.

The medical control physician agreed with the medics' assessment that the patient should be seen in the hospital. He was unsure of the degree of impairment of the patient's ability to decide for herself whether or not she needed treatment. He asked to speak to the woman's daughter and ascertained from her that the patient's behavior was truly unusual and that the change had been abrupt, over only a few days. He then ordered the paramedics to bring the patient to the hospital against her will, stating "You're a lot bigger than she is."

In the ambulance, the medics placed an oxygen mask on the patient. Shortly after, she stated that she felt better and that she was glad they were taking her to the hospital. Evaluation in the emergency department disclosed a bilateral pneumonia and hypoxemia. She made an uneventful recovery.

Do all patients have a right to refuse treatment?

When can patients be held against their will for treatment?

What constitutes assault in the medical setting?

DISCUSSION

This patient presented with an acute organic brain syndrome secondary to hypoxia. Her daughter helped make this diagnosis by noticing that her behavior was different from usual. In older patients, this may be the only clue to an acute underlying medical problem and should never be passed off as being dementia until all treatable causes of acute mental status changes have been ruled out.

In this case, the first two ambulance crews allowed this woman to sign herself out from medical care against medical advice (AMA). In the prehospital setting, this is commonly referred to as *refusal of medical attention (RMA)*. Allowing patients who have requested medical care to sign out without receiving an evaluation by a physician is a potentially dangerous practice. The legal liability for abandonment is great, especially if it can be proven that the patient did not fully understand the ramifications of refusing care.

Patients, in general, have the right to refuse any medical care offered. In order to refuse medical help, the patient must be "competent" to make this decision. Legally, competency or the lack of it can only be determined by a judge. An operational medical definition known as "capacity" requires that the patient fully understand the ramifications of his or her decision to refuse care. Most patients can be given the facts, asked questions to determine their understanding of the facts, and then they can sign a statement attesting to this understanding. The documentation of these cases is extremely important, and the signing of the AMA statement should be witnessed by at least one other staff person and, if possible, a member of the patient's family. The documentation should include the procedures or tests that the patient is refusing, the risks of refusal, and the potential benefits of treatment.

Some patients cannot be assumed to be able to understand all the ramifications of their refusals. These patients include any who are intoxicated or who have hypoxia, acidosis, or another metabolic derangement. These patients should be held for treatment against their will. Of course the problem at the scene is knowing which patient has these problems. We can seldom be sure. An abnormal vital sign might alert us to the presence of a worrisome metabolic or cardiovascular-pulmonary derangement, but what angry person, resisting unwarranted intrusion, would not have a tachycardia or elevated blood pressure?

A mental status exam should always be documented. Patients who are suicidal or homicidal may also be held against their will until a psychiatrist says that they no longer represent a threat to themselves or others. Physical restraint may be needed in these cases.

A patient can bring suit against a physician for treatment rendered against the patient's wishes. The complaint is a civil charge of assault, but the plaintiff must prove that the physician acted with wanton disregard for the patient's safety or in a malicious manner. The patient must also prove that damages resulted from this treatment. The damages that can result from *proper restraint* of a patient are less than damages resulting from *not treating* the patient. Lack of treatment can result in a poor outcome and lead to a suit for medical malpractice. This has occurred in cases of intoxicated patients being allowed to leave the emergency department AMA without adequate diagnosis (e.g., subdural hematomas, cervical spine fractures) who then have progression of their illness or injury resulting in impairment or death.

REFERENCES

Review Article

Mayer, D. Refusal of care and discharging "difficult" patients from the emergency department. *Ann. Emerg. Med.* 1990;19:1436–1446.

Additional References

Fastow, J. Medical malpractice and emergency medicine: The crisis of the 1980's (editorial). *Am. J. Emerg. Med.* 1985;6:571–573.

Holroyd, B., et al. Pre-hospital patients refusing care. *Ann. Emerg. Med.* 1988;17:957–963.

Lipowski, Z. J. Delerium in the elderly patient. *N. Engl. J. Med.* 1989;320:578–582.

Appelbaum, B. S., and Roth, L. H. Patients who refuse treatment in medical hospitals. *J.A.M.A.* 1983;250:1296–1301.

Dunn, J. D. Risk management in emergency medicine. *Emerg. Med. Clin. North Am.* 1987;5:51–69.

Stark, G., and Hedges, J. R. Patients who initially refuse prehospital evaluation and/or therapy. *Ann. Emerg. Med.* 1990;8(6):509–511.

Alicandro, J., et al. Impact of interventions for patients refusing emergency medical services transport. *Acad. Emerg. Med.* 1995;2:480–486.

Case 96 THE EXPLODING CAR BATTERY

A 23-year-old man was improperly charging his automobile battery when it exploded in his face. His face was struck by the top of the battery and splashed with acid. On arrival at the emergency department, he complained of not being able to see. We took him to a large sink, where we washed his face with cool water. He had redness and blistering on his cheeks, under both eyes, and on his eyelids. Swelling and ecchymosis were evident around his left eye.

Topical anesthetic drops were instilled in both eyes, and within 30 seconds he had less pain. Each eye was irrigated with 1 liter of normal saline. He was given 4 mg intravenous morphine for pain relief, and then his eyes were examined with a slit lamp. His right eye showed a superficial corneal abrasion over the center of the visual field. The left showed a small hyphema that could only be seen with the slit lamp. He was referred for ophthalmologic evaluation.

What problems can result in a sudden loss of vision?

Which types of eye trauma require specialty care by an ophthalmologist?

Is this patient likely to develop orbital cellulitis?

Discussion

Sudden loss of vision is most commonly caused by blunt or penetrating trauma. Less commonly, it can be due to retinal artery occlusion, temporal arteritis, retinal or vitreous hemorrhages, retinal vein occlusion, optic neuritis, or retinal detachment. All patients with visual complaints need to have a visual acuity performed, and almost all of those with true sudden loss of vision require a prompt ophthalmologic consultation for help with diagnosis and treatment.

Almost all serious chemical burns to the eye are caused by strong acids or alkalis. Alkaline burns are more dangerous, because the alkaline material seeps into the corneal epithelium, and this results in both deeper injury and greater potential for scarring. In any chemical burn, the eye should be *immediately* and copiously irrigated. Using a few drops of topical anesthetic was essential in helping this patient keep his eye open during irrigation. Either water or normal saline could have been used. Following irrigation the pH of the conjugational sack should be checked, and irrigation should be continued until it returns to normal (pH 7.3 to 7.7). The eye should then be examined using a slit lamp and a "blue light" with fluorescein dye. If a thorough eye examination is normal except for conjunctival irritation, we generally do not obtain ophthalmologic consultation, although follow-up in 12 to 24 hours is recommended in all but minor cases.

Blunt trauma to the eye can cause acute vision loss from globe rupture, retinal detachment, and hyphema (blood in the anterior chamber). If the trauma is deeper than the cornea, immediate ophthalmologic consultation is required. If a thorough examination shows that the injury is limited to a superficial corneal abrasion, treatment with a topical antibiotic and close follow-up usually suffice.

This patient certainly had the potential to develop an orbital cellulitis (heralded by a warm, red, proptotic eye), but that syndrome occurs mostly in children or the immunocompromised and usually is not preceded by obvious external trauma. This patient was more likely to develop a superficial cellulitis of the lids and periorbital tissue. In the end, he received good follow-up care, followed his discharge instructions carefully, and recovered uneventfully.

REFERENCES

Review Article

Linden, J. A., and Renner, G. S. Trauma to the globe. *Emerg. Med. Clin. North Am.* 1995;13:581–606.

The entire volume 13 number 3 issue is devoted to emergency treatment of the eye.

Additional References

Schein, O. D. Contact lens abrasions and the nonophthalmologist. *Am. J. Emerg. Med.* 1993;11:606–608.

Gossman, M. D., Roberts, D. M., and Barr, C. C. Ophthalmic aspects of orbital injury: A comprehensive diagnostic and management approach. *Clin. Plast. Surg.* 1992;19:71–85.

Zun, L. S. Acute vision loss. *Emerg. Med. Clin. North Am.* 1988;6:57–72.

Case 97 BROKE THE STEERING WHEEL WITH HIS CHEST

A 67-year-old man was in a motor vehicle accident. His car struck a tree at a high rate of speed, breaking the steering wheel and shattering the windshield. When the EMS unit arrived, he was combative, with a blood pressure of 100/60. They placed him in a MAST suit, started two large-bore intravenous lines, and applied a cervical collar. He was taken to the nearest hospital. On examination in that emergency department his blood pressure was 110/60, and he was given Valium because of his agitation. A chest x-ray showed seven rib fractures, and he was promptly transferred to the local trauma center.

On arrival there he was still quite agitated and complained of chest pain. He had received oxygen via nasal cannula during transfer, and his initial arterial blood gas results at the trauma center were pH 7.14, pO_2 55, and pCO_2 46. He was intubated and placed on a ventilator. Thirty minutes later his pO_2 had risen to 180, and his mental status had improved. A repeat chest x-ray showed a hemothorax on the right side and a slightly widened mediastinum. A chest tube was inserted and 150 ml of blood returned. A peritoneal lavage was positive. A repeat chest x-ray done after the chest tube was inserted showed a further widening of the mediastinum to over 12 cm, with obliteration of the aortic knob and displacement of his nasogastric tube to the right. Because of those signs, the doctors caring for him thought he had a traumatic aortic tear. Signs of diaphragmatic rupture (hazy diaphragm shadow, air fluid levels in the chest) were absent. The patient was taken to the operating room, where an aortic angiogram was performed. When the angiogram was normal, the surgeon proceeded with a laparotomy, during which the patient's ruptured spleen was removed. He was admitted to the intensive care unit for continued ventilation therapy.

What was the significance of this man's initial acidosis?

Why did he need to be intubated and mechanically ventilated?

DISCUSSION

Acidosis on an initial arterial blood gas frequently is the first noted sign of shock in a patient who is still able to maintain a relatively normal blood pressure. It is a key sign of occult internal hemorrhage and borderline hypovolemic shock in the trauma patient.

This patient's hypoxia was caused by his hemothorax and inadequate ventilation from chest wall trauma. He had a flail chest—multiple ribs were broken in two locations, rendering a section of his chest wall unstable. He needed to be intubated and mechanically ventilated because of his hypoxia and because positive pressure ventilation is the most effective way to keep a flail segment moving with the rest of the chest wall.

The most dramatic injuries from blunt chest trauma are ruptures of the aorta or the heart. They usually produce immediate exsanguination. A laceration of the aorta still encapsulated by clot, the vessel adventitia, or both typically presents with no symptoms and must be suspected when a widened mediastinum is seen on a chest x-ray. A partial tear of the aorta can result in delayed rupture, so it is important to promptly do an aortogram to rule in or out the diagnosis when it is suspected.

Myocardial contusion is another potentially fatal complication of blunt chest trauma. It can cause any of the same complications myocardial infarction (MI) can, and like an MI it can be difficult to diagnose. It is a poorly understood condition. Major blunt chest trauma patients are always admitted to an intensive care setting, but we often do not know which "minor" chest injury patients need to be admitted for cardiac monitoring.

REFERENCES

Review Article
Jackimczyk, K. Blunt chest trauma. *Emerg. Med. Clin. North Am.* 1993;11:81–96.

Additional References
Marconha, K. E., et al. Blunt chest trauma and suspected aortic rupture: Reliability of the chest radiographic findings. *Ann. Emerg. Med.* 1985;14:644–649.

Healey, M. A., et al. Blunt cardiac injury: Is this diagnosis necessary? *J. Trauma* 1990;30:137–145.

Camp, P. C., et al. Blunt traumatic thoracic aortic lacerations in the elderly: An analysis of outcomes. *J. Trauma* 1994;37:418–421.

McLean, J. F., et al. Significance of myocardial contusion following blunt chest trauma. *J. Trauma* 1992;33:240–243.

Case 98 VD

A young man in his twenties walked into the emergency department and told the triage nurse that he was not feeling well and wanted to see the doctor. He was very vague about his complaints and finally said he thought he had something wrong with his kidneys. He was triaged to the nonacute area of the department. The nurse on duty took his vital signs (which were normal) and asked him a few questions about his illness. He refused to give her any information and said he would tell only the doctor about his problem.

When the physician came in, the patient admitted to burning on urination and a yellow-white discharge from his penis. He also admitted to recent sexual intercourse with a woman who was not his usual sexual partner. The remainder of his history was unremarkable. Examination revealed some discharge at the penile meatus that was sent off for culture, with a small amount smeared on a slide for gram staining. The patient had some shotty inguinal lymph nodes, and his prostate and epididymis were normal. The gram stain demonstrated many WBCs, some of which were loaded with gram-negative intracellular diplococci.

He was treated with one dose of 250 mg ceftriaxone intramuscularly and 100 mg of oral doxycycline bid for 10 days. Blood was drawn for syphilis serology, and he was instructed to go to the state VD clinic 6 weeks later for repeat serology, culture, and HIV counseling. He was also told to have his recent sexual contacts examined and treated for gonorrhea and *Chlamydia* infections and to avoid sexual intercourse for a week to 10 days.

What diagnostic techniques are used to detect sexually transmitted diseases?

If this patient's sexual partners are not clearly identified and diagnosed, will they be sure to seek therapy because of their own symptoms? If not, what will happen to them?

Could this have been syphilis? Herpes?

Discussion

In most men with either gonorrhea or *Chlamydia*, there is symptomatic evidence of VD, although the patient may be reluctant to describe the symptoms, even to the physician. In contrast, most women with gonococcal or chlamydial cervicitis show no symptoms, perhaps for months or years. Nonetheless, if therapy is withheld the patient may well go on to develop acute pelvic inflammatory disease (PID), distant septic spread such as gonococcal arthritis, or infertility.

The patient should be examined. In men, the urethra should be cultured by taking a specimen from the vault just inside the meatus. In women, the cervical os should be cultured (after an initial swabbing to remove as much cervical mucus as possible). The next most useful sites for culture are the anal canal and the urethra, in that order. A gram stain of the cervix is not very helpful, for it is often negative when cultures are positive and sometimes falsely read as positive because of the presence of pleomorphic gram-negative rods that are normal flora *Neisseria vaginalis*.

Males presenting with penile discharge should have a gram stain made of their discharge. This may demonstrate the classic gram-negative intracellular diplococci and sheets of white blood cells typical of gonorrhea. If only white cells are present, the patient is presumed to have nongonococcal urethritis, usually caused by *Chlamydia*.

All men with symptoms suggestive of gonorrhea or *Chlamydia* need to be aggressively treated. Delaying treatment until culture results are available risks progression of the infection and nontreatment because of noncompliance. So, "Treat 'em while you got 'em." Treatment for both gonococcus and *Chlamydia* is recommended, as more than one-fourth of patients with gonococcus also have *Chlamydia*. Because penicillin-resistant gonorrhea is becoming more frequent, our initial treatment of choice is now a single dose of cefixime (Suprax), 400 mg orally, or ceftriaxone 250 mg intramuscularly, followed by either a one-time dose of 1 g of azithromycin or doxycycline 100 mg orally bid for 7 days. Because the incidence of syphilis is rising and it is not adequately treated with this regimen, a VDRL or equivalent serologic test for syphilis should be obtained at the time of treatment.

The most common complication of untreated or inadequately treated gonorrhea in either sex is a persistent subclinical infection, with the patient still able to transmit the disease. Female carriers may at any time become acutely ill with PID and develop nausea, vomiting, lower abdominal pain, tenderness, fever, leukocytosis, or rebound tenderness with peritonitis, all of which make differentiation from appendicitis difficult. This acute pelvic inflammatory disease may require hospitalization with parenteral high-dose antibiotic therapy and may render the female patient sterile thereafter. It will also predispose her to future ectopic pregnancies. This kind of acute illness may develop weeks or months after the initial contact with gonorrhea; thus, treatment of asymptomatic gonorrhea is essential. In fact, therapy without a pelvic examination would be acceptable, though not optimal. We automatically treat known sexual contacts of patients who have gonorrhea. We do not wait for the results of the culture to begin therapy when there is a suggestive history, as in this case.

Occasionally syphilis or herpes genitalis can be diagnosed in the ED, and the incidence of both infections has increased dramatically over the past few years. Syphilis can be detected in the early stage by the presence of a painless ulcer (chancre) in the genital area. Confirmation by dark-field microscopy can be difficult for most labs, and presumptive treatment with benzathine penicillin is often undertaken. A more common cause of venereal ulceration is herpes genitalis. It usually presents with a small cluster of vesicles or ulcers that are extremely painful. The diagnosis can be confirmed by a Tzank smear (which is much like a PAP smear) or by culture. Early treatment with acyclovir topically, systemically, or both can shorten the duration of the symptoms in some cases, especially first episodes. In patients like this man, with a discharge but no ulcerations, we do not pursue diagnostic testing for herpes, but we do routinely check a VDRL syphilis serology.

REFERENCES

Review Articles
Drugs for sexually transmitted diseases. *Med. Lett.* 1994;36:1–6.
Stewart, C., and Bosker, G. The diverse and challenging spectrum of sexually transmitted diseases (STDs): Current diagnostic modalities and treatment recommendations. *Emerg. Med. Rep.* 1994;15: 251–260.

Additional References

Horsburgh, C. R., Douglas, J. M., and Haraforce, F. M. Preventative strategies in sexually transmitted diseases for the primary care physician. *J.A.M.A.* 1987;258:815–821.

McNabney, W. K., and Barnes, W. G. Urethral and endocervical cultures: Gonorrhea and chlamydia. *Ann. Emerg. Med.* 1986;15:333–336.

Weinstock, H., et al. Chlamydia trachomatis infections. *Infect. Dis. Clin. North Am.* 1994;8:797–819.

Doll, L. S., et al. Failure to disclose HIV risk among gay and bisexual men attending sexually transmitted disease clinics. *Am. J. Prev. Med.* 1994;10:125–129.

Wendell, D. A., et al. Youth at risk: Sex, drugs, and human immunodeficiency virus. *Am. J. Dis. Child.* 1992;146:76–81.

Upchurch, D. M., et al. Interpartner reliability of reporting of recent sexual behaviors. *Am. J. Epidemiol.* 1991;134:1159–1166.

Case 99 CEREBROVASCULAR ACCIDENT

A 79-year-old man was brought to the emergency department of a community hospital by his worried wife. She said that he had awakened that morning and come down to breakfast but his speech made no sense and he seemed as frustrated by the trouble as she was. He had been able to walk and could make words, but they seemed "all wrong." As the day progressed, he developed a clumsiness and began to drop things. Finally, after dinner, she was so worried that she brought him into the hospital.

The patient had been well prior to that day. He was a retired air-conditioner repairman. He had not smoked, drank rarely, and was not noted to be allergic to any medicines. His usual physician, not yet called, had been treating him with digoxin and hydrochlorothiazide for "an irregular heartbeat."

On examination, the patient was well nourished and appeared well except for the neurologic system. His blood pressure was 170/95, pulse 88 and largely regular, with a few irregularities that the emergency physician thought to be atrial premature beats. He was afebrile, and his respiratory rate was 16. He was having a great deal of difficulty with his speech, making no sense at all. He could not name common objects (pen, comb, book) that were shown to him and seemed exasperated by his own difficulty. He managed to articulate "God damn it!" several times. His right arm and leg were both weak compared to his left side. There was a slight droop to the right side of his mouth, but when he tried to close his eyes very tightly his mouth actually pulled up higher on the right side. He could follow simple commands but had difficulty with more complex requests such as "Touch your right ear with your left hand."

The ECG showed atrial fibrillation with a well-controlled ventricular rate.

The emergency physician called the patient's primary care doctor, and they agreed that this patient was suffering a "stroke in evolution." The atrial fibrillation was a long-standing problem. The patient had also been noted to have mild hypertension in the past, well controlled with a small dose of a diuretic.

The primary care physician asked the ED doctor to admit her patient to the hospital. She would be in to visit in the morning. In the meantime, she asked, should the patient be anticoagulated?

What of anticoagulation for a "stroke in evolution"?

Where is this patient's lesion?

His blood pressure was 170/95. Should it have been lowered?

Discussion

This patient does seem to be suffering from a cerebrovascular accident, probably an infarction in the region of the left middle cerebral artery. In a patient with atrial fibrillation, the stroke may be of embolic origin or may just as likely be thrombotic. This patient has right-sided hemiparesis and aphasia. The aphasia seems to be more expressive than receptive but has elements of both, as aphasia usually does. It is still somewhat fluent; the patient can make words, even if they are inappropriate and make little sense. He is aware of his difficulty and distressed by it and will be appreciative of his doctor's recognition of that distress.

Differentiating aphasia from confusion can be difficult but is important because aphasia is a local, usually left-sided phenomenon, and confusion usually denotes diffuse brain disease. The aphasic patient may be aware of his or her difficulty and may express awareness and distress quite emphatically and quite verbally. Even if the patient is not able to express it, he or she may still be receptive to your recognition of and comments on the difficulty; your saying, "You seem to be having a great deal of trouble with speech right now" may be met with vigorous nodding and a smile of relief. The aphasic patient may be able to pick the right word out of a list and then will have a tendency to use that word over and over, incorrectly, as new objects are shown or new questions posed. The aphasic patient will have more trouble following complex requests than simple ones, and requests that oblige the patient to cross the midline will be still more difficult.

99. CEREBROVASCULAR ACCIDENT

Current dogma suggests that we should be gentle in treating hypertension after a stroke has occurred. The patient may have considerable brain swelling and may need a high pressure to perfuse the brain. In fact, plasma expanders are currently being used with some success to limit brain damage in such patients. We would not suggest decreasing this patient's blood pressure further during the acute phase of the cerebral infarction.

Anticoagulation therapy in such patients has been long debated and the data remain confusing. Of course, the patient in atrial fibrillation has another reason for anticoagulation: not to affect this stroke, but to prevent another embolic event. The big question is whether treatment with anticoagulants prevents progression of a stroke in the midst of its usual evolution. The data are mixed, and experts are divided in their opinions. This patient was treated with heparin and then warfarin sodium (Coumadin), as well as oxygen. His initial CT scan was entirely normal. The hemiparesis developed further during his first three days in the hospital, and the clinical diagnosis remained that of a left cerebral infarction. The radiologist commented that early CT scans are often normal in such strokes and that it would probably show an infarction if repeated in a week or two.

Ten days after the onset of the stroke, while in a rehabilitation program, with a prothrombin time of 18 seconds from Coumadin therapy, the patient suddenly worsened. He became stuporous and developed Cheyne-Stokes respiration. A repeat CT scan of his brain at that time showed a large hemorrhagic infarction in his left frontoparietal cerebral cortex. There was a slight midline shift to the right. The lateral ventricles were distorted by mass effect. A consulting neurologist thought that an initial ischemic infarction had hemorrhaged, partly from the anticoagulation, and recommended stopping the Coumadin and perhaps reversing its effect with fresh frozen plasma. The patient did not improve and was eventually discharged to a nursing home. Unfortunately, we have also seen a similar patient who was *not* anticoagulated then proceed to throw a second, more massive clot to his brain and do equally poorly. That is what makes the decision whether to anticoagulate or not so difficult.

A national trial looking at the use of thrombolytic therapy such as streptokinase or tPA in patients like this is currently underway.

REFERENCES

Review Article

Starkman, S., and Barron, D. Stroke: Emergency evaluation and management. *Emerg. Med. Rep.* 1994;15:75–82.

Additional References

Jonas, S. Anticoagulant therapy in cerebrovascular disease: Review and meta-analysis. *Stroke* 1988;19:1043–1048.

A Working Group on Emergency Brain Resuscitation. Emergency brain resuscitation. *Ann. Intern. Med.* 1995;122:622–627.

Adams, H. P., Jr., et al. Guidelines for the management of patients with acute ischemic stroke. A statement for healthcare professionals from a special writing group of the Stroke Council, American Heart Association. *Stroke* 1994;25:1901–1914.

Barnaby, W. Stroke intervention. *Emerg. Med. Clin. North Am.* 1990;8:267–280.

Case 100 MEDICAL MALPRACTICE

A 15-year-old student from a local boarding school was brought into the emergency department complaining of neck pain. She was accompanied by the school nurse, who presented a signed consent from the youth's parents (both of whom were physicians) allowing treatment in case of emergency.

The student said that she had experienced intermittent neck pains in the past and an exacerbation over the past two days without any trauma or other precipitating cause. Examination revealed no abnormalities except pain on palpation of the neck. In fact, the patient jumped when the paraspinous muscles were palpated. Treatment with acetaminophen, bedrest, and a cervical collar was recommended. She was discharged to the care of the school nurse.

Four years later, the physician was presented with a charge of malpractice against this patient claiming that because of his failure to take cervical spine x-rays and to perform proper treatment the patient had continuous, unremitting pain and was unable to pursue her chosen career as a surgeon.

What is the most appropriate ED workup and treatment for nontraumatic neck pain?

What are the elements of medical malpractice, and who gets sued?

What are the best defenses against a successful malpractice suit?

Discussion

Any physician can be sued for malpractice. The shock of being sued in this case came from the fact that there was no question about the appropriateness of the treatment rendered. Malpractice accusations can come at any time and about any case. Sometimes suits are brought by patients who do not get better or who get worse and are angry about the outcome. Sometimes a patient who did not get the anticipated result or who had a poor outcome wants to be paid for a perceived wrong, such as a poor attitude on the part of the treating physician or nurse.

The elements of a successful medical malpractice suit are (1) preexisting duty to treat, (2) breach of that duty, (3) damage has occurred, and (4) *"proximate cause."* Duty exists whenever any person presents to the ED for treatment. Breach of duty includes any action that the physician takes that is below a set standard of treatment for the problem. The standard may be local or national. Damages are whatever the patient alleges to have suffered. *Proximate cause* means that the damage was caused by the breach of duty. All four of these elements must be proven in court in order for a malpractice charge to be upheld. (Where good samaritan acts apply, e.g., when a physician stops by the side of the road to aid an accident victim, different standards apply and malpractice is harder to prove). In any case, the job of the lawyer arguing a malpractice case is to convince a panel of ordinary citizens that his or her client's damages are severe and will interfere with the client's life, and that the physician in question may be at least partly to blame for the damages.

Although many paint a dismal picture of the physician's ability to defend against a malpractice case, many defensive measures can be taken to prevent a bad outcome. *The most important defense that the physician has is the medical record.* A well-written and comprehensive description of the events involved in the encounter will allow the physician to reconstruct long-forgotten events and explain the reasons for the treatment given. This suit was begun four years after the incident (the statute of limitations began again when the patient became 18). By that time the facts were far from the memory of the practitioner. Equally important are the nursing notes and prehospital care provider notes. These can all help corroborate the physician's information. The importance of the medical record cannot be overemphasized, and it is reasonable to treat every chart as if you were going to have to go to trial with it in the future.

Poor outcomes in medical practice do occur, and these should be documented along with the reasons for their occurrence. An active departmental quality assurance program will help to discover which types of cases have the greatest potential for malpractice action and will allow the physicians to improve their treatment and documentation of these cases. In this case, the physician and nurse had both documented the case carefully, and, although the case went to trial, the ED physician won. Had the documentation been poor, the outcome might have been different.

The workup for acute nontraumatic neck pain in an otherwise healthy young person depends on the setting. If increasing pain, neurologic signs, or hard, matted lymph nodes are present, an x-ray may be useful to look for underlying neoplastic disease of the spine. Otherwise, physical examination including range of motion, areas of tenderness, distal sensation, strength, and circulation is all that is necessary for a presumptive diagnosis. In older age groups x-rays should be taken more freely, because the incidence of bony metastases is higher and the presence of osteoporosis increases the likelihood of cervical spine fracture with otherwise minimal trauma. Treatment is the same for acute muscle spasm or a herniated disc without cord or nerve root involvement. The treatment prescribed in this case was reasonable. We recommend follow-up in a week if needed. Further evaluation may then be performed on an outpatient basis.

REFERENCES

Review Articles

Cailliet, R. *Neck and Arm Pain.* Philadelphia: Davis, 1964. Pp. 40–44, 86–90.

Wood, C. L. Historical perspectives on law, medical malpractice, and the concept of negligence. *Emerg. Med. Clin. North Am.* 1993;11: 819–832.

The entire volume 11 number 4 issue is devoted to medicolegal issues.

Additional References

Gore, D. R., et al. Neck pain. A long term follow-up of 205 patients. *Spine* 1987;12:1–5.

Medical Malpractice Statutes. Arizona Revised Statutes. St. Paul, MN: West, 1982. Pp. 357–370.

Describes a model malpractice statute.

Fish, R., and Ehrhardt, M. Review of medical negligence cases: An essential part of residency programs. *J. Emerg. Med.* 1992;10(4):501–504.

Case 101 RULE OUT MI

A man drove himself to the emergency department and presented at the triage desk complaining of a "spasm of his breast bone." He was a very physically active 52-year-old man who had first noticed discomfort early that morning at his gym. He had done his usual 12 minutes on the treadmill, followed by a walk around the track and stretching exercises. He then lifted weights for 30 minutes, and, while cooling down after finishing, he noticed some mid-sternal discomfort and right-sided chest wall tenderness. The discomfort went away, and he went home from the gym. When he had another "spasm" later that morning, he became concerned and went to the ED. He had experienced similar but less extensive discomfort in the past. He was in good health otherwise, except for a recent prostatitis for which he was taking Bactrim.

On arrival at the ED, the patient was very anxious. In fact, he was shaking so hard when he got to the stretcher that his electrocardiogram was unreadable and the nurse had to reinsert his IV because he shook it loose the first time. His vital signs were normal, including a pulse 52 and blood pressure 140/70. The rest of his physical examination was normal except for right-sided chest wall tenderness to palpation, which the patient said reproduced his pain. Both the ED physician and the patient's private attending physician, who happened to be passing through the department, saw him almost immediately after arrival. The second electrocardiogram, taken after the patient said he could calm down, showed J-point elevation in leads V_2, V_3, and V_4. While the two physicians were discussing what to do with the patient, he developed a recurrence of his discomfort and the ED physician asked that the electrocardiogram be repeated. At this point, the ED physician wanted to admit the patient as a "Rule out MI." The private attending disagreed and audibly grumbled that the patient had "obvious costochondritis." Nevertheless, he reluctantly agreed to admit the patient, although when the ED physician went to the patient's bedside to see the most recent ECG the private attending said loudly to a group of ED nurses and clerks, "Let's get the patient out of here before he (the ED doctor) ECG's him to death."

The patient was soon seen in the coronary care unit by the attending cardiologist, who agreed with the private attending physician and wrote as his diagnosis "Probable chest wall musculoskeletal tenderness." The initial CPK and CPK-MB were normal, but subsequent tests later that day confirmed that the patient was having a myocardial infarction. He was transferred stat. to the nearest hospital with cardiac catheterization and angioplasty capability. The patient survived.

How unusual is "atypical" chest pain in heart attack victims?

What are the implications of loud and public disagreements between two caregivers?

DISCUSSION

This case is typical of patients who present to the ED with chest pain and ischemic heart disease. The diagnosis of ischemia is often difficult in such patients, as they often do not present with "classic" symptoms, such as substernal pressure with jaw and left arm involvement, nausea, and shortness of breath. Most studies of patients with MI show that they often present to the ED with pain that is "atypical." As many as 20% will present with sharp or stabbing pain, and another 20 to 30% will present with heartburn-like discomfort. Older patients with MI have atypical presentations even more often, with as few as 50% having a chief complaint of chest pain.

A minority of patients with documented MI will have pleuritic, positional or palpable chest pain, thus emphasizing the point that cardiac ischemia cannot be excluded on the basis of these symptoms alone. Only 50% of initial ECGs will be abnormal in patients with documented MIs, so it is not a reliable screening tool unless positive. The initial cardiac enzymes will be positive only half the time in patients who have MI, which limits this test's usefulness as well.

This patient had both typical and atypical presenting signs and symptoms. His pain was fairly characteristic but was also associated with chest wall tenderness. Of note, the pain was exertional in nature and so strongly suggestive of an ischemic etiology. His pulse of 52 may be because of a well-conditioned heart, but bradycardia is often associated with cardiac ischemia and is a potentially worrisome finding. The ECG also has some S-T and T wave abnormalities, which *could* be from a nonischemic cause such as early repolarization, but also may be ischemic in nature.

The fact that the patient had chest wall tenderness convinced the private physician that the pain was musculoskeletal in nature. It is very important to ascertain if palpating the chest wall fully reproduces the pain syndrome. If not, it may be an unrelated finding; studies have shown that up to 20% of patients with MI will have associated chest wall tenderness. Unfortunately, we have occasionally seen other patients, like this one, who, in spite of acute MI being the actual diagnosis, tell us, possibly for a variety of reasons, that they have chest wall tenderness and that our chest wall palpation reproduces their acute discomfort.

The emergency physician often has a difficult task in making the correct diagnosis of cardiac ischemia in patients who present to the ED with chest pain. This point is emphasized by the fact that missed MI remains the most frequent malpractice claim against emergency physicians. Given the potentially grave consequences of discharging a patient with myocardial ischemia or infarct, the physician must understand the various clinical presentations of this disease and not consider discharge for patients at risk for cardiac disease.

The "stage whisper" of the patient's private attending ("Let's get him out of here before he ECG's him to death") deserves some comment. Much of the difficulty doctors have is with other doctors. The best care is collaborative and respectful, yet loud public disagreements between two caregivers are all too common. They can make an already anxious patient more so and can lead one caregiver to defer to another when it's not appropriate.

REFERENCES

Review Articles

Albrich, J. M. Acute myocardial infarction: Comprehensive guidelines for diagnosis, stabilization, and mortality reduction. *Emerg. Med. Rep.* 1994;15:51–62.

American College of Emergency Physicians. Clinical policy for the initial approach to adults presenting with a chief complaint of chest pain, with no history of trauma. *Ann. Emerg. Med.* 1995;25:274–299.

Additional References

Bayer, A. J., et al. Changing presentation of myocardial infarction with increasing old age. *J. Am. Geriatr. Soc.* 1986;34:263–266.

Herr, C. H. The diagnosis of acute myocardial infarction in the emergency department. *J. Emerg. Med.* 1992;10:455–461.

Rusnak, R. A., Stair, T. O., Hansen, K., and Fastow, J. S. Litigation against the emergency physician: Common feature in cases of missed myocardial infarction. *Ann. Emerg. Med.* 1989;18:1029–1034.

Wears, R. L., et al. How many myocardial infarctions should we rule out? *Ann. Emerg. Med.* 1989;18:953-963.

Case 102 THE LIAR

A 41-year-old man arrived at our ED complaining of severe right flank pain. He had a history of surgery for kidney stones four years earlier at a large metropolitan university teaching hospital. He also had undergone an appendectomy at age 12. His current flank pain had begun approximately four hours prior to his arrival. There was no radiation to the scrotum or penis. He said he had vomited twice and had severe nausea. He also stated that he had blood-tinged urine but no fever. On examination he had right costovertebral angle tenderness. An old scar was found on the right flank and back. There was no other tenderness in the back or abdomen.

He was initially medicated with intramuscular Demerol and Vistaril (hydroxyzine). He had pain relief at first, but approximately 20 minutes after receiving the narcotic injection he was screaming for the physician to come back and remedicate him. He was also screaming for the urinal and stated to the nurse that he knew we wanted a urine specimen. Because of his severe pain, the nurse felt that he should not be left alone; she thought he might become dizzy while trying to give the urine sample. When the nurse would not leave as the patient stood to urinate, the patient became angry and actually threw the urinal at the nurse. He said he didn't want anyone watching him. He was told that this was the policy of the ED, and he then agreed to give the urine sample anyway and turned away from the nurse. While the patient was giving the urine sample, the nurse observed him taking a safety pin from his pocket and pricking his finger. The nurse immediately confronted the patient and took the now filled urinal away from him.

The urine that was in the urinal tested negative for gross and microscopic blood. The physician was immediately informed. The patient continued to ask for pain medication, and the physician finally agreed to give him a very small additional dose of Demerol and Vistaril intramuscularly. When this was given, the nurse noted that there were more than six old injection sites on his buttock. When confronted with this, the patient stated that he was recently treated at the VA hospital for migraine headaches. However, he stated that he did not wish to return there. He was reevaluated 20 minutes later and stated that he had no pain and was discharged to follow up with his family physician.

102. THE LIAR

Did the nurse invade this patient's privacy by demanding to stay in the room when he gave his urine sample?

What is the best way of dealing with patients who are feigning illness in order to obtain narcotics?

What is a reasonable evaluation process for patients who have renal colic?

Discussion

The patient with renal colic always presents difficulties. They are in such severe pain that they are typically unable to sit still. Characteristically, these patients will frequently move on the stretcher, pace around the room holding their sides, or otherwise be unable to find a comfortable position. Prompt evaluation of these patients requires a good initial physical examination. The physician must then promptly decide whether it is safe to give immediate pain medication or whether it is essential to wait until further diagnostic tests are done. Giving pain medication early in the evaluation of the patient with an intra-abdominal catastrophe can cloud the diagnosis. However, waiting until extensive testing is done leaves the renal colic patient in pain for an unnecessarily long period of time. A reasonable solution is to give a small amount of medication immediately. This will make the patient's pain more tolerable and actually allow a better physical examination. Typically, parenteral Toradol or Demerol, neither of which cause smooth muscle colic, are used first. The physician then needs to become relatively certain that an immediately life-threatening problem (e.g., ruptured or dissecting aortic aneurysm, perforated bowel or bowel obstruction) is not present.

In this case, the nurse discovered that this patient was using deceit to obtain more narcotic drugs. This discovery occurred because she refused to leave the patient while he was urinating. The nurse's assessment of this patient was correct. He was at risk of falling and injuring himself if he were left alone to give a urine sample while in severe pain. A nurse's responsibilities include assisting patients, providing for their creature comforts, and protecting them from bodily harm. Physicians share these responsibilities and should always be available to assist the nursing staff in carrying them out. Responsibilities such as making sure that bed rails are up, sheets are covering the patient, and IVs are running properly all fall into this category. Patients who are in severe pain, dizzy, frail, or dehydrated should not be allowed to stand up without assistance. The nurse's presence in the room in this case was not an undue invasion of privacy but an assurance of safety.

When patients appear to be drug seeking they should be confronted. These patients need help. They have a severe drug abuse problem, which is a medical illness that can be treated. Patients should be offered treatment for their drug abuse problems. In most cases, the patients initially deny that there is a drug problem and often become angry at the physician. However, if the physician is certain that the patient is seeking drugs and does not have another bona fide medical illness, the physician would do more harm by giving in to the patient and giving drugs. Some clues to drug seeking behavior, such as needle track marks, are obvious. Additional clues are inappropriate behavior, overly demanding, obsessive requests for pain medication, multiple allergies (specifically to IVP dye, aspirin, ibuprofen (Motrin), Toradol, or codeine), requesting specific drugs by name, being *too* inquisitive about the name and dosage of the drug used, and an exam including vital signs that is grossly normal in a patient complaining of severe symptoms.

The obvious problem in these cases is the need to identify patients with a true medical illness that requires treatment and medicate them early, while also identifying and not giving inappropriate drugs to the abuser. Unfortunately, it is impossible to correctly decide which is which in all cases.

REFERENCES

Review Article
Peterson, N. E. Common urologic emergencies: A logical and practical approach to rapid diagnosis and treatment. *Acad. Emerg. Med.* 1994;1:186–189.

Additional References
Ducharme, J. Emergency pain management: A Canadian Association of Emergency Physicians consensus document. *J. Emerg. Med.* 1994;12:855–866.

Heller, M. B. Emergency management of acute pain. New options and strategies. *Postgrad. Med.* 1992; Special Number:39–47.

Chang, T. S., and Lepanto, L. Ultrasonography in the emergency setting. *Emerg. Med. Clin. North Am.* 1992;10:1–25.

Yealy, D. M. Acute pain management. *Acad. Emerg. Med.* 1994;1:186–189.

Case 103 DO NOT RESUSCITATE

An 86-year-old woman was brought to the ED at 5 A.M. by ambulance because she was unable to breathe. The patient had been in her usual state of health, had been living in a nursing home, and had no complaints when she went to bed the night before. She had a past history of congestive heart failure, GI bleeding, and Parkinson's disease. She also had a history of hiatal hernia, cholelithiasis, COPD, osteoarthritis, and arteriosclerotic heart disease with congestive heart failure and pulmonary edema. She had been admitted in the past, had been intubated and on a ventilator, and was designated as DNR (do not resuscitate) on her last admission. She had awoken in the middle of the night and was found by the nursing home staff to be diaphoretic, slightly cyanotic, and severely short of breath. She was immediately put on oxygen, and an ambulance was called to rush her to the ED.

On arrival in the ED the patient was initially unresponsive to verbal stimuli and in acute respiratory distress. There were rales on both sides of her lungs, almost up to the apices. The heart was regular, and no murmur or gallop could be heard because of the noisy breath sounds. The remainder of her exam was benign except for moderate pedal edema. An arterial blood gas obtained shortly after admission showed a pH of 7.16, pCO_2 of 60, and a pO_2 of 74. The patient was immediately treated with a high dose intravenous furosemide, nitroglycerin paste, and sublingual nitroglycerin. After a short period of time, she had not increased her urine output. The chest x-ray showed acute pulmonary edema. The patient was still in extremis.

The ED physician initiated a discusison with the patient's son, requesting some guidance on the issue of intubation. As the son went to discuss this issue with other members of the family, the respiratory therapist was called to apply continuous positive airway pressure (C-PAP) to the patient in order to assist her respirations. This was applied, and, within a short period of time (approximately 30 minutes), the patient was feeling better. She was more alert, her skin dried up, and she was able to respond by nodding her head. The patient was admitted to intensive care but did not require intubation.

103. DO NOT RESUSCITATE

How are DNR orders interpreted in the ED setting?

If someone has a valid DNR, why would they come to the ED?

What alternatives are there for treating patients in acute pulmonary edema other than immediate intubation?

DISCUSSION

This patient presented with the classic signs of acute pulmonary edema. This condition is usually treated with intravenous diuretics, topical nitroglycerin paste, sublingual nitroglycerin, and occasionally the addition of intravenous vasodilators, such as low-dose dopamine. The goal is to reduce the "preload" of fluid entering the heart by dilating peripheral blood vessels. Additional treatment to increase the end expiratory pressure essentially forces the edema fluid back into the capillaries. This usually requires intubation, with continuous end expiratory pressure on the ventilator.

A relatively new method for treating pulmonary edema and exacerbations of COPD is the use of C-PAP. This is a way of maintaining elevated expiratory pressures in the unintubated patient through the use of a mask applied tightly to the nose and mouth. The patient will require some time in intensive care for the increased nursing care involved in monitoring this treatment.

In this particular case, the patient had previously expressed a desire not to be resuscitated. She had vocalized (although not written down) a desire to *not* be intubated. Because there was no written documentation of this, we asked the family to discuss intubation amongst themselves and determine whether they would feel comfortable attesting to this wish of the patient while we tried to temporize by using C-PAP. Had this measure not been successful, and had the family been unable to come to a conclusion about the patient's true wishes, we would have been obligated to intubate the patient. An alternative would have been to ask the patient if she wanted to be intubated and then follow her wishes if she were able to respond to us, but in this case she was initially unable to respond thoughtfully to verbal stimuli.

Patients are DNR for various reasons. The most common is that they do not wish to be maintained for long periods of time on external life support. These patients' willingness to accept various forms of relatively short-term, immediate treatment for life-threatening illnesses varies widely. For example, a patient with severe pneumonia may not want CPR done but may want to be intubated and to have intravenous antibiotics for a short period of time if an almost full recovery can probably be made. In most cases, we commence with the lifesaving treatment and then deal with the ethical issue of what level of resuscitation should be continued or added later on.

Patients in the field who are DNR may pose a more difficult problem. If there is a valid signed DNR form available documenting the DNR status, the family usually calls EMS because they don't know who else to call. They often need to have a medical professional tell them when their family member is indeed deceased. In most cases, when a properly signed DNR order is present the EMTs are not obligated to perform CPR. If no DNR order is available, then the EMTs are obligated to begin CPR and all other possibly lifesaving interventions. This should be done in spite of what anyone at the scene may say. This policy protects the patient from a situation where the family member is mistaken about his or her DNR status or the even more serious situation where the family member is trying to prevent a previously capable patient from making his or her own decision. The rules for prehospital DNRs vary from state to state, and EMTs and emergency physicians should be acquainted with the rules in their state. Most states now require that prehospital providers withhold CPR if a valid DNR form is present at the bedside. Each state's health department is a source for information on that state's unique DNR laws and regulations.

REFERENCES

Review Article

Arras, J. Ethical issues in emergency care. *Clin. Geriatr. Med.* 1993;9: 655–664.

Additional References

Newberry, D. L., et al. Noninvasive bilevel positive pressure ventilation in severe acute pulmonary edema. *Am. J. Emerg. Med.* 1995;13: 479–482.

Meyer, T. J., and Hill, N. S. Noninvasive positive pressure ventilation to treat respiratory failure. *Ann. Intern. Med.* 1994;120:760–770.

Iserson, K. V. Foregoing prehospital care: Should ambulance staff always resuscitate? *J. Med. Ethics* 1991;17:19–24.

Becker, B. M. Physicians' and nurses' knowledge of and attitude towards advance directives: Experience and preference. *Acad. Emerg. Med.* 1995;2:439. Abstract.

Johnson, D. R., and Maggiore, W. A. Resuscitation decision making by New Mexico emergency medical technicians. *Am. J. Emerg. Med.* 1993;11:139–142.

Case 104 "THE WORST HEADACHE OF MY LIFE"

A 64-year-old man arrived at a small community hospital emergency department on Thanksgiving morning. He complained of a severe frontal headache that had begun a few hours earlier. He had minimal nausea and no vomiting. He could not recall any unusual activity at the start of the headache and said it had begun shortly after waking.

He had a history of high blood pressure and was on an ACE inhibitor. There were no other medical problems that he was aware of, and he was on no other medications. He had been a career military non-commissioned officer and had retired to this small community for the past several years. He did not smoke and drank alcohol rarely.

On physical examination his pupils were equal and reactive to light. His facial exam showed a mild weakness of the right side of his face, with normal evaluation of his eyebrows bilaterally. The heart and lung exam was normal, and the remainder of his examination was completely benign. His vital signs were normal with the exception of a slightly elevated blood pressure at 160/98.

The ED physician had an immediate CT scan ordered. This was read as normal, showing no evidence of bleeding or of a stroke. A spinal tap was then performed. The fluid was grossly bloody and did not clear from the first to the fourth tube. Cell counts were the same in both tubes, with approximately 10,000 RBCs per mm^3 in each tube.

Immediate consultation was obtained from a nearby medical center, and arrangements were made to transfer the patient to the care of a neurosurgeon. Before being transferred, the patient confided to the nurse that he had had sexual intercourse with his wife immediately before the onset of this headache.

He had several angiograms done during his stay at the medical center that were all negative. He was discharged with a diagnosis of acute subarachnoid brain hemorrhage of undetermined cause.

Who should get a full workup for subarachnoid hemorrhage?

What is the correct sequence of diagnosis and treatment for it?

What are other causes of a severe headache?

Discussion

The management of the *worst headache of the patient's life* should always be directed towards diagnosing possible subarachnoid hemorrhage. This piece of information is key to picking up the "sentinel bleed"—a small leak that sometimes precedes a catastrophic bleed that results in a hemorrhagic stroke. The mortality of hemorrhagic stroke is extremely high (up to 70% in some reports). It often affects young people and is a potentially preventable cause of severe morbidity and mortality.

In this patient, the subsequent evaluation did not disclose a leak, and we can hypothesize that he had a small aneurysm that leaked and then thrombosed. This probably will not give him any further problems, but he must constantly be under surveillance for other bleeds secondary to his hypertension. In the past, headache has frequently been linked to sexual intercourse. However, more recent studies have showed that this kind of exertion is no more likely than any other kind of activity to precipitate SAH, and many subarachnoid hemorrhages also occur at rest. A common mistake is to do the CT scan and not follow it with a spinal tap. This is a dangerous strategy because approximately 15% of subarachnoid hemorrhages are not visible on CT scans.

The immediate treatment of this patient was with Compazine. This actually resulted in a dramatic reduction of his headache discomfort. Nevertheless, this improvement should not be totally relied on as a test of etiology, because some people who have brain hemorrhages also get relief with Compazine, Toradol, or narcotic medications.

References

Review Article
Silberstein, S. D. Evaluation and emergency treatment of headache. *Headache* 1992;32:396–407.

Additional References
Reichman, O. H., and Karlman, R. L. Berry aneurysm. *Surg. Clin. North Am.* 1995;75:115–121.

Kumar, K. L., and Reuler, J. B. Uncommon headaches: Diagnosis and treatment. *J. Gen. Intern. Med.* 1993;8:333–341.

Juvela, S. Minor leak before rupture of an intracranial aneurysm and subarachnoid hemorrhage of unknown etiology. *Neurosurgery* 1992;30:7–11.

Case 105 "I THINK I HAVE PNEUMONIA"

A 30-year-old man arrived at our emergency department saying, "I think I have pneumonia." Four days earlier, after an eight-hour drive to another state, he had noted sharp right-sided chest pain that worsened on deep inspiration. He was somewhat short of breath and had a nonproductive cough. There was no fever or hemoptysis, and he denied any history of trauma. His past medical history was unremarkable, but he did smoke a pack of cigarettes daily.

While still away from home, he had presented himself to the local ED with these complaints. His workup there revealed a right basilar infiltrate that "did not look like a pneumonia" according to the physician on duty. On returning home, he received a call from the hospital informing him that the radiologist had reviewed his chest film and thought that it was consistent with pneumonia. They suggested that he go to the closest ED for treatment.

His symptoms had persisted unchanged despite treatment with ibuprofen. Vital signs at our hospital revealed a pulse of 120, blood pressure of 120/80, respiratory rate of 28, and an oral temperature of 100.2°F. Physical exam was unremarkable except for decreased breath sounds at the right base and absence of obvious respiratory distress. Repeat chest x-ray revealed elevation of the right hemidiaphragm, right basilar atelectasis, and a small right-sided pleural effusion. His arterial blood gas results were pH 7.50, pCO_2 30, and pO_2 70 on room air. Because of the possibility of a pulmonary embolus, a lung scan was performed that revealed a matched ventilation-perfusion defect at the right base. It was interpreted as an indeterminate-probability lung scan.

What is the most common clinical sign or symptom of pulmonary embolism?

Is an arterial blood gas helpful in ruling in or out the diagnosis of anxiety with "hyperventilation syndrome?"

What are the clues that you might be dealing with a pulmonary embolism?

What are the common causes of pleuritic chest pain?

DISCUSSION

Pulmonary embolism is a common illness. Estimates claim that there are approximately 300,000 cases in the United States each year. It is also a common cause of death, although it is probably underreported because we often don't get postmortems on elderly patients who have sudden death outside the hospital.

The common primary risk factors for pulmonary embolism include deep vein thrombosis, recent surgery, recent prolonged bed rest or prolonged travel without moving around (such as long airplane trips), obesity, malignancy, smoking, and birth control pill use.

Patients usually present with pleuritic chest pain and shortness of breath. This is also the presentation of many other medical problems, from the relatively benign to the much more serious. The differential diagnosis includes: viral pleurisy (pleurodynia, the Devil's Grippe), pneumonia, chest trauma, and pneumothorax. The initial step is to determine whether a pulmonary embolism is likely. If embolism is the correct diagnosis, the danger is that another larger embolism may be forthcoming and may prove fatal. The problem usually is not *this* embolus but the next one.

The diagnosis is difficult to make in many cases. In a patient with pulmonary embolism's symptoms and with any risk factors, a reasonable screening test is an arterial blood gas. We look at the alveolar-arterial (a-A) oxygen gradient, which is a way of looking at the patient's ability to transfer oxygen from inhaled air (in the alveoli) to the bloodstream. The a-A gradient at sea level can be estimated by the formula.

$$\text{a-A gradient} = 145 - (pO_2 + pCO_2)$$

This should be less than 10 to 20 mm Hg in normal persons. If the gradient is greater than expected, then a pulmonary embolism is more likely. Other causes of an elevated a-A gradient are smoking, chronic obstructive pulmonary disease, congestive heart failure, and pneumonia. There will be some patients with a small pulmonary embolism who have a normal a-A gradient, and, if there are other clues to this

105. "I THINK I HAVE PNEUMONIA"

diagnosis, a normal blood gas does not totally exclude it. In the hyperventilation syndrome there is no a-A oxygen gradient, because the patient's lung physiology is not made abnormal by anxiety.

The ECG may be helpful in showing some degree of right heart strain, as in this patient, who had an incomplete right bundle branch block, but the most common electrocardiographic sign of pulmonary embolism is sinus tachycardia. The classic S1-Q3-T3 (S wave in lead I, Q in lead III, and inverted T in lead III) is uncommonly seen but very suggestive when present. The chest x-ray in pulmonary embolism is usually abnormal. It may show an area with characteristic lack of vascular markings (Westermark's sign) or a dome-shaped opacity pointing towards the hilum (Hampton's hump). Usually it only shows nonspecific abnormalities, such as a small effusion, infiltrate, or atelectasis.

The next step is often to obtain a ventilation-perfusion (V/Q) nuclear scan. Because it has many variations, only one of which is totally characteristic of a pulmonary embolism, the V/Q scan is not particularly sensitive or specific. The high-likelihood scans show a normal ventilation scan with an abnormal perfusion scan; the perfusion defect being at the site of the embolism. Indeterminate or low-probability scans frequently occur in patients with and without pulmonary emboli and require further evaluation. A totally *normal* V/Q scan almost totally excludes the diagnosis of pulmonary embolism.

In some cases, such as in the presence of a DVT, the diagnosis is clinically obvious despite an indeterminate V/Q scan. If the patient is at a high enough risk, an alternative strategy for management is to immediately start the patient on intravenous heparin. In hospitals that do not have 24-hour availability for V/Q scans, this strategy actually may be the most effective and may result in timely treatment of these patients. A new test that is becoming more frequently used, particularly in hospitals without 24-hour V/Q scanning capability, is D-dimer measurement. D-dimer is a fragment produced when plasmin acts on a clot's cross-linked fibrin, and measuring D-dimer has been shown to be useful for ruling out deep venous thrombosis (DVT) or pulmonary embolism. The initial data suggests that D-dimer measurement is a very effective screening tool, and that a level less than 500 mg/dL makes the possibility of DVT or pulmonary embolism extremely unlikely.

The patient in this case did quite well, and was discharged from the hospital on oral Coumadin the next week.

REFERENCES

Review Article

Henschke, S. I., et al. Changing practice patterns in the workup of pulmonary embolism. *Chest* 1995;107:940–945.

Additional References

Valenzuela, T. D. Pulmonary embolism. *Ann. Emerg. Med.* 1988;17:209–213.

PIOPED Investigators. Value of the ventilation/perfusion scan in acute pulmonary embolism. *J.A.M.A.* 1990;263:2753–2795.

Stein, P. D., et al. Untreated patients with pulmonary embolism: Outcome, clinical, and laboratory assessment. *Chest* 1995;107:931–935.

de Moerloose, P., et al. D-dimer determination to exclude pulmonary embolism: A two-step approach using later assay as a screening tool. *Thromb. Haemost.* 1994;72(1):89.

Matsumoto, A. H., and Tegtmeyer, C. J. Contemporary diagnostic approaches to acute pulmonary emboli. *Radiol. Clin. North Am.* 1995;33:167–183.

Manganelli, D., et al. Clinical features of pulmonary embolism: Doubts and certainties. *Chest* 1995;107(Suppl. 1):25S–32S.

Case 106 KEYHOLE MEDICINE

A nurse hands you the phone and says that some woman is calling about her husband; could you please see what you can do with her? You introduce yourself, and the woman on the other end of the telephone explains that she is Mrs. Grey and is calling about her husband, who is in terrible pain. Indeed, in the background you can hear a man bellowing and moaning in pain. She says that he is too sick to come to the phone and then tells you this story: Her husband is 54 years old and began to have pain in the middle of his stomach about ten days ago. Four days ago it got worse, and she took him to another hospital's emergency department, where the doctor took off the husband's shirt and examined him. The doctor also ordered an upper GI x-ray series, which was done and was normal. The doctor diagnosed "stomach flu" and sent him home with some Pepto-Bismol. Despite that therapy his pain had not improved, and she now thought he was going to die if something was not done soon. You agree that he sounds pretty badly off and transfer the phone to your ambulance section so that the husband can be picked up and brought in.

When he arrives at the ED 30 minutes later, an orderly undresses him and comes out to tell you the diagnosis. The orderly has noticed a swelling in the man's scrotum, mostly on the left side, that is, according to the orderly, melon sized. You go to see your patient and find that, although he says his pain is periumbilical, the scrotal mass is very tender, not reducible, and refers pain on palpation to the middle of his abdomen. He tells you that the doctor at the other ED loosened his belt but never removed his pants during the examination four days ago. You diagnose an incarcerated inguinal hernia and call for a surgeon, who takes your patient off to the operating room and solves the problem.

What is "stomach flu?"

What must the physical examination contain when the patient has pain in the midabdomen?

What is "keyhole medicine?"

351

DISCUSSION

Influenza is, of course, an epidemic respiratory disease caused by a virus. It often appears in the winter and causes a self-limited illness with fever, cough, malaise, and other respiratory symptoms in young people but may be the last illness for older or chronically ill people.

The lay public may refer to almost any sort of illness as "flu" and have extended the term to acute gastroenteritis by calling it "stomach flu." If we are to make that lay term even slightly more specific, we ought to limit it to presumed viral infections lasting no more than a few days and presenting with nausea, vomiting, diarrhea, and weakness. We surely ought to be very careful applying such a term to any illness wherein steady abdominal pain is a cardinal symptom. Constant pain is often a symptom of serious intra-abdominal catastrophe and should be taken much more seriously.

Because of lack of time, we seldom can do as thorough a physical examination as we would like on many of our ED patients. However, whatever we do, we must pay careful attention to vital signs, and we must examine the area of the body that the patient is complaining of. We must undress the patient and be sure that we consider what is connected to what. For example, a respiratory complaint should lead to a careful examination of the neck, the chest, and the entire circulatory system. An abdominal complaint should lead to examination not just of the abdomen but also of the chest, genitalia, pelvis, and rectum. Zachary Cope's dictum, "Semper per rectum," should not be forgotten. If we are rushed for time, we should remember that there is not enough time to do the job badly and never enough time to warrant wasting it on "keyhole examinations" through partly unbuttoned or partially removed clothing. Take it off, take it all off. You are not likely to miss a coconut in the scrotum if you uncover it and look at it. Again, to quote Zachary Cope, "More harm is done by those who do not look than by those who do not know what is in the book."

REFERENCES

Review Article
Nyhus, L. M., and Bombeck, C. T. Hernias. In D. C. Sabiston (ed.), *Textbook of Surgery*. Philadelphia: Saunders, 1986. Pp. 1231–1252.

Additional References

Janzon, L., Ryden, E. I., and Zederfeldt, B. Acute abdomen in surgical emergency room: Who is taking care of when for what? *Acta Chir. Scand.* 1982;148:141–148.

Rusnak, R. A., et al. Misdiagnosis of acute appendicitis: Common features discovered in cases after litigation. *Ann. Emerg. Med.* 1994;12:397–402.

Zeta (Zachary Cope). *The Acute Abdomen In Verse.* London: H. K. Louis, 1962.

Appendix A NURSING LITERATURE REFERENCES

Case 1

Kinkle, S. L. Violence in the ED: How to stop it before it starts. *Am. J. Nurs.* July 1993;93:22–24.

Wagner, M. M. The patient with abdominal injuries. *Nurs. Clin. North Am.* March 1990;25(1):45–55.

Lanza, M. L., et al. Predicting violence: Nursing diagnosis versus psychiatric diagnosis. *Nurs. Diagn.* October–December 1994;5(4): 151–157.

Case 2

Roberts, S. J. Somatization in primary care: The common presentation of psychosocial problems through physical complaints. *Nurse Pract.* 1994;19:50–56.

Davidhizar, R., and Vance, A. The management of the suicidal patient in a critical care unit. *J. Nurs. Manage.* March 1993;1(2):95–102.

Case 3

Rourke, K. The evaluation and treatment of acute ankle sprains. *J. Emerg. Nurs.* 1994;20:528–539.

Case 4

Haney, S. A., et al. Iowa EMS law: EDNA involved in legislative process. EMT scope of practice. *J. Emerg. Nurs.* 1984;10(4):19A–23A.

Johnson, R. I., et al. Regulation of prehospital nursing practice: A national survey. *J. Emerg. Nurs.* 1993;19(5):437–440.

George, J. Potential liability for the patient signing out against medical advice. *J. Emerg. Nurs.* 1985;11(2):110.

CASE 5

Muhrer, J. C. Diagnostic considerations in the evaluation and treatment of sore throat. *Nurse Pract.* 1991;16:33–41.

CASE 6

Holt, J. How to help confused patients. *Am. J. Nurs.* August 1993;93:32–36.

Drake, D. K., and Nettina, S. M. Recognition and management of heat related illness. *Nurse Pract.* 1994;19(8):43–47.

CASE 7

Davidhizar, R., et al. Emergency room nurses: Helping families cope with sudden death. *J. Pract. Nurs.* 1993;43:14–19.

Tye, C. Qualified nurses' perceptions of the needs of suddenly bereaved families in the accident and emergency department. *J. Adv. Nurs.* 1993;18:948–956.

CASE 8

Cassidy, E. Vital signs. *J. Emerg. Nurs.* December 1992;18(6):36A.

Muir, R. A 15 year old girl with abdominal pain, vomiting, tachycardia, and tachypnea . . . diabetic ketoacidosis. *J. Emerg. Nurs.* August 1992;18(4):357–358.

Epifanio, P. C. Diabetic ketoacidosis—the hidden danger. *Emerg. Nurs. Rep.* July 1986;1(4):1–8.

CASE 9

Ledray, L. E. Sexual assault evidentiary exam and treatment protocol. *J. Emerg. Nurs.* 1995;21:355–359.

Ruckman, L. Rape: How to begin the healing. *Am. J. Nurs.* September 1992;92:48–51.

Case 10

Morelli, J. The prescription drugs most toxic to children. *Am. J. Nurs.* July 1993;93:26–29.

Lammon, C. A., et al. Organophosphate overdose: Nursing strategies. *Dimens. Crit. Care Nurs.* 1992;11:310–317.

Case 11

Moss, V. A. Battered women and the myth of masochism. *J. Psychosoc. Nurs. Ment. Health Serv.* July 1991;29(7):18–23.

Snyder, J. A. ED protocols for domestic violence. *J. Emerg. Nurs.* 1994;20:65–68.

Grunfeld, A. F., et al. Detecting domestic violence against women in the ED: A nursing triage protocol. *J. Emerg. Nurs.* 1994;20:271–274.

Case 12

Dubiel, D. Ectopic pregnancy in the ED. *Adv. Clin. Care* 1991;6:22–23.

Case 13

Walsh, E. A., et al. Childhood near drowning: Nursing care. *Pediatr. Nurs.* 1994;20:265–292.

Case 14

Fredrickson, J. M., et al. Emergency nurses' perceived knowledge and comfort level regarding pediatric patients. *J. Emerg. Nurs.* 1994;20:13–17.

ANA supports "Back to sleep" campaign to combat SIDS. *Am. Nurse* 1994;26:35.

APPENDIX A. NURSING LITERATURE REFERENCES 357

Devlin, B. K., and Reynolds, E. Child abuse: How to recognize it, how to intervene. *Am. J. Nurs.* March 1994;94(3):26–32.

Case 15

Knight-Macheca, M. K. Diabetic hypoglycemia: Keeping the threat at bay. *Am. J. Nurs.* April 1993;93:26–41.

Case 16

Endicott, P., and Watson, B. Interventions to improve the AMA discharge rate for opiate-addicted patients . . . against medical advice. *J. Psychosoc. Nurs. Ment. Health Serv.* August 1994;32(8):36–40, 48–49.

Cooper, D. B. Substance misuse: Withdrawing gracefully. *Nursing Times* 1993;89(17):42–44.

Case 17

Hayden, R. A. What keeps oxygenation on track? *Am. J. Nurs.* December 1992;92:32–41.

Case 18

Tan, N., et al. Acute gouty arthritis: Modern approaches to an ancient disease. *Postgrad. Med.* 1993;94:73–84.

Case 19

Garrison, M. W., and Campbell, R. K. Identifying and treating common and uncommon infections in the patient with diabetes. *Diabetes Educ.* November–December 1993;19(6):522–531.

Case 20

DellaBella, L. A. Steroidphobia and the pulmonary patient. *Am. J. Nurs.* February 1992;92:26–29.

Reinke, L. F., et al. Breathing space: Teaching asthma co-management. *Am. J. Nurs.* October 1992;92:40–51.

Case 21

Boyes, A. P. Repetition of overdose: A retrospective 5-year study. *J. Adv. Nurs.* September 1994;20(3):462–468.

Weinman, S. A. Emergency management of drug overdose. *Crit. Care Nurse* December 1993;13(6):45–51.

Bell, K. Identifying the substance abuser in clinical practice. *Orthop. Nurs.* March–April 1992;11(2):29–36.

Case 22

Westlake, C., and Funkhouser, S. W. Cardiovascular effects of recreational cocaine use. *AACN Clin. Issues Crit. Care Nurs.* 1990;1:65–71.

Case 23

Al-Saden, P. Anticoagulation-induced epistaxis. *Nursing* December 1994;24(12):33.

Lockhart, J. S. Action STAT! Epistaxis. *Nursing* November 1986;16(11):33.

Case 24

Propulsid-associated dystonia. *Nurses Drug Alert* March 1995;19(3):23.

Case 25

Stiesmeyer, J. K. A 4-step approach to pulmonary assessment. *Am. J. Nurs.* August 1993;93:22–31.

Case 26

Talbert, S. R. Inhalation injuries: Review and two case studies. *J. Emerg. Nurs.* December 1993;19(6):482–485.

Faldmo, L., and Kravitz, M. Management of acute burns and burn shock resuscitation. *AACN Clin. Issues Crit. Care Nurs.* May 1993;4(2):351–356.

Case 27

Usher, K. Carbon monoxide poisoning: Nursing priorities and treatment. *J. Psychosoc. Nurs. Ment. Health Serv.* 1994;32:7:71–75.

Case 28

Childs, S. G. Syncope: Categories and considerations of practice. *J. Emerg. Nurs.* 1995;21:125–134.

Case 29

Stiesmeyer, J. K. A 4-step approach to pulmonary assessment. *Am. J. Nurs.* August 1993;93:22–31.

Myers, M. B., et al. Standing orders for trauma care. *J. Emerg. Nurs.* 1994;20:111–117.

Case 30

Parker, C. D. Fast action for subarachnoid hemorrhage. *Am. J. Nurs.* January 1995;95(1):47.

Foley, J. J. Pharmacologic treatment of acute migraine and related headaches in the emergency department. *J. Emerg. Nurs.* June 1993;19(3):225–230.

Case 31

Lause, L. D. Bringing your patient through the DTs. *RN* August 1988;51(8):58–59.

Mattera, C. J. American traditions . . . Alcohol-related crashes. *J. Emerg. Nurs.* August 1994;20(4):317–319.

George, J. E., and Quattrone, M. S. The problem of alcohol abuse. *J. Emerg. Nurs.* October 1993;19(5):454.

Warden, V. D. Blood and breath alcohol testing. *J. Emerg. Nurs.* June 1992;18(3):278–283.

CASE 32

Beachley, M., et al. Abdominal trauma: Putting the pieces together. *Am. J. Nurs.* November 1993;93:26–35.

CASE 33

Hardick, M. Foreign body removal in the gastrointestinal tract. *Gastroenterol. Nurs.* Spring 1989;11(4):227–234.

CASE 34

Handerhan, B. Managing a perforated viscus. *Nursing* February 1993;23(2):92–93, 95.

Perforated peptic ulcer. *Am. J. Nurs.* September 1990;90(9):28.

CASE 35

Knight-Macheca, M. K. Diabetic hypoglycemia: Keeping the threat at bay. *Am. J. Nurs.* April 1993;93:26–41.

CASE 36

Foster, T. M. Emergency nurse encounters man with seizure at 20,000 feet. *J. Emerg. Nurs.* April 1995;21(2):181–183.

Rich, J. Action STAT: Generalized motor seizure. *Nursing* April 1986;16(4):33.

Novotny-Dinsdale, V., and Miller, M. Evaluation of two reusable wound irrigation systems. *J. Emerg. Nurs.* August 1993;19(4):329–331.

CASE 37

Rush, C. Action STAT! Gastrointestinal bleeding. *Nursing* August 1995;25(8):33.

Mattera, C. J. American traditions . . . Alcohol-related crashes. *J. Emerg. Nurs.* August 1994;20(4):317–319.

George, J. E., and Quattrone, M. S. The problem of alcohol abuse. *J. Emerg. Nurs.* October 1993;19(5):454.

Warden, V. D. Blood and breath alcohol testing. *J. Emerg. Nurs.* June 1992;18(3):278–283.

Case 38

Boriskin, M. I. Primary care management of wounds: Cleaning, suturing, and infection control. *Nurse Pract.* November 1994;19(11):38, 40, 45–46.

Case 39

Vaughn, L. Help—Just a phone call away . . . "Barbiturate overdose." *Nursing* May 1995;25(5):6.

Alexander, J. G., Marshall, E., and Hambright, F. D. Would you recognize this toxic emergency? *RN* 1991;1:26–30.

Laskowski-Jones, L. First-line emergency care: What every nurse should know. *Nursing* January 1995;25(1):34–45.

Beards, S. C., and Nightingale, P. Aspiration. *Care Crit. Ill.* September–October 1994;10(5):198–202.

Case 40

Blouin, A. M. Munchausen syndrome. *J. Emerg. Nurs.* 1993;19:513–515.

Case 41

Acorn, S. Use of the brief psychiatric rating scale by nurses. *J. Psychosoc. Nurs. Ment. Health Serv.* May 1993;31(5):9–12, 34–35.

Perry, M. V., and Anderson, G. L. Assessment and treatment strategies for depressive disorders commonly encountered in primary care settings. *Core Nursing* 1992;17(6):25, 29–30, 33–36.

Case 42

Childs, S. G. Syncope: Categories and considerations for practice. *J. Emerg. Nurs.* April 1995;21(2):125–134.

Molitor, L. Syncope in an elderly woman. Septicemia. *J. Emerg. Nurs.* June 1994;20(3):245–246.

Case 43

Scher, H. E. Chest pain: Developing rapid assessment skills. *Orthop. Nurs.* May–June 1995;14(3):30–34.

Bonnono, C., Hedges, J. R., Peterson, C., and Collings, J. L. Initial nursing impression in patients with chest discomfort. *J. Emerg. Nurs.* 1992;18(1):28–33.

Case 44

Holt, J. How to help confused patients. *Am. J. Nurs.* August 1993;93:32–36.

Case 45

Baer, C. L. Investigating dysuria. *Nursing* 1989;19:108–110.

Gibbons, P. Cystitis in the sexually active female. *Nursing Times* 1990;86:33–35.

Case 46

Bender, P. Deceptive distress in the elderly. *Am. J. Nurs.* October 1992;92:28–33.

Johannsen, J. M. Update: Guidelines for treating hypertension. *Am. J. Nurs.* March 1993;93:42–53.

Trottier, D. J., et al. Managing isolated systolic hypertension. *Am. J. Nurs.* October 1993;93:50–55.

Case 47

Stringfield, Y. N. Back to basics: Acidosis, alkalosis, ABG's. *Am. J. Nurs.* November 1993;93:43–50.

Case 48

Bourn, M. K. Multisubstance overdose: Nursing assessment and management. *Emerg. Nurs. Rep.* 1987;2(1):1–8.

Case 49

Brown, J. Commentary on the etiology of missed cervical spine injuries. *Enas. Nurs. Scan Emerg. Care* September–October 1993;3(5):13. *Original article by Davis, J., et al. appears in* J. Trauma *1993;34(3): 342–346.*

Ohman, K., and Spaniol, D. Halo immobilization: Discharge planning and patient education. *J. Neurosci. Nurs.* December 1990;22(6): 351–357.

Case 50

Moncada, G. A. Traumatic injuries of the face and hands. *Nurs. Clin. North Am.* 1994;29:777–789.

Case 51

Krasner, P. R. Treatment of tooth avulsion by nurses. *J. Emerg. Nurs.* 1990;16:29–35.

Case 52

Herron, D. G., and Nance, J. Emergency department nursing management of patients with orthopedic fractures resulting from motor vehicle accidents. *Nurs. Clin. North Am.* March 1990;25(1):71–83.

Case 53

O'Brien, L. M., and Bartlett, K. A. TB plus HIV spells trouble. *Am. J. Nurs.* May 1992;92:28–35.

Case 54

Hauswald, M., and Kerr, N. L. Gynecologic causes of abdominal pain. *Emerg. Care Q.* 1989;5:37–48.

Case 55

Catania, U. Monitoring coumadin therapy. *RN* 1994;57:29–34.

Case 56

DellaBella, L. A. Steroidphobia and the pulmonary patient. *Am. J. Nurs.* February 1992;92:26–29.

Ward, J. D., et al. Penetrating head injury. *Crit. Care Nurs. Q.* 1994; 17:79–89.

Case 57

Cosgriff, J. A., and Anderson, D. L. A man with abdominal and back pain. *J. Emerg. Nurs.* March–April 1986;12(2):109–110.

Case 58

de la Cour, J. Neuroleptic malignant syndrome: Do we know enough? *J. Adv. Nurs.* May 1995;21(5):897–904.

Stewart, K. B. What's wrong with this patient? . . . Neuroleptic malignant syndrome (NMS). *RN* February 1995;58(2):45–46, 48.

Case 59

Aragon, D., et al. What you should know about thrombolytic therapy for acute MI. *Am. J. Nurs.* September 1993;93:24–31.

Eleven, R. F. Caring for the cardiac spouse. *Am. J. Nurs.* November 1993;93:50–53.

Case 60

Noel, N. L., and Yam, M. Domestic violence: The pregnant battered woman. *Nurs. Clin. North Am.* 1992;27:871–884.

Moss, V. A. Battered women and the myth of masochism. *J. Psychosoc. Nurs. Ment. Health Serv.* July 1991;29(7):18–23.

Case 61

Boriskin, M. I. Primary care management of wounds: Cleaning, suturing, and infection control. *Nurse Pract.* November 1994;19(11):38, 40, 45–46.

Novotny-Dinsdale, V., and Miller, M. Evaluation of two reusable wound irrigation systems. *J. Emerg. Nurs.* August 1993;19(4):329–331.

James, H. Wound dressings in accident and emergency departments. *Accid. Emerg. Nurs.* April 1994;2(2):87–93.

Laskowski-Jones, L. First-line emergency care: What every nurse should know. *Nursing* January 1995;25(1):34–45.

Case 62

Ross, D. G. Altered bowel elimination patterns among hospitalized elderly and middle-aged persons: Quantitative results. *Orthop. Nurs.* January–February 1995;14(1):25–31.

Van der Horst, M., Sykula, J., and Lingley, K. L. The constipation quandary. *Can. Nurse* January 1994;90(1):25–27, 29–30.

Case 63

Derkay, C. S., et al. Retrieving foreign bodies from upper aerodigestive tracts of children. *AORN-J.* 1994;60:53–61.

Kitay, G., et al. Cafe coronary: Recognition, treatment, and prevention. *Nurse Pract.* 1989;14:36–43.

Case 64

Patten, V. C., et al. When your patient is allergic. *Am. J. Nurs.* September 1992;92:58–61.

Case 65

Patterson, R. J., et al. Head injury in the conscious child. *Am. J. Nurs.* August 1992;92:22–31.

Devlin, B. K., and Reynolds, E. Child abuse: How to recognize it, how to intervene. *Am. J. Nurs.* March 1994;94(3):26–32.

Case 66

Ramsden, C. A. Miscarriage counselling. An accident and emergency perspective. *Accid. Emerg. Nurs.* April 1995;3(2):68–73.

Allan, A. Types and causes of miscarriage. *Mod. Midwife* March 1995; 5(3):27–30.

Stockman, M. Patient teaching in the emergency department: Vaginal bleeding during early pregnancy. *J. Emerg. Nurs.* December 1991; 17(6):424–426.

Case 67

Starr, L. M. Emergency oxygen: What? Who? When? *AAOHN-J.* 1994;42:15.

Hayden, R. A. What keeps oxygenation on track? *Am. J. Nurs.* December 1992;92:32–41.

Freichels, T. Orchestrating the care of mechanically ventilated patients. *Am. J. Nurs.* October 1993;93:26–35.

Stringfield, Y. N. Back to basics: Acidosis, alkalosis, ABG's. *Am. J. Nurs.* November 1993;93:43–50.

Case 68

Beachley, M., et al. Abdominal trauma: Putting the pieces together. *Am. J. Nurs.* November 1993;93:26–35.

Laskowski-Jones, L. Meeting the challenge of chest trauma. *Am. J. Nurs.* September 1995;95(9):22–30.

Hammond, S. G. Chest injuries in the trauma patient. *Nurs. Clin. North Am.* March 1990;25:35–43.

Turner, J. A. Cardiovascular trauma. *Nurs. Clin. North Am.* March 1990;25:119–130.

Case 69

A differential for pleuritic pain. *Emerg. Med.* 1984;16:97.

Scher, H. E. Chest pain: Developing rapid assessment skills. *Orthop. Nurs.* May–June 1995;14(3):30–34.

Bonnono, C., Hedges, J. R., Peterson, C., and Collings, J. L. Initial nursing impression in patients with chest discomfort. *J. Emerg. Nurs.* 1992;18(1):28–33.

Case 70

Ammons, A. M. Cerebral injuries and intracranial hemorrhages as a result of trauma. *Nurs. Clin. North Am.* March 1990;25(1):23–33.

Hilton, G. Diffuse axonal injury. *J. Trauma Nurs.* January–March 1995;2(1):7–14.

Case 71

George J. E., Quattrone, M. S., and Goldstone, M. Phone consultations with the ED physician: Is there nursing liability? *J. Emerg. Nurs.* April 1995;21(2):163–164.

Horsley, J. E. A hostile doctor? Don't lose your cool. *RN* April 1987; 50(4):77–78.

Brown, J. Commentary on the etiology of missed cervical spine injuries. *Enas. Nurs. Scan Emerg. Care* September–October 1993;3(5):13. Original article by Davis, J., et al. appears in J. Trauma *1993;34(3): 342–346.*

CASE 72

Tepry, J. The major electrolytes: Sodium, potassium, and chloride. *J. Intravenous Nurs.* 1994;17:240–247.

Rainer, F. How to identify electrolyte imbalances on your patient's ECG. *Nursing* 1994;24:54–58.

CASE 73

Staff, L. M. Emergency oxygen: What? Who? When? *AAOHN-J.* 1994; 42:15.

CASE 74

Foster, T. M. Emergency nurse encounters man with seizure at 20,000 feet. *J. Emerg. Nurs.* April 1995;21(2):181–183.

Rich, J. Action STAT: Generalized motor seizure. *Nursing* April 1986; 16(4):33.

CASE 75

Prescott, P. A. Nursing: An important component of hospital survival under a reformed health care system. *Nurs. Econ.* 1993;11:192–199.

Miller, C. A., Kondrotis, A. M., and Roy, J. C. Determination of the cost of operation for one emergency department. *J. Emerg. Nurs.* February 1993;19(1):38–44.

Case 76

Stopping ureteral colic at its source. *Emerg. Med.* 1990;22:104–107.

Case 77

Keis, N. A. Cardiotoxic side effects associated with TCA overdose. *AACN Clin. Issues Crit. Care Nurs.* 1992;3:226–232.

George, J. Potential liability for the patient signing out against medical advice. *J. Emerg. Nurs.* 1985;11(2):110.

Case 78

Kolb, S. E. Reye's syndrome in adults. *Crit. Care Nurse* January 1991;11(1):73–74.

Case 79

Loken, E. Giardiasis: Diagnosis and treatment. *Nurse Pract.* 1986;11:20–26.

Case 80

Childs, S. G. Syncope: Categories and considerations for practice. *J. Emerg. Nurs.* 1995;21:125–134.

Case 81

Halpern, J. S. Respiratory syncytial virus (RSV): A common health problem. *J. Emerg. Nurs.* February 1992;18(1):61–63.

Schwartz, R. The diagnosis and management of sinusitis. *Nurse Pract.* December 1994;19(12):58–63.

Case 82

Berg, E. E. Posterior shoulder (glenohumeral) dislocation. *Orthop. Nurs.* January–February 1995;14(1):47–49.

Berg, E. E. Anterior shoulder dislocation. *Orthop. Nurs.* May–June 1993;12(3):51–53, 60.

CASE 83

Ziglar, M. K., and Parrish, R. S. An 18 year old male patient with multiple trauma including an open pelvic fracture. *J. Emerg. Nurs.* August 1994;20(4):265–270.

Harrahill, M. Open pelvic fracture: The lethal injury. *J. Emerg. Nurs.* June 1994;20(3):243–245.

Dunwoody, C. J. Pelvic fracture patient care: Reflections on the past, implications for the future. *Nurs. Clin. North Am.* March 1991; 26(1):65–72.

CASE 84

Tonetti, J. A. Testicular torsion or acute epididymitis? Diagnosis and treatment. *J. Emerg. Nurs.* March–April 1990;16(2):96–98.

CASE 85

Byars, F. K., Gunter, M., and Henry, L. L. What's wrong with this patient? . . . epiglottitis. *RN* February 1990;53(2):43–45.

CASE 86

Anastasi, J. K. Why give corticosteroids for pneumocystis carinii pneumonia? *Am. J. Nurs.* February 1992;92:30–33.

O'Brien, L. M., and Bartlett, K. A. TB plus HIV spells trouble. *Am. J. Nurs.* May 1992;92:28–35.

Laskowski-Jones, L. Meeting the challenge of chest trauma. *Am. J. Nurs.* September 1995;95(9):22–30.

Hammond, S. G. Chest injuries in the trauma patient. *Nurs. Clin. North Am.* March 1990;25:35–43.

Case 87

Beards, S. C. Nightingale-P: Aspiration. *Care Crit. Ill.* September–October 1994;10(5):198–202.

Case 88

Brown, D. L. Fighting an infant's fever: "Febrile seizure." *Nursing* April 1995;25(4):6.

Thomas, V., et al. National survey of pediatric fever management practices among emergency department nurses. *J. Emerg. Nurs.* December 1994;20(6):505–510.

Case 89

Ritchie, S. R., and Thompson, P. J. Primary bacterial skin infections. *Dermatol. Nurs.* August 1992;4(4):261–268.

Case 90

Biggers, V. T. Codes for a code. *Am. J. Nurs.* May 1992;92:56–61.

Lewis, F. H., et al. Revisiting CPR knowledge and skills among registered nurses. *J. Contin. Educ. Nurs.* 1993;24:174–179.

Case 91

Brown, J. Commentary on the etiology of missed cervical spine injuries. *Enas. Nurs. Scan Emerg. Care* September–October 1993;3(5):13.
Original article by Davis, J., et al. appears in J. Trauma 1993; 34(3):342–346.

Brown, J. Commentary on head injury and facial injury: Is there an increased risk of cervical spine injury? *Enas. Nurs. Scan Emerg. Care* November–December 1993;3(6):13.
Original article by Hills, M., et al. appears in J. Trauma 1993; 34(4):549–554.

Ohman, K., and Spaniol, D. Halo immobilization: Discharge planning and patient education. *J. Neurosci. Nurs.* December 1990;22(6): 351–357.

CASE 92

Meurer, M. K. A 21 year old woman with rapid atrial fibrillation after adenosine administration. *J. Emerg. Nurs.* June 1991;17(3):135–136.

Owens, M. W., and Daniel J. L. IV magnesium sulfate in the treatment of ventricular tachycardia and acute myocardial infarction. *Crit. Care Nurse* 1993;13:83–85.

Schuster, D. M. Patients with an implanted cardioverter defibrillator: A new challenge. *J. Emerg. Nurs.* May–June 1990;16 (Suppl. 3):219–225.

CASE 93

Lanza, M. L., et al. Predicting violence: Nursing diagnosis versus psychiatric diagnosis. *Nurs. Diagn.* October–December 1994;5(4): 151–157.

Advice, P. R. N. Difficult patient: Master of manipulation. *Nursing* July 1995;25(7):9–10.

Mikan, L. Difficult patient: Were Frank's salty sauces killing him? *Nursing* April 1995;25(4):44–46.

CASE 94

Noel, G. E. The role of women and NNAs in disaster management. *Int. Nurs. Rev.* November–December 1990;37(6):363–367.

Berglin, S. L. Emergency nurses in community disaster planning. *J. Emerg. Nurs.* July–August 1990;16(4):290–292.

Sloan, K. A. Volcano! Disaster management. *J. Emerg. Nurs.* July–August 1990;16(4):263–268b.

Case 95

Laskowski-Jones, L. Meeting the challenge of chest trauma. *Am. J. Nurs.* September 1995;95(9):22–30.

Hammond, S. G. Chest injuries in the trauma patients. *Nurs. Clin. North Am.* March 1990;25:35–43.

Case 96

Boyd-Monk, H. Eye trauma: A close-up on emergency care. *RN* December 1989;52(12):22–30.

Case 97

Stringfield, Y. N. Back to basics: Acidosis, alkalosis, ABG's. *Am. J. Nurs.* November 1993;93:43–50.

Daleiden, A. Clinical manifestations of blunt cardiac injury: A challenge to the critical care practitioner. *Crit. Care. Nurs. Q.* August 1994;17(2):13–23.

Laskowski-Jones, L. Meeting the challenge of chest trauma. *Am. J. Nurs.* September 1995;95(9):22–30.

Turner, J. A. Cardiovascular trauma. *Nurs. Clin. North Am.* March 1990;25:119–130.

Case 98

Nettina, S. L., and Kauffman, F. H. Diagnosis and management of sexually transmitted genital lesions. *Nurse Pract.* 1990;15:20–39.

Alexander, L. L. Sexually transmitted diseases: Perspectives on this growing epidemic. *Nurse Pract.* October 1992;17(10):31, 34, 37–42.

Case 99

Macabasco, A. C., and Hickman, J. L. Thrombolytic therapy for brain attack. *J. Neurosci. Nurs.* June 1995;27(3):138–151.

Licata-Gehr, E. E. Etiology of stroke subtypes. *Nurs. Clin. North Am.* 1991;26:943–955.

CASE 100

Mandel, M. S. Surviving cross-examination. *Am. J. Nurs.* June 1993; 93:22–24.

George, J. E., and Quattrone, M. S. Professional malpractice or simple negligence? *J. Emerg. Nurs.* December 1993;19(6):532–533.

CASE 101

Green, E. Solving the puzzle of chest pain. *Am. J. Nurs.* January 1992;92:32–40.

Bender, P. Deceptive distress in the elderly. *Am. J. Nurs.* October 1992;92:28–33.

Hochrein, M., et al. Heart smart: A guide to cardiac tests. *Am. J. Nurs.* December 1992;92:22–26.

CASE 102

Jacox, A., et al. Managing acute pain: A guideline for the nation. *Am. J. Nurs.* May 1992;92:49–55.

CASE 103

Meyer, C. "End of life" care: Patients' choices, nurses' challenges. *Am. J. Nurs.* February 1993;93:40–47.

Edwards, B. S. When the physician won't give up. *Am. J. Nurs.* September 1993;93:34–37.

Jacobson, B. S. Ethical dilemmas of do-not-resuscitate orders in surgery. *AORN-J* September 1994;60(3):449–452.

Case 104

Parker, C. D. Emergency! Fast action for subarachnoid hemorrhage. *Am. J. Nurs.* January 1995;95(1):47.

Case 105

Corry, J. C. Identifying the patient with tuberculosis and protecting the ED staff. *J. Emerg. Nurs.* 1994;20:293–304.

Case 106

Zeta (Zachary Cope). *The Acute Abdomen in Verse.* London, H. K. Lewis, 1962.

Appendix B PREHOSPITAL CARE REFERENCES

Case 1

Meade, D. M. Create the carnage and we will come. *Emerg. Med. Serv.* 1995;24(5):31.

McManus, D., and Phan-Gruber, M. Scene of the crime. *Emerg. Med. Serv.* 1994;23(7):60.

Machenheimer, B. A. Stat wounds: The BLS approach. *Emerg. Med. Serv.* 1994;23(8):39.

Case 2

Ford, C. V., et al. Managing somatization and hypochodriacis. *Patient Care* 1993;27(2):31–40.

Case 3

Stewart, C. E. Orthopedic emergencies. *Emerg. Med. Serv.* 1991;20(9):10.

Case 4

Rhoads, J. Restraint restrictions. *Emerg. Med. Serv.* 1993;22(1):16.

Koenig, K. L. *Quo vadis:* "Scoop and run," "stay and treat," or "treat and street?" *Acad. Emerg. Med.* 1995;2:477–480.

Case 5

Rauch, S. D. ENT Emergencies: When to call for help. *Emerg. Med.* 1989;21:16–30.

Elizondo, E. Streptococcal pharyngitis: An update. *Physician Assistant* 1992;16:79–85.

All about mono. *Emerg. Med.* 1988;20(9):89–93.

Case 6

Foose, T. L. Diagnosing and treating the elderly. *Emergency* 1986; 18:40–43.

Case 7

Norton, R. L., et al. Survey of EMT's ability to cope with the deaths of patients during prehospital care. *Prehosp. Disaster Med.* 1992; 7:233–242.

Case 8

Bartos, B. J. Assessing diabetic emergencies. *Emergency* 1992;24(2):36.

Rothenberg, M. A. Diabetic emergencies. *Emerg. Med. Serv.* 1991; 29(10):18.

Case 9

Card, D. R. What every EMT needs to know about rape. *Emerg. Med. Serv.* 1994;22(4):45.

Case 10

Kirk, M. A., et al. Clueing in on the acutely poisoned patient. *JEMS* 1991;16(5):64.

Daniels, P. Organophosphates. *JEMS* 1991;16(11):76.

Case 11

Blauch, J. D. Commentary on hitting close to home: Domestic violence and the EMS responder. *JEMS* 1994;19:112–231.

Case 12

Copass, M. K., Soper, R. G., and Eisenberg, M. S. Gut reactions. *Emerg. Med. Serv.* 1991;20(3):54.

Dickinson, E. T. Gynecological emergencies—when pain calls for quick action. *JEMS* 1990;13(3):20–22.

Case 13

Grandy, J. T. Hypothermia. *Emergency* 1995;27(1):28–31.

Werdmann, M. J. Pediatric drowning. *Emergency* 1994;26(8):28.

Case 14

Pike, K. M. When a child cries. *Emergency* 1993;25(9):39.

Costello, L. When children die. *Emerg. Med. Serv.* 1990;19(4):16.

Case 15

Hunt, D. Seizures. *Emerg. Med. Serv.* 1990;19(6):66.

Case 16

Schoen, S. T. Case review: Heroin overdose. *Emerg. Med. Serv.* 1993;22(11):53.

Kirk, M. A., et al. Clueing in on the acutely poisoned patient. *JEMS* 1991;1(5):64.

Cahill, J. J. Drug watch: Treatment of opioid overdose. *Emergency* 1993;25(12):20.

Shade, B. Ventilating via bag-valve device. *Emergency* 1992;24(3):18.

Case 17

Greiff, S. Blind nasotracheal intubation. *Emergency* 1991;23(11):53.

Peppers, M. Drug watch: Inotropes for heart failure. *Emergency* 1995;27(7):18.

Murphy, P. M., et al. Successfully treating congestive heart failure. *JEMS* 1991;16(9):48.

Case 18

Tan, N., et al. Acute gouty arthritis: Modern approaches to an ancient disease. *Postgrad. Med.* 1993;94:73–84.

Case 19

Rothenberg, M. A. Diabetic emergencies. *Emerg. Med. Serv.* 1991;29(10):18.

Case 20

Nixon, R. G. A sigh of relief: Pharmacologic interventions for respiratory distress. *Emerg. Med. Serv.* 1993;22(6):39.

Matera, P. M. Breathe easy: Diagnosing and treating asthma in the field. *JEMS* 1993;18(11):40.

Case 21

Cahill, J. J. Drug watch: Treatment of opioid overdose. *Emergency* 1993;25(12):20.

Stewart, C. E. Puppy love. *Emerg. Med. Serv.* 1995;24(9):25.

Case 22

Kirk, M. A., et al. Clueing in on the acutely poisoned patient. *JEMS* 1991;1(5):64.

Case 23

Stewart, C. E. EMT review discussion: Epistaxis. *Emerg. Med. Serv.* 1991;20(8):36.

Case 24

Cahill, J. J. A twist of face: Acute dystonic reactions. *JEMS* 1993; 18(7):46.

Case 25

Bartos, B. J. Assessing diabetic emergencies. *Emergency* 1992;24(2):36.

Rothenberg, M. A. Diabetic emergencies. *Emerg. Med. Serv.* 1991;29(10):18.

Case 26

Manoguerra, A. S. Drug watch: Fire toxicology. *Emergency* 1994;26(7):20.

Guyette, M. J. Emergency burn care. *Emerg. Med. Serv.* 1993;22(9):47.

Fontanarosa, P. B. Taking charge of patients with electrical injuries. *JEMS* 1992;17(3):50.

Case 27

Ball, R. A. Carbon monoxide poisoning. *Emergency* 1992;24(1):23.

Case 28

Taigman, M, and Canan, S. Cardiology practicum: Precursors to complete heart block. *JEMS* 1991;16(9):87.

Case 29

Burton, B., and Grandy, J. Skills primer: Needle decompression. *Emergency* 1995;27(8):18.

Corey, E. C. Blunt and penetrating chest trauma. *Emergency* 1994; 26(4):34.

Case 30

Peppers, M. Drug watch: Emergency treatment of migraines. *Emergency* 1995;27(5):18.

Case 31

McKinney, H. E. Drug watch: Ethanol emergencies. *Emergency* 1991; 23(5):22.

Peppers, M. P. Drug watch: Alcohol withdrawal syndrome. *Emergency* 1991;23(12):47.

Judd, R. L. Altered mental status. *Emerg. Med. Serv.* 1991;20(9):39.

Case 32

Cox, D. M. Drug watch: Trauma fluid resuscitation. *Emergency* 1994;26 (4):22.

Klofas, E. S. Pumping up the volume: A case for pre-hospital IV therapy. *JEMS* 1991;16(5):60.

Case 33

Stewart, C. E. Sexually related trauma: Anorectal injuries. *Emerg. Med. Serv.* 1995;24(5):36.

Case 34

Copass, M. K., Soper, R. G., and Eisenberg, M. S. Gut reactions. *Emerg. Med. Serv.* 1991;20(3):54.

Case 35

Bolin, A. Drug watch: Glucagon hydrochloride. *Emergency* 1995; 27(5):24.

Bartos, B. J. Assessing diabetic emergencies. *Emergency* 1992;24(2):36.

Rothenberg, M. A. Diabetic emergencies. *Emerg. Med. Serv.* 1991; 29(10):18.

CASE 36

Gaull, E. S. Are you overlooking O_2? *Emerg. Med. Serv.* 1993;22(6):31.

CASE 37

Judd, R. L. Altered mental status. *Emerg. Med. Serv.* 1991;20(9):39.

Alcouloumre, E. The intoxicated patient. *Emerg. Med. Serv.* 1990;19(4):65.

CASE 38

Stewart, C. E. The booze blues. *Emerg. Med. Serv.* 1992;21(4):38–45.

CASE 39

Bourn, S. Treating the unconscious patient: Who's in the coma? *JEMS* 1992;17(11):27.

CASE 40

Erenreich, B. Silent Munchausen epidemic. Advent of insurance unleashes "orgy" of health care consumption. *Nurse Health Care* 1993;14:316–317.

CASE 41

Meade, D. M., Lynch, T. G., and Fuller, G. Adolescent suicide. *Emerg. Med. Serv.* 1995;24(3):27.

Nordberg, M. Suicidal callers: The dispatcher's dilemmas. *Emerg. Med. Serv.* 1995;24(3):36.

CASE 42

Deliere, H. M., et al. A study of CPR technical skill retention among EMT-As. *Emerg. Med. Tech.* 1980;4:57.

Case 43

Alcouloumre, E. The intoxicated patient. *Emerg. Med. Serv.* 1990; 19(4):65.

Case 44

McKinney, H. E. Drug watch: Ethanol emergencies. *Emergency* 1991; 23(5):22.

Alcouloumre, E. The intoxicated patient. *Emerg. Med. Serv.* 1990;19 (4):65.

Case 45

Gibbons, P. Cystitis in the sexually active female. *Nursing Times* 1990;86:33–35.

Case 46

Hunt, D. Hypertensive crises. *Emerg. Med. Serv.* 1993;22(10):42.

Judd, R. L. Altered mental status. *Emerg. Med. Serv.* 1991;20(9):39.

Case 47

Judd, R. L. Altered mental status. *Emerg. Med. Serv.* 1991;(20)9:39.

Kirk, M. A., et al. Clueing in on the acutely poisoned patient. *JEMS* 1991;1(5):64.

Case 48

Kirk, M. A., et al. Clueing in on the initially poisoned patient. *JEMS* 1991;1(5):64.

Case 49

Peppers, M. P. Drug watch: Spinal cord injury and methylprednisolone. *Emergency* 1992;24(6):56.

Case 50

Kelleher, J. Action STAT! Partial hand amputations. *Nursing* 1985; 15(8):25.

Case 51

Saving a tooth. University of California Berkeley. *Wellness Letter* 1995; 11(4):6–7.

Ronis, D. L. Updating a measure of dental anxiety. *J. Dent. Hyg.* 1994;68:228–233.

Case 52

Stewart, C. E. Orthopedic emergencies. *Emerg. Med. Serv.* 1991;20 (9):10.

Case 53

National Foundation for Infectious Diseases. Hepatitis B. *Emerg. Med. Serv.* 1992;21(8):64.

Stull, J. O. Hands on protection. *Emergency* 1994;26(11):34–37.

Hallinan, L. Personal protection products. *Emergency* 1994;26(11):38–41.

Smith, S. J. The path to safety. *Emergency* 1993;25(5):32.

Stehlin, D. Hepatitis B: Available vaccine safe, but under used. *Emerg. Med. Serv.* 1990;19(7):45.

Case 54

Copass, M. K., Soper, R. G., and Eisenberg, M. S. Gut reactions. *Emerg. Med. Serv.* 1991;20(3):54.

Case 55

Tagamet potentiated coumadin anticoagulation. *Nurses Drug Alert* 1982;6:94.

Case 56

Hartzog, M. Drug watch: RSI and intubation. *Emergency* 1995;27(1):9–17.

Davis, E. Prehospital paralytics. *Emerg. Med. Serv.* 1994;23(3):56.

Case 57

Grubbs, T. C. The ultimate emergency: Managing aortic aneurysms. *JEMS* 1991;16(10):56.

Case 58

Tkach, T. Psychiatric emergencies. *Emerg. Med. Serv.* 1993;22(1):21.

Case 59

Handberg, E., Keith, T., and Rucinski, P. Clot busters: The future of EMS thrombolytics. *JEMS* 1992;17(4):74.

Stewart, C. Prehospital thrombolysis. *Emerg. Med. Serv.* 1993;22(10):46.

Mercer, S. Thrombolysis for the acute myocardial infarction. *Emergency* 1992;24(2):29.

Case 60

Lee, M. J., and Martinez, A. J. Focusing on facial and ocular injuries. *JEMS* 1992;17(2):28.

Drake, A. A. Portrait of a batterer. *Emerg. Med. Serv.* 1994;23(4):40.

Case 61

Taylor, M., and Washko, J. "Ouch!" *Emerg. Med. Serv.* 1993;22(7):27.

Case 62

Copass, M. K., Soper, R. G., and Eisenberg, M. S. Gut Reactions. *Emerg. Med. Serv.* 1991;20(3):54.

Case 63

Kitay, G., et al. Café coronary: Recognition, treatment, and prevention. *Nurse Pract.* 1989;14:36–43.

Case 64

Corey, E. C. Drug watch: Anaphylactic shock. *Emergency* 1993;25(10):48.

Ball, R. A. Hot stuff: Assessing and treating burns. *JEMS* 1993;18(2):9.

Case 65

Connor, L., and Light, J. Child abuse calls. *Emergency* 1995;27(8):30.

Thomas, J. L., and Towberman, D. B. Responding to the child within: Child abuse and the EMS provider. *JEMS* 1992;17(3):98.

Pike, K. M. When a child cries. *Emergency* 1993;25(9):39.

Case 66

Murphy, P. M. Problem pregnancies: Hemorrhagic complications in the third trimester. *JEMS* 1992;17(9):44.

Flattum-Riemers, J. OB emergencies. *Emerg. Med. Serv.* 1994;23(4):51.

Case 67

Greiff, S. Blind nasotracheal intubation. *Emergency* 1991;23(11):53.

Gaull, E. S. Are you overlooking O_2? *Emerg. Med. Serv.* 1993;22(6):31.

Heimback, L. J., and Newman, J. G. In quest: Oxygen and the COPD patient. *Emergency* 1993;25(11):63.

Auerbach, J. Expanding the choices in COPD cases. *JEMS* 1991; 16(3):66.

Jay, F. D. Pulse oxymetry. *Emerg. Med. Serv.* 1992;20(5):40.

Case 68

Corey, E. C. Blunt and penetrating chest trauma. *Emergency* 1994; 26(4):34.

Brown, K., et al. Trauma rounds: The case of the penetrating chest wound. *JEMS* 1991;16(3):83.

Case 69

A differential for pleuritic pain. *Emerg. Med.* 1984;16:97.

Case 70

McKinney, H. E. Drug watch: Ethanol emergencies. *Emergency* 1991;23(5):22.

Bourn, S. Treating the unconscious patient: Who's in the coma? *JEMS* 1992;17(11):27.

Case 71

Platt, F. W. *Conversation Failure.* Tacoma, WA: Life Sciences, 1992.

Case 72

Can the ECG detect hyperkaloma? *Emerg. Med.* 1992;24:119.

Case 73

Gaull, E. S. Are you overlooking O_2? *Emerg. Med. Serv.* 1993;22(6):31.

Case 74

Klepser, M. E., Levy, D. B. Drug watch: Status epilepticus. *Emergency* 1993;25(7):59.

Case 75

Kirkwood, S., et al. Make your voice heard. EMS directors comment on health care reform. *Emergency* 1994;26(7):54–70.

Case 76

Stopping ureteral colic at its source. *Emerg. Med.* 1990;22:104–107.

Pekkanen, J. I am Joe's kidney stone. *Reader's Digest* 1990;137(823):147–150.

Stone, L. Percutaneous lithotripsy: An advancement in kidney stone extraction. *AORN-J.* 1984;39(4):773–780.

Case 77

Shanaberger, C. J. The legal file: The trials of no transport. *JEMS* 1992;17(2):75.

Spiro, D. C. Tricyclic troubles. *Emerg. Med. Serv.* 1992;21(4):25–37.

Neely, K. "No Way": How should you handle patients who refuse prehospital care? *Emerg. Med. Serv.* 1992;21(11):29.

Schiffman, M. A. Managing the toxic ingestion. *Emerg. Med. Serv.* 1992;21(4):28–32.

Kirk, M. A., et al. Clueing in on the acutely poisoned patient. *JEMS* 1991;1(5):64.

Case 78

Judd, R. L. Altered mental status. *Emerg. Med. Serv.* 1991;20(9):39.

Case 79

What causes diarrhea in HIV disease? *Emerg. Med.* 1994;26:37.

Case 80

Syncope: Distrust the easy answer. *Emerg. Med.* 1992;24:163.

Case 81

Just a viral syndrome? Ruling out drug problems. *Emerg. Med.* 1989; 21:67.

Case 82

Gormley, P. On the scene: The dislocation dilemma. *Emerg. Med. Serv.* 1993;22(9):75.

Stewart, C. E. Orthopedic emergencies. *Emerg. Med. Serv.* 1991;20(9):10.

Case 83

McGraw, S. Pelvic problems. *Emerg. Med. Serv.* 1994;23(1):39.

Case 84

Blank, B. H., et al. Acute scrotal problems. *Patient Care* 1990;24(11): 152–163.

Case 85

Bledsoe, B. E. Pediatric respiratory emergencies. *JEMS* 1994;19(2):38–49.

Case 86

Simmons, M., et al. Bench evaluation: Three face shield CPR barriers. *Resp. Care* 1995;40(6):618–623.

Case 87

First aid for a choking child. *Patient Care* 1987;21(13):223–224.

Case 88

Wertz, E. On guard for meningitis. *Emergency* 1995;27(8):36.

Littrell, K. A., and Contwell, G. P. Pediatric status epilepticus: Managing the complexities. *JEMS* 1991;16(2):71.

Crabb, J. J. In the hot seat: Managing febrile seizures. *JEMS* 1993;18(1):50.

Case 89

Rigby, D. African diary. *Br. J. Theatre Nurs.* 1994;3:26.

Case 90

Greiff, S. Blind nasotracheal intubation. *Emergency* 1991;23(11):53.

Stapleton, E. S. Cardiopulmonary resuscitation during ambulance transport. *JEMS* 1991;16(9):63.

Case 91

Mistreated by EMS. *Emerg. Med. Serv.* 1994;23(11):14.

Case 92

Duffy, S. P., Murphy, P. M., and Schatzle, J. C. Adenosine: An old drug learns a new trick. *JEMS* 1992;17(4):58.

Case 93

Blum, L. A. Rude awakenings: Prickly patients. *Emerg. Med. Serv.* 1995;24(5):31.

Meade, D. M. Create the carnage and we will come. *Emerg. Med. Serv.* 1994;23(7):57.

Case 94

Holliman, G. J., et al. Comparison of interventions in prehospital care by standing orders versus on line medical command. *Prehosp. Disaster Med.* 1994;9(4):202–209.

Case 95

Shanaberger, C. J. The legal file: The trials of no transport. *JEMS* 1992;17(2):75.

Rhoads, J. Restraint restrictions. *Emerg. Med. Serv.* 1993;22(1):16.

Neely, K. "No Way": How should you handle patients who refuse prehospital care? *Emerg. Med. Serv.* 1992;21(11):29.

Case 96

Lee, M. J., and Martinez, A. J. Focusing on facial and ocular injuries. *JEMS* 1992;17(2):28.

Case 97

Corey, E. C. Blunt and penetrating chest trauma. *Emergency* 1994;26(4):34.

Case 98

Swanson, J. M. Clinical features and psychosocial factors in young adults with genital herpes. *Image J. Nurs. Sch.* 1995;27:16–22.

Case 99

Springer, C. Stroke. *Emerg. Med. Serv.* 1992;21(11):49.

Case 100

Cohn, B. M., and Cohn, E. Limiting liability in pre-hospital care. *Emergency* 1994;26(1):54.

Page, J. The portrait of EMS liability. *JEMS* 1991;16(7):6.

Case 101

Bledsoe, B. E., and Clayden, D. E. Recognizing and managing angina pectoris. *JEMS* 1993;18(4):22.

Case 102

Blazer, L. K. A comparison of substance abuse rates among female nurses, clerical workers, and blue collar workers. *J. Adv. Nurs.* 1995;21(2):305.

Case 103

Norton, R. L., et al. Survey of EMT's ability to cope with the deaths of patients in prehospital care. *Prehosp. Disaster Med.* 1993;7(3):235–242.

Forgues, M. In the best interest of the patient. *Emergency* 1991;23(12):34–56.

Iserson, K. V. Foregoing prehospital care: Should ambulance staff always resuscitate? *J. Med. Ethics* 1996;17:19–24.

Crager, D. Do not resuscitate. Society's recognition of the right to die with dignity has accelerated state and local passage of prehospital DNR legislation or protocols. *Emergency* 1995;27(2):42–45.

Case 104

Segatore, M. Thrombolysis after stroke: Hope for the future. *Axon* 1995;16(3):71–77.

Different strokes for younger folks: Causes of CVA in patients under 45. *Emerg. Med.* 1985;17(18):65–68.

Case 105

Reilly, A., et al. Factors influencing prehospital delay in patients experiencing chest pain. *Am. J. Crit. Care* 1994;3(4):300–306.

West, K. Multidrug resistant TB. *Emerg. Med. Serv.* 1992;21(9):54.

Case 106

Zeta (Zachary Cope). *The Acute Abdomen in Verse*. London, H. K. Lewis, 1962.

INDEX

ABCs (airway, breathing, circulation), 1, 90–92, 101, 291–297. *See also* Trauma, multiple
Abdomen, acute, 107–109
Abdominal aortic aneurysm, 234
   ruptured, 183–186
Abdominal injuries, in blunt trauma, evaluation of, 103
Abdominal pain, 22–24, 29–30, 173–176, 233–235, 351–353
   crampy, 4, 259–262
   groin kick and, 274–276
   left lower quadrant, 35–37
   in perforated duodenal ulcer, 107–109
Abdominal trauma
   blunt, 2
   penetrating, 1–3
Aberrancy, description of, 301
Abortion, threatened, 212–214
Abscess(es), in drug abusers, 289–291
Abuse
   alcohol. *See* Alcohol abuse
   child, 209–211
   cocaine. *See* Cocaine, abuse of; Drug abuse
   narcotic. *See* Heroin, abuse of; Methadone
   physical, 31–34, 195–197
Abusive patient, 303–306
Acetaminophen, overdose of, 49, 252
Ache(s). *See* Pain
Acid(s), eye burns due to, 315–317
Acidosis
   metabolic, causes of, 78–79, 151
   in motor vehicle accidents, 318–320
ACLS. *See* Advanced cardiac life support
Acquired immunodeficiency syndrome (AIDS), 169–172
   Pneumocystis carinii pneumonia in, 225
Acute abdomen, 107–109
Acute dystonic reaction, 74–76
Acute organic brain syndrome. *See* Organic brain syndrome, acute
Adenosine, 79
Advanced cardiac life support (ACLS)
   in cardiac arrest, 292–297
   defibrillation, 234
Agitation, 325–328. *See also* Confusion; Delirium tremens (DTs); Organic brain syndrome
   following overdose, 251

AIDS. *See* Acquired immunodeficiency syndrome
Airway, breathing, and circulation (ABCs). *See* ABCs (airway, breathing, circulation)
Airway management. *See also specific types, e.g.,* Intubation
Albuterol, for COPD, 217. *See also* Bronchodilators
Alcohol, withdrawal from, 98–100, 117–120, 150–152
   patient evaluation form, 118
   seizures due to, 240
Alcohol abuse, 31–34, 140–142, 150–152, 187–190, 195–197, 227–229
   falling due to, 137–139
   in perforated duodenal ulcer, 107–109
Alcohol withdrawal syndrome, 98–100
Alcohol-Antabuse reaction, 140–142
Alcoholic stupor, 124–126
Alkalis, eye burns due to, 315–317
Allergens, reactions to, 206–208
Allergic reactions, 206–208
AMA (against medical advice), 32
Aminophylline, in acute pulmonary edema, 53–54
Amoxicillin, and clavulinic acid, 16
Ampicillin, mononucleosis and, relationship between, 16
Anaphylaxis, 206–208
Aneurysm, abdominal aortic, 234
   ruptured, 183–186
Angina, intestinal, 234
Anorexia
   with diarrhea, 259–262
   in HIV infection, 280–282
   in viral hepatitis, 169–172
Antabuse, in alcoholics, 140–142
Anterior spinal cord injury, 158
Antibiotics, in urinary tract infection, 144–145
Anticoagulants, 177–179
   in stroke patients, 327
Antidepressants
   seizures due to, 49
   tricyclic, overdose of, 250–255
Anxiety, 127–129
   in depression, 7
   hyperventilation due to, 77–79
Aphasia, 325–328
   versus confusion, 326

Appetite
  changes in, 7
  loss of, 169–172
Arm, soreness of, 289–291
Arrhythmia(s), 133–136
  in cocaine abusers, 69
  reperfusion, 193
  syncope due to, 264
Arterial blood gases (ABGs), cost of, 245. *See also* Acidosis
Arthritis
  gonococcal, 56, 322, 323
  monoarticular, 55–57
Aspiration, of foreign bodies, in children, 283–285
Aspirin, in Reye's syndrome, 257
Assault, civil charge of, by patient, 311–314
Asthma, 61–64, 215–218
  "cardiac," heart failure with, 63
ATO$_2$MIC^5, 189–190
Atrial fibrillation, 325–328
Atrioventricular (AV) block, and right bundle branch block, 87–89
Atropine
  in cardiac arrest, 293–294
  in food poisoning, 30
Automobile accidents. *See* Motor vehicle accidents
Automobile battery, exploding, 315–317
Azithromycin, in sexually transmitted diseases, 322
AZT, in AIDS, 171

Back pain, 143–146
  low, 303–306
Bacterial enteritis, viral, diarrhea due to, 260
Bacterial meningitis, versus seizures, 286–288
Bag-valve-mask
  in acute respiratory failure, 236–238
  in cardiac arrest, 293–294
Bat bites, 122
Battery(ies), car, exploding, 315–317
Behavior
  altered, in Reye's syndrome, 257
  change in, 311–314
  inappropriate, 336–339
"Bell-clapper" deformity, 274–276
Benzodiazepines
  in abscess drainage, 289–290
  in anxiety disorders, 128–129
  for seizures, 240
Beta-blockers, in acute pulmonary edema, 53–54

Bicarbonate, in tricyclic antidepressant overdose, 253. *See also* Advanced cardiac life support (ACLS)
Bilirubin, in viral hepatitis, 169–172
Binge drinker, 98–100
Bite(s)
  bat, 122
  cat, 121–123
  dog, 121–123
  human, 123
  leopard, 121–123
  skunk, 122
  snake, 122–123
Bleeding
  on coumarin, 177–179
  gastrointestinal, 117–120
  during pregnancy, 212–214
  stopping, 198–200
  vaginal, 35–37
Blisters, burn-related, 80–83
Blood, coughing up, 127–129
Blood pressure
  acute evaluation of, 147–149
  arterial, low, 22–24
"Body packer," cocaine overdose in, 68
Body writhing, total, 75
Boil, 289–291
Bone(s)
  breast, spasm of, 332–335
  navicular, fracture of, 10
Borderline personality disorder, 130–132
Botulism, 29
"Bounce back," 298–299
Bowel, near-necrotic, 107–109. *See also* Abdominal pain
Brain failure, following overdose, 47–50
Breach of duty, 330
Breath, shortness of. *See* Shortness of breath
Breathing
  cessation of, 47–50, 51–54
  difficulty in, 215–218, 243–246, 277–279, 340–343, 347–350
  in cardiac arrest, 292–297
Bretylium, for ventricular tachycardia, 134
Bromide, hallucinations due to, 151
Bronchitis, 243–246, 280–282
  in alcohol withdrawal, 98–100
Bronchodilators
  in acute pulmonary edema, 53–54
  in asthma, 62–63
  in COPD, 217
  inhaled, in asthma, death due to, 62
Bronchopneumonia, 267

INDEX

Bronochitis, 215–218, 266–268
Brown-Séquard syndrome, 158
Bruise, blue, 177–179. *See also* Myocardial contusion
Burn(s), 80–83
  chemical, ocular, 315–317
  electrical, 82
  first-degree, 82
  respiratory complications of, 81
  second-degree, 82
  third-degree, 82
"Burn sheet," 81

Café coronary, 204
Cancer, testicular, 275
Capacity, medical definition of, 312
Car battery, exploding, 315–317
Carbon monoxide, 81, 190
  carboxyhemoglobin level, 85
  description of, 85
  poisoning, 29, 84–86
Cardiac arrest, 292–297
  ACLS in, 292–297
Cardiac tamponade, 221
Cardiogenic shock, 140–142
Cardiopulmonary resuscitation (CPR), in cardiac arrest, 293–294
Cardioversion
  for tachyarrhythmia, 301
  for ventricular tachycardia, 134
Carotid sinus massage, in supraventricular tachycardia, 301–302
Cat bites, 121–123
CAT scan. *See* Computed tomography (CT)
Cefixime, in sexually transmitted diseases, 322
Ceftriaxone, in PID, 175
Cefuroximine axetil, in bronchitis, 281
Cellulitis, orbital, 315–317
Central cord syndrome, 158
Cephalexin, in HIV infection, 280–282
Cephalosporin, in oral infections, 163–165
Cerebrovascular accidents (CVAs), 325–328
Cervical spine fractures, 230–232
Cervical spondylolisthesis, 156–159
Charcoal, in overdose patient, 252
Chemical burns, ocular, 315–317
Chemstrips, in diabetic ketoacidosis diagnosis, 23
Chest
  flail, 319
  pounding in, 300–302
  trauma to, 219–223

Chest pain, 4, 137–139, 191–194, 224–226
  in cardiac arrest, 292–297
  cocaine use and, 67–70
  costochondritis, 332–335
  in heart attack victims, 332–335
  following motor vehicle accidents, 102
  in motor vehicle accidents, 318–320
  pleuritic, 347–350
Chest tubes, 90–91, 219–223
Chest wall, tenderness of in acute MI, 332–335
Cheyne-Stokes respiration, 327
Child abuse, 209–211
Children
  choking in, 283–285
  cough in, 277–279, 283–285
  croup in, 277–279
  diarrhea in, 261
  fever in, 283–285
    causes of, 287
  runny nose in, 283–285
  seizures in, 286–288
Chills, 143–146
  abscess and, 289–291
Choking, sudden, in children, 283–285
Cholinesterase levels, 29–30
Chronic obstructive pulmonary disease (COPD), 215–218
  oxygen therapy in, 237
Clavulinic acid, amoxicillin and, 16
Clumsiness, 325–328
Cluster headache, 93–97
Cocaine
  abuse of, abscess in, 289–291
  chest pain due to, 67–70
  overdose of, 67–70
  seizures due to, 49
Cold, common, 266–268
Colic
  renal, 337
  ureteral, 247–249
Coma, 124–126
  in gunshot wound victim, 180–182
  in overdose patient, 153–155
  patient positioning in, 124
  in Reye's syndrome, 257
Common cold, 266–268
Computed tomography (CT), 228
  in abdominal injuries, 103
  in cervical spine injury evaluation, 230–232
  in head injuries, 210
Confusion, 18–19, 147–149, 187–190
  versus aphasia, 326

Confusion—*Continued*
   in diabetics following motor vehicle accidents, 110–113
      differential diagnosis of, 188–189
      following motor vehicle accidents, 271–273
      in scrotal infection, 58–60
Congestion, nasal, 277–279
Consciousness
   fluctuating levels of, in overdose patient, 153–155
   lapses of, 44–46
Constipation, 201–202
Continued positive airway pressure (CPAP), 340–343
Contusion, myocardial, following chest trauma, 319
COPD. *See* Chronic obstructive pulmonary disease
Coronary artery bypass graft, 300–302
Coronary artery disease, 135
Corticosteroids
   in COPD, 217
   in HIV infection, 280
Costochondritis, 332–335
Costs, of ED care, 243–246
Cough, 215–218, 224–226, 236–238, 266–268
   barking, in children, 277–279
   blood with, 127–129
   in children, 283–285
   in HIV infection, 280–282
   nonproductive, 347–350
   in pneumonia, 138
Coumarin, bleeding while on, 177–179
Crack, description of, 68, 69
Crib death, 41–43
Croup, in children, 277–279
Crying spells, changes in, 7
CT scan. *See* Computed tomography (CT)
CVAs. *See* Cerebrovascular accidents
Cyanide, 81
Cyanosis, 236–238
Cystitis, in postmenopausal women, 145
Cystoscopy, in urinary tract infection, 143–146

Damages, description of, 330
Defibrillation, in cardiac arrest, 293–294
Dehydration, 259–262
Delayed neuropsychiatric syndrome, 86
Delirium
   in acute organic brain syndrome, 257
   in alcoholic, 187–190

Delirium tremens (DTs), 98–100
   in alcoholic, 150–152
Dental infection, 163–165
   mandibular, 164
   maxillary, 164
Dental problems, headache following, 96
Depression, 5, 130–132
   in alcoholics, 150–152
   symptoms of, 7
Dextrostix, in diabetic ketoacidosis diagnosis, 23
Diabetic(s)
   acute myocardial infarction in, 191–194
   confusion in, following motor vehicle accidents, 110–113
Diabetic ketoacidosis (DKA), 22–24
   scrotal swelling in, 58–60
Diaphoresis, 117–120, 169, 280–282
Diarrhea, 29–30, 201–202, 259–262
   acute causes of, 260
   in children, 261
Diazepam, for seizures, 239–242, 240
Digitalis
   in acidotic patient, 78–79
   side effects of, 79
Diltiazem, 79
Direct pressure, in bleeding cessation, 198–200
Disaster(s), EMS, 308
Disaster plan, elements of, 307–310
Disc, "slipped," 303–306
Dislocations, 10, 269–270
Distention, in acute abdomen, 107–109
Diuretics, loop, in hypertensive emergencies, 149
Diving reflex, in supraventricular tachycardia, 301–302
Divorce, stress due to, hyperventilation due to, 77–79
Do not resuscitate (DNR), 340–343
Dog bites, 121–123
Domestic violence, 195–197
   victim of, 31–34
Doxycycline
   in PID, 175
   in sexually transmitted diseases, 322
Drowning, 38–40
Drug(s)
   failure of, 143–146
   schizophrenic on, 187–190
Drug abuse, 6. *See also* Cocaine; Heroin; Alcohol abuse
   abscess in, 289–291
   presentation of, 303–306
   seekers, 336–339

INDEX

399

DTs. *See* Delirium tremens
Dysphasia, 188, 189
Dyspnea, in acute respiratory failure, 236–238
Dystonic reaction, acute, 74–76

Ectopic pregnancy, 35–37, 173–176
Edema, pulmonary. *See* Pulmonary disorders, pulmonary edema
Elbow, "nursemaid's," 270
Elderly
  confusion in, 18–19
  fainting in, 263–265
Electrical burns, 82
Electrical countershock, 79
Embolism, pulmonary, 347–350
Emergency department, leaving without being seen, 31–34
Emergency medical services (EMS)
  in cardiac arrest, 292–297
  costliness of, 243–246
  disaster, definition of, 308
  prehospital care, 183–186
  radio call, 183–186
Emergency medical technicians (EMTs)
  information to be obtained by, 111–112
  training of, 13
  treatment provided by, 13
Emphysema, 215–218, 237
EMS. *See* Emergency medical services
EMTs. *See* Emergency medical technicians
Encephalopathy, acute, causes of, 189–190
Endometriosis, 175
Enemas, 201–202
Enteritis, bacterial, diarrhea due to, 260
Enterocolitis, pseudomembranous, 260
Epidural hematoma, 227–229. *See also* Computed tomography (CT), in head injuries
Epiglottitis, 266–268
  in children, 277–279
Epinephrine
  in anaphylaxis, 207
  in asthma, 61–62
  in cardiac arrest, 293–294
Epistaxis, 71–73
Erythromycin, in oral infections, 163–165
Esophageal obstruction, 203–205
Esophageal-obturator airway, 38–40
Ewald tube, 252
Extrapyramidal diseases, 74–76
Eye(s), trauma to, 315–317

Face, trauma to, 195–197
  following motor vehicle accident, 44–46
Fainting. *See* Syncope
Falling
  from bed, 209–211
  down stairs, 137–139
  hip pain following, 166–168
Fatigue, 4, 127–129, 236–238
  in asthma, 63
  in depression, 7
Fentanyl, in abscess drainage, 289–290
Fever, 29–30, 277–279
  abscess and, 289–291
  in alcohol withdrawal, 98–100
  in children, 283–285
    causes of, 287
  headaches with, 94
  in HIV infection, 280–282
  in pneumonia, 137–139, 224–226
  seizure-related, in children, 286–288
  sore throat and, 15–17
Fiber, for constipation, 201–202
Fibrillation, atrial, 325–328
Flail chest, in motor vehicle accidents, 319
Flank pain, 247–249, 336–339
Flexor tenosynovitis, 161
Flu, stomach, 351–353
Food poisoning, 29–30
  diarrhea due to, 260
Foot (feet), swelling of, 4
Forcible treatment of trauma patients, 12–14
Foreign bodies
  gastrointestinal, 203–205
  in hand, 160–162
  nasal, epistaxis due to, 72
  in rectum, 105–106
  respiratory, 283–285
  in wounds, 198–200
Fracture(s)
  cervical spine, 230–232
  of hip, 167
  mandibular, 196
  nasal, 195–197
  of navicular bone, 10
  "no fracture," 166–168
  pelvic, 167, 271–273
  rib, 137–139
    in motor vehicle accidents, 318–320
  spinal, 156–159
Furosemide, 53, 149

Gangrene, gas, 58–60
Gastroenteritis, viral, 29–30

Gastrointestinal bleeding
  lower, 119
  upper, 117–120
Gastrointestinal tract, foreign bodies in, 203–205
Giardiasis, 259–262
Glass fragments, in hand, 160–162
Glucagon, in foreign body ingestion, 204
Gonococcal arthritis, 56, 322, 323
Gonorrhea, *Chlamydia*, 321–324
Gout, 56
Groin, kicked in, 274–276
Gunshot wound, 219–223, 307–310
  to head, 180–182

Hallucinations, 130–132
  in alcohol withdrawal, 98–100
  in alcoholic, 150–152
Haloperidol, movement disorders due to, 75
Hand(s)
  laceration of, 160–162
  swelling of, 4
Head
  gunshot wound to, 180–182. *See also* Gunshot wound
  sandbagging of, 156–159
  trauma to, headache following, 95–96
Head trauma, 227–229. *See also* Computed tomography (CT), in head injuries
  in alcoholics, 98–100
  in children, 209–211
Headache(s), 4, 84–86, 93–97, 344–345
  dental problems and, 96
  eye problems and, 96
  febrile, 94
  hypertension, 95
  muscular, 94
  post–head-trauma, 95–96
  sinus, 95
  vascular, 94–95
Hearing aid, in motor vehicle accidents, 230–232
Heart failure, with "cardiac asthma," 63
Heat stroke, 18–19
Heimlich maneuver, 204
Hematoma
  epidural, 227–229
  subdural, 227–229
Hematuria, 247–249
Hemiparesis, right-sided, 325–328
Hemorrhage, subarachnoid, 344–345
  in cocaine abusers, 69
Heparin, in acute myocardial infarction, 193

Hepatitis
  contacts of patients with, 170–171
  viral, 169–172
Hereditary hemorrhagic telangiectasia, epistaxis due to, 72
Hernia, inguinal, 351–353
Heroin
  abuse of, abscess in, 289–291
  addict, 65–66
  withdrawal from, 65–66
Herpes genitalis, detection of, 323
Hip(s), fractures of, 167
Hip pain, following fall, 166–168
HIV infection. *See* Human immunodeficiency virus (HIV) infection
Hives, alergies and, 206–208
Hoarseness, 266–268
"Horse," 66
Horton's histamine cephalalgia, 93–97
Human bites, 123
Human immunodeficiency virus (HIV) infection, 169–172, 280–282
  counseling about, for rape victims, 27
  Pneumocystis carinii pneumonia in, 280–282
  positive testing for, 280–282
Hyperbaric oxygen, in carbon monoxide poisoning, 84–86
Hyperkalemia, 233–235
Hyperpyrexia, in cocaine abusers, 69
Hypertension
  in acute myocardial infarction, 191–194
  in cocaine abusers, 69
  headaches with, 95
  following stroke, 327
Hypertensive emergencies, 147–149
Hypertensive urgency, 148
Hyperthermia, 18–19
Hyperventilation, 77–79
  differential diagnosis of, 79
  in gunshot wound victim, 180–182
Hypoglycemia
  in diabetics, 112–113
  in heat stroke, 19
  presentation of, 112–113
  in seizure patient, 115
Hyponatremia, in seizure patient, 115
Hypotension, 22–24
  in alcohol-Antabuse reaction, 140–142
  in gunshot wound victims, 219–223
  in penetrating thoracic trauma, 220
Hypothermia, 19
Hypoxemia, 311–314

INDEX

Immobilization
  following motor vehicle accidents, 156–159
  wrist, 10
Infants, nonbreathing, 41–43. *See also* Fever
Infection
  with acute organic brain syndrome, 189
  dental, 163–165
  oral, 163–165
  pharyngeal, 163–165
  scrotal, 58–60
Infertility, 322, 323
Influenza, 352
Inguinal hernia, 351–353
Insomnia, in depression, 7
Insulin, in diabetic ketoacidosis, 23
Intestinal angina, 234
Intravenous pyelogram (IVP), in urinary tract infection, 143–146
Intubation, 219–223
  in acute respiratory failure, 237
  in COPD, 217–218
  in gunshot wound victim, 181
Ipecac, syrup of, for induction of vomiting in overdose patient, 252
Ischemia, cardiac, 295, 332–335
Isoniazid, seizures due to, 49

Kaopectate, for diarrhea, 259
Keflex. *See* Cephalexin
Kemadrin, overdose of, 153–155
Ketoacidosis
  diabetic, 22–24
  scrotal swelling in, 58–60
"Keyhole medicine," 351–353
Knees, swelling of, 55

Labetalol, in hypertensive emergencies, 149
Laceration(s), 198–200
  facial, 44–46
  of hand, 160–162
  of wrist, 130–132
Laparoscopy, in PID, 175
Laryngeal trauma, 195
Lawsuits, malpractice, 245–246
  threat of, 303–306
Leopard bite, 121–123
Lethargy, 147–149
Lidocaine
  in abscess drainage, 289
  in acute myocardial infarction, 191–194
  in cardiac arrest, 293–294
  in facial lacerations, 46
  in ventricular tachycardia, 134

Lockjaw, 74–76
Loop diuretics, in hypertensive emergencies, 149
Lorazepam, for seizures, 240
LSD. *See* Lysergic acid
Lung, diseases of. *See specific types and* Pulmonary disorders
LWBS (leave without being seen), 32
Lysergic acid (LSD), hallucinations due to, 151

Malpractice, 329–331
Malpractice lawsuits, 245–246
  threat of, 303–306
Mandibular fractures, 196
Mannitol, in gunshot wound victim, 181
Marital problems, 5
Mechanical ventilation
  in COPD, 217
  in motor vehicle accidents, 318–320
Medical record, in malpractice defense, 330
Megacode, 295
Memory loss, in carbon monoxide poisoning, 84–86
Meningitis, bacterial, versus seizures, 286–288
  description of, 287
Menstrual cycle
  changes in, 4
  late, 35–37
Mental status, altered, 18, 147–149, 256–258. *See also* Overdose
  agitation, 325–328
  in carbon monoxide poisoning, 84–86
  in intoxicated patients, 100
  panic attack, 127–129
  in rape victim, 26
  secondary to hypoxia, 311–314
  in suicidal patient, 130–132
Meperidine, seizures due to, 49
Mescaline, hallucinations due to, 151
Metabolic acidosis, 22–24
  causes of, 78–79
Metaproterenol, for COPD, 217
Methadone
  in heroin addicts, 66
  request for, 65–66
Methylprednisolone
  for COPD, 217
  in spinal cord injuries, 158
Metronidazole, in alcoholics, 141
Midazolam, in abscess drainage, 289–290
Migraine, 93–97

Military antishock trousers (MAST)
  in gunshot wound victims, 222
  in motor vehicle accident victim, 318–320
  in pelvic fracture, 271–273
Monoarticular arthritis, 55–57
Mononucleosis, 15–17
Morphine, description of, 53
Motor vehicle accidents, 12–14, 44–46, 156–159, 271–273, 318–320
  diabetic in, 110–113
  evaluation following, 101–104
  hearing aid in victim of, 230–232
Motorcycle accident, 90–92
Multiple-casualty incident, 307–310
Mycoplasma pneumonia, 224–226
Myocardial contusion, 319
Myocardial infarction, 133–136, 332–335
  acute, 191–194
  in cocaine abusers, 69
Myocardial ischemia, acute, 192–193

Narcan, 65, 125
  in overdosed patient, 47–50
Nasal congestion, 277–279
Nasopharyngeal tumors, epistaxis due to, 72
Nausea, 4
  abdominal pain with, 173–176
  in alcohol withdrawal, 98–100
  with diarrhea, 259–262
  with flank pain, 336–339
  groin kick and, 274–276
Near-necrotic bowel, 107–109
Neck, immobilization of, 156–159
Neck pain, 298–299
  following motor vehicle accident, 230–232
  nontraumatic, 329–331
Neurologic examination, following single car accidents, 45
Nifedipine, in hypertensive emergencies, 149
Night sweats, 169–172
  in HIV infection, 280–282
Nitroglycerin
  in acute pulmonary edema, 53
  in cardiac ischemia, 292
Nitroprusside, in hypertensive emergencies, 148–149
Nose
  foreign body in, 283–285
  fracture of, 195–197
  runny, in children, 283–285
  trauma to, 72
Nosebleed, 71–73
"Nursemaid's" elbow, 270

Observed, definition of, 154
Ocular problems, headache following, 96
Oculogyric crisis, 75
Oral infections, 163–165
Orbit
  blowout fractures of, 196
  cellulitis, 315–317
Organic brain syndrome, 18
  acute, delirium in, 257
  secondary to hypoxia, 311–314
  workup for, 257
  versus schizophrenia, 188, 189
Organophosphates, in food poisoning, 30
Osler-Weber-Rendu disease, 72
Otitis media, bilateral, 286–288
Overdose, 47–50, 153–155
  of acetaminophen, 252
  cocaine, 67–70
  of tricyclic antidepressants, 250–255
Oxygen therapy
  in acute respiratory failure, 236–238, 311–314
  in gunshot wound victim, 181
  hyberbaric, in carbon monoxide poisoning, 84–86

Pacemakers, 88–89
Pain
  abdominal. See Abdominal pain
  back, 143–146
    low, 303–306
  chest. See Chest pain
  flank, 247–249
  hip, following fall, 166–168
  neck, 298–299
    following motor vehicle accident, 230–232
    nontraumatic, 329–331
  pleuritic, 224–226
  shoulder, 269–270
  testicular, 185
  tooth-related, 163–165
  on urination, 143–146
Palm, laceration of, 160–162
Panic attack, 127–129
Paramedics. See Emergency medical services
Parkinson's disease, 201–202
Paroxysmal atrial tachycardia (PAT), 77–79
Pasteurella multicoda, 121–123
Pelvic inflammatory disease (PID), 322, 323
  acute, 173–176
  agents causing, 174
Pelvis, fractures of, 167, 271–273

INDEX

Penicillin, in oral infections, 163–165
Penile discharge, 321–324
Pentamidine, in HIV infection, 280
Pericardial tamponade, 221
Peripheral neuropathy, in alcoholic, 150–152
Peripheral vascular disease, with hypotension and vasoconstriction, poorly palpable pulses due to, 234
Peritoneal lavage
  in abdominal trauma, 2, 103–104
Peritonitis, 107–109
Pharyngeal infection, 15–17, 163–165. *See also* Throat, sore
Phenothiazines
  movement disorders due to, 75
  overdose of, 153–155
Physical abuse, 31–34, 195–197
Physostigmine
  in agitation, 251
  in anticholinergic toxicity, 253
  in hyperventilation, 79
PID. *See* Pelvic inflammatory disease
Pleuritic pain, 224–226
Pneumococcal pneumonia, 224–226
Pneumocystis carinii pneumonia, 225, 280–282
Pneumonia, 137–139, 187–190, 347–350
  bilateral, 311–314
  diagnosis of, 225
  mycoplasma, 224–226
  pneumococcal, 224–226
  Pneumocystis carinii, 225, 280–282
Pneumothorax, tension, 90–92, 220
Poison control centers, 254
Poisoning
  carbon monoxide, 29, 84–86
  following tricyclic antidepressant overdose, 253–254
  food, 29–30
    diarrhea due to, 260
  hepatitis due to, 169–172
Pregnancy
  bleeding during, 212–214
  ectopic, 35–37, 173–176
  prevention of, in rape victim, 27
Procainamide, in tachycardia, 134, 302
Prochlorperazine, movement disorders due to, 75
Propoxyphene
  overdose of, 47
  seizures due to, 49
Prothrombin time, 177–179
Proximate cause, 330
Pseudomembranous enterocolitis, 260

Pseudoseizures, 241
Psilocybin, hallucinations due to, 151
Psychiatric disorders, 31–34, 130–132. *See also* Agitation; Schizophrenia
  versus organic brain syndrome, 188
Psychoses, 105–106
Pulmonary disorders
  acute respiratory failure, 47–50, 51–54
  breathing difficulty, 215–218
  COPD, 215–218
  pneumocystis lung infection, 281–282
  pneumothorax, 90–92, 219–220, 223
  pulmonary edema, 216
    acute, 51–54, 340–343
    in burn victim, 80
  pulmonary embolism, 347–350
  respiratory infection, 266–268
Pulse, lack of, 233–235
Pupils, unequal, 114–116
Pyelonephritis, 145
Pyuria, 143–146

Quadraplegia, following motor vehicle accidents, 158
Quinine, 66

Rabies, 121–123
  animals carrying, 122
Radio, EMS, 183–186
Rape, 25–28
Rape crisis center, 26–27
Rapid sequence intubation (RSI), 181
Rash(es), ampicillin and, 16
Rectal injuries, 105–106
Refusal of medical attention (RMA), 311–314
Refusal of treatment, 250–255, 311–314
Renal colic, 337
Repeat visits, 130–132
Reperfusion arrhythmia(s), 193
Respiration, Cheyne-Stokes, 327
Respiratory arrest, in children, 277–279
Respiratory failure, acute, 51–54, 236–238
  following overdose, 47–50
Respiratory infection, 266–268
  upper, symptoms of, 267
Respiratory system, evaluation of, 102
Restraint, of patient, 13–14
Reye's syndrome, 256–258
Rib, fracture of, 137–139
  in motor vehicle accidents, 318–320
Right bundle branch block (RBBB), and first-degree atrioventricular (AV) block, 87–89
Rigidity, in acute abdomen, 107–109

Salicylate toxicity, 151–152
Sandbag, 156–159
Schizophrenia, 105–106
   drug-related, 187–190
   versus organic brain syndrome, 188
   paranoid, 153–155
Scopolamine, hallucinations due to, 151
Scrotum, swelling of, 58–60, 351–353
Seconal, overdose of, 153–155
Seizure(s), 44–46, 239–242
   in cocaine abusers, 68
   drugs causing, 49
   versus faint, 264
   febrile, versus bacterial meningitis, 286–288
      in children, 286–288
   first, 241
   following overdose, 251
   in overdose patient, 47–50
   status, 240–241
   types of, 239
   unequal pupils due to, 114–116
Sexual assault, 25–28
Sexual deviancy, 105–106
Sexually transmitted diseases (STDs), 321–324
   in rape victim, 25–28
Shellfish, allergic reaction to, 206–208
Shock, 118–119, 183–186
   anaphylactic, 206–208
   cardiogenic, 140–142
   following motor vehicle accidents, 103, 318–320
   poorly palpable pulses due to, 234
   treatment of, 237
Shortness of breath, 61–64, 102, 127–129, 215–218, 243–246, 340–343, 347–350
   in cardiac arrest, 292–297
Shoulder, dislocation of, 10, 269–270
"Sick all over," 4–8, 22–24
SIDS. See Sudden infant death syndrome
Sinus headache, 95
Skin, edematous, 4, 15–17
Skunk bites, 122
Sleep patterns, abnormalities in, 5
Slipped disc, 303–306
SLUDGE (salivation, lacrimation, urinary incontinence, diarrhea, gastrointestinal irritability, and emesis) syndrome, 30
Smoke inhalation injury, burns and, 81

Smoking
   alcohol abuse and, 98–100
   breathing difficulties due to, 215–218
   cough due to, 266–268
   pneumonia due to, 137–139
   and pulmonary embolism, 347–350
Snake bites, 122–123
Sodium bicarbonate, in tricyclic antidepressant overdose, 253
Sodium nitroprusside, in hypertensive emergencies, 148–149
Somatic complaints, multiple, 4–8
Sore throat. See Throat, sore
Speech, slurred, 325–328
Spinal cord injuries
   anterior, 158
   incomplete, types of, 158
   steroids in, 158
Spine, fracture of, 156–159
   cervical, 230–232
Splinters, in wounds, 198–200
Spondylolisthesis, cervical, 156–159
Sprain, 9–11
Stab wounds, 1–3, 221
Stable, definition of, 14, 154
Status epilepticus, 240–241
Sternum, discomfort in, 332–335
Steroids
   in head trauma, 181
   in spinal cord trauma, 158
Stokes-Adams attacks, 88
Stomach, emptying of, in overdose patient, 252
Stomach flu, 351–353
Strain, definition of, 10
Strep throat, treatment of, 267. See also Throat, sore
Streptokinase, in acute myocardial infarction, 193
Stress, 5
   hyperventilation due to, 77–79
Stroke, 325–328
   in cocaine abusers, 69
   hypertension following, 327
   "stroke in evolution," 325–328
"Stuffer," cocaine overdose in, 68
Stupor
   in alcoholics, 227–229
   in Reye's syndrome, 257
Subarachnoid hemorrhage, 344–345
   in cocaine abusers, 69
Subdural hematoma, 227–229
Submersion, prolonged, outcome following, 38–40

INDEX

Sudden death
  asthma and, 62
  prevention of, in acute myocardial infarction, 192
Sudden infant death syndrome (SIDS), 41–43
Suicidal, 31–34, 130–132, 219–223, 250–255
Suppositories, for constipation, 202
Supraventricular tachycardia, 300–302
Sutures, in wound healing, 199–200
Swallowing, difficulty with, 203–205
Sweatiness. *See* Diaphoresis
Swelling
  abdominal, 4
  of hands and feet, 4
  scrotal, 58–60
  skin, 15
Sympathomimetics, seizures due to, 49
Syncope, 87–89, 133–136
  causes of, 264
  death following, 20–21
  definition of, 88
  in diabetic ketoacidosis patients, 22–24
  in the elderly, 263–265
  emergency department evaluation of, 263–265
  following motor vehicle accidents, 44
  versus seizure, 264
Syphilis, detection of, 323

Tachyarrhythmia(s), 300–302
Tachycardia
  in alcoholic, 150–152
  in cocaine abusers, 69
  narrow complex, 300–302
  paroxysmal atrial, 77–79
  at rest, 58–60
  supraventricular, 300–302
  ventricular, 133–136, 191–194, 300–302
Telangiectasia, hereditary hemorrhagic, epistaxis due to, 72
Tenosynovitis, 161
Tensilon, 79
Tension pneumothorax, 90–92, 220
Testicular
  cancer, 275
  pain, 185
  swelling, 58–60, 274–276
  torsion, 274–276
Theophylline
  in asthma, 62–63
  seizures due to, 49

Thiamine, 19, 125
Thigh, bruise on, 177–179
Thorazine, overdose of, 153–155
Throat, sore, 15–17, 163–165, 266–268, 277–279
Thrombolysis, in acute myocardial infarction, 193
Tissue plasminogen activator (TPA), 191–194
Toothache, 163–165
Torticollis, 75
Tourniquets, in bleeding cessation, 198–200
Toxidrome, 30, 68, 151, 253
TPA. *See* Tissue plasminogen activator
Trauma. *See also* Fracture(s); Laceration(s); Wound(s)
  abdominal
    blunt, 2
    penetrating, 1–3
  blunt, 101–104
  chest, in motor vehicle accidents, 318–320
  deaths, preventable, 90–92
  dislocations, shoulder, 269–270
  facial, 195–197
    following motor vehicle accident, 44–46
  forcible treatment following, 12–14
  from gunshot wound. *See* Gunshot wound
  head
    in alcoholics, 98–100
    in children, 209–211
    computed tomography in, 210
    epidural hematoma, 227–229
    headache following, 95–96
    subdural hematoma, 227–229
  laryngeal, with facial trauma, 195
  multiple, care in, 1–3, 12–14, 90–92, 101–104, 220–223
  nasal, 72
  ocular, 227–229, 315–317
Tremors, in alcohol withdrawal, 117–120
Triage nurse, function of, 303–306
Trimethoprim/sulfamethoxazole (TMP/SMZ), in bronchitis, 281
Tumor(s), nasopharyngeal, epistaxis due to, 72
Tzank smear, 323

Ulcer(s) duodenal, 107–109
Upper respiratory infection, 266–268
Ureteral colic, 247–249
Urethritis, recurrent, in postmenopausal women, 145

Urinalysis, white blood cell count in, 144
Urinary tract infection, 143–146
Urination
  burning on, 321–324
  pain during, 143–146

Vaccine, rabies, 121–123
Vaginal bleeding, 35–37, 212–214
Valium. *See* Diazepam
Valsalva maneuver, in supraventricular tachycardia, 301–302
Venereal disease, 321–324
  in rape victim, 25–28
Ventilation
  in gunshot wound victim, 181
  mechanical, in COPD, 217
    in motor vehicle accidents, 318–320
Ventilation/perfusion (V/Q) nuclear scan, in pulmonary embolism detection, 349
Ventricular tachycardia, 133–136, 191–194, 300–302
Violence
  domestic, 195–197
  victim of, 31–34
Vision
  changes in, 4
  loss of, 315–317
Visual acuity, following facial trauma, 195–196
Vital signs, 12–14, 59, 72, 78, 92, 102–103, 264, 272
Vitamin C, for alcohol-Antabuse reaction, 141

Vomiting, 169–172
  abdominal pain with, 173–176
  in alcohol withdrawal, 98–100
  in alcoholics, 124–126
  in diabetic ketoacidosis patients, 22–24
  with diarrhea, 259–262
  with flank pain, 336–339
  with head injuries, 209–211
  with perforated duodenal ulcer, 107–109
  in Reye's syndrome, 257

Weight loss, 4, 280–282
Wheezes, in acute respiratory failure, 52, 61–64, 215–218
Withdrawal, alcohol. *See* Alcohol, withdrawal from
Wood's lamp, in rape victim examination, 26
Wound(s)
  bleeding from, treatment of, 198–200
  closure of, 199
  foreign body in, 198–200
  gunshot, 219–223, 307–310
    to head, 180–182
  infection, of hand, 160–162
  lacerations
    facial, 44–46
    of hand, 160–162
  stab, 1–3, 221
Wrist
  slashed, 130–132
  sprained, 9–11

Zidovudine, in AIDS, 171
Zygomatic arch, fracture of, 196